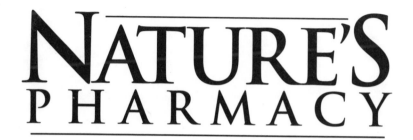

NATURE'S PHARMACY

LYNNE PAIGE WALKER, Pharm.D.
ELLEN HODGSON BROWN, J.D.

FOREWORD BY EARL MINDELL, R.Ph., Ph.D.

PRENTICE HALL PRESS

Library of Congress Cataloging-in-Publication Data

Brown, Ellen Hodgson.
    The alternative pharmacy : break the drug cycle with safe, natural alternative treatments for over 200
  common health conditions / Ellen Hodgson Brown and Lynne Paige Walker : foreword by Earl Mindell.
      p.   cm.
    Includes bibliographical references (p.   ) and index.
    ISBN 0-7352-0021-1 (jkt/case). — ISBN 0-13-907254-3 (preprint) — ISBN 0-7352-0122-6 (pbk.)
    1. Naturopathy—Encyclopedias.   2. Alternative medicine—Encyclopedias.   I. Walker, Lynn Paige.
  II. Title.
  RZ433.B76 1998
  615.5'35—dc21
                                    98-21512
                                       CIP

Acquisitions Editor: *Doug Corcoran*
Production Editor: *Eve Mossman*
Formatting/Interior Design: *Robyn Beckerman*

Previously published as *The Alternative Pharmacy*

© *1998 by Prentice Hall, Inc.*

All rights reserved. No part of this book may be reproduced in any form or by any means,
without permission in writing from the publisher.

Printed in the United States of America

10 9 8 7 6 5 4 3 2 1

ISBN 0-7352-0122-6

PRENTICE HALL PRESS
Paramus, NJ 07652

On the World Wide Web at http://www.phdirect.com

ALSO BY ELLEN BROWN AND LYNNE WALKER

The Informed Consumer's Pharmacy (New York: Carroll & Graf, 1990).

Menopause and Estrogen: Natural Alternatives to Hormone Replacement Therapy (formerly *Breezing Through the Change*) (Berkeley: Frog Ltd., 1994, 1996).

ALSO BY ELLEN BROWN

With the Grain: Eat More, Weigh Less, Live Longer (New York: Carroll & Graf, 1990).

The Key to Ultimate Health, with Richard Hansen, D.M.D. (La Mirada, California: Advanced Health Research Publishing, 1998).

Forbidden Medicine (Murrieta, CA: Third Millenium Press, 1989).

FOREWORD

by Earl Mindell

In the vast world of natural remedies, consumers are left feeling perplexed about the many choices available to them. These "cure-alls" are often not only scientifically unproven, but simply ineffective. When consulting a doctor or pharmacist, most people walk away with no real advice. Finally, we have a book that not only points out the side effects and hazards of prescription medication, but offers effective natural alternatives. As a pharmacist, with extensive knowledge in the field of natural supplementation, I am impressed with the thorough research and sound treatments offered in *Nature's Pharmacy* by Ellen Brown and Dr. Lynne Walker. In a straightforward, easy-to-read format, it lists over 200 diseases and discusses over 700 safe and natural alternative remedies.

Ellen Brown is an experienced researcher, writer, and attorney, who has thoroughly explored both the therapeutic and legal ramifications of alternative remedies. She includes reviews of current research and incorporates the latest information and techniques available. Dr. Walker has accumulated over 20 years experience as a pharmacist and naturopath, operating a successful practice and retail store—The Sun Valley Herb Company—in Sun Valley, Idaho for the last four years. It is through Dr. Walker's vast hands-on experience with her customers that she has been able to compile this impressive, tried and true compendium of what works and what doesn't.

Every disease is listed alphabetically, with a corresponding alternative treatment plan, outlining a step by step procedure for successful recovery. A brief description of each ailment and its underlying causes, signs, and symptoms, diagnosis, and conventional treatment are also covered. Dr. Walker cites many actual cases based on her experiences with her customers and their positive feedback. On a recent visit to The Sun Valley Herb Company, I was privileged to witness the interactive relationship Dr. Walker has with her customers and clients. These relationships have formed the basis of many of her successful remedies.

I strongly believe that every person should have the opportunity and be armed with the knowledge to give natural medicine a try, particularly when traditional methods, including prescription drugs have failed to deliver positive results. This book does exactly what it promises. It offers the reader an in-depth, honest evaluation of alternative forms of medication. Backed up by extensive research, case histories, and Dr. Walker's credentials as a pharmacist, homeopath, and herbalist, delivered in a clear and engaging style.

An invaluable addition to the holistic medicine cabinet.

Earl Mindell, R.Ph., Ph.D.,
Author of the following books:

Earl Mindell's Vitamin Bible, Warner Books (December 1979), updated 1985 & 1991. 87 printings. (A national best seller; on best-seller list of *The New York Times*, *Publisher's Weekly*, and *The Washington Post*.) Sold more than 8.5 million copies in hard cover, trade, and paperback, worldwide. Most recent and revised printing through Warner Books, 1991. Published in 30 languages.

Earl Mindell's Vitamin Bible for Kids, Bantam Books (September 1981); paperback Bantam Books (1983).

Pill Bible, Bantam Books (1982); updated version (May 1988).

Shaping Up With Vitamins, Warner Books (1986); 12th printing.

Safe Eating, Warner Books (May 1987); paperback (May 1988); 6th printing.

Parents Nutrition Bible, Hay House (January 1992); 4th printing.

Earl Mindell's Herb Bible, Simon & Schuster (February 1992); 20th printing. Over 500,000 copies in print.

Earl Mindell's Food as Medicine, Simon & Schuster (February 1993); 5th printing. 135,000 copies in print.

Earl Mindell's Soy Miracle, Simon & Schuster (February 1995); 4th printing. 200,000 copies in print.

Earl Mindell's Anti Aging Bible, Simon & Schuster (February 1996); Over 125,000 copies in print.

Earl Mindell's Secret Remedies, Simon & Schuster (February 1997); Over 50,000 copies in print.

Earl Mindell's Supplement Bible, Simon & Schuster (January, 1998).

Earl Mindell's Nutrition and Health for Dogs, Simon & Schuster (April 1998).

Earl Mindell's Prescription Alternative, Keats Publishing (September 1998).

CONTENTS

ENDNOTES   355

APPENDIX:
NATURAL REMEDY HEALTH ADVISOR   387

INDEX   399

INTRODUCTION

Reliable data exist about the safety and efficacy of herbal remedies, but finding, reading, and evaluating these data is difficult and confusing. There are no statistics about the number of medical doctors who prescribe herbal remedies, but they are clearly in the minority and difficult to find; and government regulation forbids manufacturers of natural products from making claims about their products. The manufacturer can't tell you on the label what to expect or even how the product should be taken. You need a good book to guide you through.

I came to appreciate the value of a good book when my children were small. They suffered from one ear infection after another and seemed to be continually on antibiotics. I questioned whether these remedies were doing any good when my daughter developed yet another ear infection while she was still on a prior course of the drugs. My suspicions were confirmed by a book—*How to Raise a Healthy Child in Spite of Your Doctor*, by Robert Mendelsohn, M.D.—which warned mothers of the hazards of antibiotics and advised us to resist giving them except in certain narrow circumstances. I followed Dr. Mendelsohn's advice, which proved to be invaluable. For both of my children there was a "healing crisis"—a single traumatic episode of the condition—after which they never suffered from ear infections again.

In this book, we hope to give you the confidence and the resources to break the drug and surgery cycles for your own common health conditions. Catering to the recent surge of interest in natural medicines are a number of books that aid enthusiasts in choosing remedies for their particular conditions, but these can leave you confused, taking a shotgun approach not necessarily calculated to direct you to the specific remedy that will work for your particular condition. The approach of this book is to narrow your choices to what really works as reported by users. We will also discuss why the commercially popular options may *not* be your best choices for particular conditions. Our discussion is liberally supported throughout with research and actual case histories. We'll be drawing from and comparing a number of approaches—drugs, herbs, nutritional supplements, homeopathic remedies, Chinese patent medicines, flower essences, and essential oils.

Dr. Lynne Walker has eclectic experience with all of these options. Her first doctorate was in pharmacy. But after working for a number of years as a hospital pharmacist, she became aware of the limitations of pharmaceuticals. She got interested in natural alternatives after she was diagnosed at the early age of 33 with a large fibroid tumor and was told she needed a hysterectomy. When alternative approaches saved her from that surgery, she was so impressed that she went on to acquire doctorates in Chinese medicine and homeopathy. Besides ten years as a hospital pharmacist, her experience now includes five years as pharmacist at Capitol Drugs, the largest and busiest homeopathic pharmacy in the country; ten years in private practice as a homeopath and acupuncturist and three years as proprietor of an herb company in Sun Valley, Idaho. As a result of this varied experience, she has seen the effects and side effects of drugs and the benefits of a broad range of natural remedies in virtually all of the ailments discussed in the following pages.

My own professional background is in law. As an attorney, I have followed cases in court involving both conventional medicine gone wrong and the legal vicissitudes of several "alternative" pioneers. As a woman and a mother, I've also had to make personal choices among the health approaches of different disciplines. Like Dr. Walker, I've been advised by several gynecologists (seven, to be exact) that I needed a hysterectomy— first for a prolapsed uterus, then for a large fibroid tumor, then for cysts on the ovaries. All three conditions eventually resolved without surgery, through natural means to be discussed hereafter. Another invasive surgery I managed to avoid was for carpal tunnel syndrome, a swelling of the wrists that numbs the hands and increasingly afflicts computer operators and other workers with stressed wrists. As far as we know, we are the first investigators to report the simple remedy that has cured this condition in a number of cases, including mine.

Our respective interests prompted us to co-author an earlier book on the hazards of drugs, called *The Informed Consumer's Pharmacy*. The question we most frequently got in response was, "Then what *should* I use?" This sequel undertakes to answer that question, comparing the drug and natural options for nearly 200 common ailments, listed alphabetically. The recommended remedies are not merely theoretical selections. They have been tested on hundreds of people and found to work, often when conventional remedies have failed.

An unbiased approach would warrant omitting brand names, but the fact is that some brands simply work better than others. In order to tell you what really works, we feel we have to name names. Our recommendations include a combination of remedies from different disciplines that have been found to give optimum results for specific conditions.

Please make frequent use of the Natural Remedy Health Advisor in the appendix of this book. It contains detailed information about the products we recommend including brand names, company names, types of remedies, and dosages. The appendix will prove most useful in shopping for remedies of your choice.

For more information, see our Web site at

www.alternativepharmacy.com

Or write

PO Box 913
Agoura, CA 91376

For a personalized consultation, call

1-818-865-8694

I

REFURBISHING YOUR MEDICINE CABINET

CHAPTER 1

BREAKING THE DRUG HABIT

The well-stocked medicine cabinet that graces nearly every home is a tribute to Madison Avenue advertisers, who have convinced us that everything that ails us can be cured by something in a bottle. What advertisers haven't stressed are the adverse reactions and side effects of their pharmaceuticals and how the drugs can interfere with natural bodily processes.

Take a recent television commercial for an H2-blocker, a type of drug that includes Tagamet and Zantac and was until recently a prescription-only ulcer medicine. A father takes his robust-looking son aside at the son's wedding and advises him to take this medicine preventatively, to make sure his first night of connubial bliss won't be disturbed by an upset stomach. What the advertisers refrain from mentioning is that the stomach acid blocked by this drug has beneficial functions, including killing unwanted bacteria in the stomach. Without the acid, you run the risk of infection by a variety of organisms, including those responsible for typhoid, salmonella, chlorella, dysentery, and giardia.[1] Ironically, another side effect of H2-blockers can be impotence. These risks might be worth taking for a person in excruciating ulcer pain with no other relief in sight, but for a healthy groom on his honeymoon, taking H2-blockers would seem to be asking for unnecessary trouble.

Natural, nontoxic remedies are available for indigestion that have no side effects and that that aid rather than inhibit the body's functions. But you aren't likely to hear about the healing properties of these remedies in television commercials. Only FDA-approved drugs can be advertised as "safe and effective" for curing disease. Not that natural remedies aren't safe and effective enough to pass the FDA's tests; they just aren't lucrative enough to fund the massive studies needed for FDA approval, which now requires an average investment of more than $100 million per drug or device.[2] Products found naturally in plants or animals can't be patented and are therefore unlikely to generate this type of revenue. Research discussed hereafter indicates that these nontoxic products are actually *more* safe and effective than their patented, FDA-approved counterparts, for

3

the very reason that they can't be patented: they are found naturally in living things. Unnatural substances are perceived by the body as foreign and can provoke allergic reactions, anaphylactic shock, even death. Even when synthetic drugs are accepted by the body, they are liable to block or disrupt its functions, since they don't "fit" like its natural keys—natural hormones, enzymes, vitamins, minerals, and so forth. Yet manufacturers have been known to alter a perfectly good natural hormone just to render the product patentable, and it is these unnatural, patentable substances with protected markets that are in a position to fund FDA approval. These drugs get advertised, reach mass markets, and tend to compose the armamentarium of conventional treatment.

According to the September 1997 issue of *U.S. News & World Report*, as many as 140,000 people die annually from adverse reactions to prescription drugs approved as "safe and effective" by the FDA. A University of Toronto study reported in April of 1998 found toxic reactions to drugs *taken improperly* to be the leading cause of U.S. deaths after heart disease, cancer, and strokes.[3] By contrast, deaths due to terrorism, which prompted a furor and immediately mobilized Congress after the Oklahoma City bombing, have never exceeded 200 a year.[4] The General Accounting Office estimates that 51 percent of FDA-approved drugs have major unwanted side effects that aren't detected until the drugs have been on the market long enough for them to show up. More people now die from taking legal, government-approved drugs than from auto accidents; and deaths from infections picked up in hospitals is equal to the number of deaths from auto accidents.[5]

INSIDIOUS SIDE EFFECTS

Besides the reported cases ending in death, drugs can be responsible for remote diseases and long-term side effects that are hard to detect and may go unreported. Take the case of a patient named Mary, reported by British authors Arabella Melville and Colin Johnson. Mary was a healthy woman in her late twenties who was under a lot of stress. She started suffering heart palpitations, for which her doctor prescribed a beta-blocking drug called practolol. The heart palpitations stopped, but Mary's periods became very heavy and she was often dizzy. Once, she went completely blind for several hours. Her doctor prescribed tinted glasses. Gradually, it got so Mary ached all over and was in constant pain. Her doctor prescribed painkillers. When she got a severe pain in her neck that kept her in bed for three days, he prescribed a surgical collar and more painkillers.

Yet Mary's eyes continued to hurt. Her ears ached and rang. Her skin itched. She cried frequently. She couldn't sleep, although her doctor prescribed a battery of sleeping pills. Her stomach became upset, and her nose and throat were sore and dry. When her stomach pains became severe, her doctor finally took her off practolol.

The rash cleared up, but her other troubles persisted. Her abdomen grew huge. She had a hysterectomy, and a grapefruit-sized mass of fibrous tissue was removed. She tried to hold down a job but couldn't, because she kept falling. She was given medicines for vertigo, along with sleeping pills, painkillers, and tranquilizers. She had to undergo another operation, after which she was kept in the hospital for six weeks for extensive testing. Her doctors diagnosed multiple sclerosis. Mary was convinced she did not have this disease, and her suspicion was subsequently confirmed. Her condition has now been diagnosed as systemic lupus erythematosus ("lupus"), a complicated syndrome resulting from her treatment with the drug practolol. The drug led her body to reject its own tissues as foreign.[6]

Lupus is a connective tissue disease whose specific cause is unknown, but an estimated 10 percent of the 500,000 American cases are drug-related. Known offenders include the drug procainamide, an antiarrythmic used to regulate erratic heart beats; the antiarrhythmic quinidine; the blood-pressure-lowering drugs hydralazine and methyldopa; the tuberculosis drug isoniazid; and the tranquilizer chlorpromazine. A probable association has also been shown with the antipsychotic lithium, many anticonvulsant agents, antithyroid drugs, penicillamine (used to treat rheumatoid arthritis), sulfasalazine (used to treat ulcerative colitis), and the beta-blockers (used to lower blood pressure). A possible association has been shown with estrogens, the antibiotics penicillin and tetracycline, para-aminosalicylic acid (used to treat tuberculosis), gold salts (used for arthritis), griseofulvin (used for fungal infections), and reserpine (used to lower blood pressure).[7]

As for practolol, it was never introduced in the United States; and in Britain, where it was introduced, it has been taken off the market. Still, it illustrates what can go wrong. Its dangers weren't detected until its cumulative use totaled a million patient/years and its victims totaled 7,000.

Mary could not walk without support and had to wear a surgical collar for years after she had quit taking the drug.[8] What could she have done to avoid this result? If she had known how the drug was going to affect her, she would obviously have resisted taking it. But what if she had merely been given a technical description of its potential side effects? They don't sound so bad when couched in vague, general terms and labeled "remote"—skin rash, joint and neck problems, eye and ear problems, tinnitus.

The Informed Consumer

For most patients, whether they would choose to take their prescriptions if they knew everything that could go wrong is a moot question, since even general warnings are omitted from the bottles. Unlike over-the-counter drugs, which are boxed with circulars detailing side effects, prescription drugs are typically removed from their boxes by the pharmacist, who places them in unmarked bottles and labels them only with the names of the patient and drug and directions for use. In part, this lack of warnings is merely expedient. The druggist gets the wares in economy-sized containers that include only one warning circular, and he or she doesn't have enough to go around. But in part, the lack of warnings is intentional. Doctors know that if their patients were aware of all the known risks of the drugs they prescribe, the patients would never take them. Doctors quite reasonably feel they are more capable than their patients of weighing the risks and of determining whether the risks are justified in individual cases.

The National Council on Patient Information and Education in Washington, D.C., suggests you ask your doctor these questions about any drug he or she prescribes: What is the name of the drug, and what does it do? How and when do I take it, and for how long? What foods, drinks, other medicines or activities should I avoid while taking the drug? Are there any side effects, and what should I do if they occur? Is there any written information on the drug? Your pharmacist is another potential source of information. Although your prescription won't come with warning labels, your pharmacist is required to furnish the insert on request.

You can also do some independent research. Your local library is one source of information. The *Physicians' Desk Reference* contains information supplied by drug manufacturers that includes the side effects of their products. For a more complete discussion of side effects, see *Facts and Comparisons*, which is written by independent authorities. If you do enough reading about the hazards of the drugs you are taking, you are liable to start looking for natural, nontoxic alternatives. But that means doing more research.

This book is designed to simplify your research needs. Relying on your doctor for a prescription has one comforting advantage: It relieves you of the ominous responsibility of having to choose a remedy yourself. The consumer who takes the natural route has suddenly become her own doctor. She faces shelves of supplements that all look alike, and the information on drugs and their alternatives can be overwhelming. This book discusses a wide range of diseases, the treatments used for them, and the more interesting issues surrounding them. Then it zeroes in on the bottom line—what works and what doesn't, what's safe and what isn't, as reported by users.

CHAPTER 2

THE NATURAL APPROACH TO CURE

Alternative medicine is taking the market by storm. In 1993, a report in the *New England Journal of Medicine* suggested that, for the first time in modern history, annual visits to alternative practitioners may exceed those to primary care physicians. A growing disillusionment with pharmaceuticals has prompted a surge of interest in natural remedies. Herbal products are practically flying off the shelves. In a 1995 Gallup survey, more than 28 million Americans reported taking herbal supplements. Sales have doubled since 1985 and are predicted to exceed three billion dollars by the end of 1998.

The natural approach to cure recognizes that most common complaints will go away by themselves. The body can heal itself. Most drugs actually work to suppress the body's efforts in that direction. Drugs target the coughing, sneezing, fever and diarrhea we think of as the problem, when in fact these symptoms may be the body's attempt to get rid of the problem—the foreign toxins, microbes, or chemicals that have built up in the tissues. When these reactions are deadened with drugs, the toxins are left to accumulate in the body. And the intended effects of synthetics tend to be accompanied by unintended side effects. Alternative practitioners maintain that except in life-threatening situations, it is therefore usually better to live with your symptoms than to try to suppress them with drugs. Conventional doctors, too, are coming to recommend "watchful waiting" in many cases where drastic surgeries used to be the order of the day.

While you're waiting, excellent natural, nontoxic remedies are available to ease your symptoms and help your body heal. Remedies that support the body's efforts to do its own housecleaning and repair include nutritional supplements, Western and Chinese herbs, homeopathic remedies, aromatherapy and flower essences.

HERBAL MEDICINE

Herbs have been used for healing throughout recorded history. Many conventional drugs are derived from plants. The leaves of the foxglove plant are the source of the heart drug digitalis. Taxol, a powerful new cancer drug, is made from the Pacific yew tree. Capoten, a blood-pressure-lowering medicine, comes from snake venom. Even aspirin was originally derived from willow bark. Pharmaceutical companies start with the herb and extract the "active ingredients," but alternative practitioners maintain that the whole herb is more therapeutic than its isolated ingredients and is less likely to result in side effects. *Aromatherapy*, a form of herbal medicine, involves distillations of the essential oils of the whole plant, carrying all the plant's important information (sometimes referred to as the "blood" or "life force" of the plant).

Statistics from the American Association of Poison Control Centers confirm that while drug poisonings kill hundreds of people annually, deaths from herbal medicine are virtually unheard of. A few medicinal plants can cause bodily harm when taken in excess: comfrey, for example, has been linked to liver damage, although only in enormous overdoses. Dosings are also harder to gauge accurately for herbs than for drugs, and herbs can cause allergic reactions in the susceptible. They should be used only with professional advice by pregnant women and people with chronic medical conditions. For children, professional advice is also recommended, and doses should be diluted. But even with these provisos, herbs are far less risky than their pharmaceutical counterparts. For healthy, nonpregnant people, they are considered quite safe in recommended doses.[9]

If you think you are having an unwanted reaction to an herbal or any other oral product, you should stop taking it, drink copious amounts of water, take a hot bath to alleviate the symptoms, wait for a period of time, then consider starting the remedy again to see if it was really the cause of the problem. What is sometimes thought to be a bad reaction may not be an allergic one or a reason not to take the remedy. The dose may simply be too high (even if it's the recommended dose), or the effect may be a "healing crisis" or cleansing reaction prompted by the remedy. (See Chapter 3.)

CENTURIES-OLD TRACK RECORDS FROM VARIOUS MEDICAL TRADITIONS

Herbal remedies are important constituents of traditional Oriental medicine. Chinese doctors view health as a state of harmonious balance of the body's *Qi*, or vital force, which flows in set patterns throughout the energy systems of the body. These energy patterns are called meridians and are named for the major organs they pass through (heart, stomach, lung, kidney, liver). Disruption of the flow of the vital force to any organ causes an imbalance throughout the system. The more out of balance the system is, the more likely symptoms will result.

One way Chinese doctors correct imbalances is with acupuncture, a technique that involves placing very fine needles in specific locations to facilitate the flow of Qi through the energy meridians. Once considered akin to "voodoo," this technique is now gaining wide acceptance among doctors and hospitals in the United States. In November of 1997, a consensus panel convened by the National Institutes of Health concluded that there is clear evidence that acupuncture is effective for relieving pain in a variety of situations, including postoperative and chemotherapy nausea and vomiting, nausea of pregnancy, and postoperative dental pain.

Chinese doctors also correct imbalances with traditional herbal formulas, the safety and effectiveness of which have been proven through centuries of use. Publications from the People's Republic of China report that Chinese herbal formulas are effective in a broad range of clinical situations.[10] (NOTE: It's important to take Chinese herbs in the balanced formulas that address your whole symptom complex. If you take them singly, you run the risk of throwing your body further out of balance.)

European folk medicine, Native American medicine, and the Ayurvedic system developed in India are other herbal traditions that contain excellent botanicals proven through centuries of use.

NUTRIENTS AS MEDICINE

Drugs can mask symptoms and herbs can stimulate body functions that have gone awry, but health will elude the patient so long as there is an underlying lack of essential nutrients in the body. Health problems are increasingly being traced to nutritional deficiencies that can be corrected only by supplying the missing vitamins, minerals, amino acids, and so on.

Few people today eat a balanced diet of natural, unprocessed plant foods; and even if they did, these ideal foods can no longer be relied on to fully satisfy nutrient requirements. At one time, everything the body needed was furnished by the foods of the earth. But today, the earth seems to be as depleted as our bodies are. Canning, irradiation, and other methods of preserving shelf life have further decreased the biological value of our food. Processing removes the food's natural antioxidants. (For a discussion of antioxidants, see "Aging.") A report presented to the U.S. Department of Agriculture in 1936 concluded that our soils and the crops grown on them are so mineral deficient that the only way to prevent and cure the resulting deficiency diseases is by taking mineral supplements—and that was more than half a century ago.[11] The situation has declined significantly since.

It is the rare single nutrient that will cure a disease, on the other hand, unless the disease happens to be due to a deficiency of that nutrient. For example, rickets, which is caused by a lack of vitamin D, can be cured by supplying that vitamin. For most conditions, however, a wide range of nutritional support is required. Every disease state can be helped by a good, balanced vitamin- and mineral-supplement program; but for purposes of this book, we will be mentioning specific nutritional supplements only to the extent that studies or experience have produced results with them for particular conditions. You can determine if you are short in particular nutrients by visiting a practitioner who specializes in the field. For a complete resource on vitamins, see Earl Mindell's *Vitamin Bible*. (For a resource on herbs, he has also written an *Herb Bible*.)

When choosing basic nutritional supplements, it is important to recognize that not all brands are equally good. Natural is better than synthetic, and nutrients need to be in proper balance and in an absorbable form. We'll be mentioning particularly good brands in particular contexts.

Colloidal Versus Ionized Minerals

"Colloidal minerals" are currently popular products promoted as containing a broad range of minerals in a highly absorbable form. But researcher Dr. Alexander Schauss observes that colloidal minerals are basically clays dispersed in water. Something colloidal (suspended in water) is insoluble by definition, and insoluble minerals are generally less absorbable than soluble minerals. An analysis of five of these products showed they averaged only fifteen elements each, not the seventy or more claimed; and the mineral balance was poor. Four of the five contained aluminum (a toxic element linked to Alzheimer's disease) as their first or second element by weight. Other toxic trace elements included arsenic, barium, cadmium, mercury and lead. Colloidal mineral products contain only small amounts of calcium and magnesium, the body's main mineral requirements. Trace minerals should be taken only in trace amounts. If they overpower the macro-minerals (calcium and magnesium), they can throw mineral balance into chaos.

A better way to get your macro- and trace minerals is in ionized form, the form in which plants and mammals are designed to absorb inorganic minerals. Converting calcium requires stomach acid—something in which many people, and particularly the elderly, tend to be deficient. To be absorbed, calcium must be reduced to the ionized state (charged particles of elemental calcium). If you take your calcium in this form, it can be immediately absorbed without intermediate processing. (See "Bone Loss.")

AN OVERLOOKED NATURAL CURE

Another cheap and simple key to health that is often overlooked is plain, unadulterated *water*. F. Batmanghelidj, M.D., in his groundbreaking book, *Your Body's Many Cries for Water*, links the major chronic epidemics of modern life to water dehydration. Our mistake, he says, is in thinking we have satisfied our need for water by satisfying our thirst with other beverages. We need half our body's weight in ounces of water per day—not coffee, tea, soft drinks, or juices, but plain (filtered or bottled) water. Thus a 128-pound woman would need 64 ounces, or eight glasses of water. Diseases Dr. Batmanghelidj reports seeing reversed with this simple therapy include high blood pressure, low back pain, asthma, allergies, and ulcers, among others. The regimen is also a good way to lose weight.

Wait one-half hour before meals and two-and-a-half hours after meals for your heavy water doses, to avoid diluting your digestive juices. Dr. Batmanghelidj advises adding one-half teaspoon of *salt* to your diet daily for every ten glasses of water added. (Unheated sea salt is preferred. Table salt, which has been heated to very high temperatures in processing, can be treated by the body as a foreign toxin.) Increase your water intake gradually to make sure your kidneys are functioning properly. Output should increase proportionally with input.[12] Dr. Batmanghelidj's protocol also includes getting sufficient daily *exercise* (for example, an hour's walk), to stimulate internal movement and healing.

REMOVING BLOCKS TO HEALING

Besides giving the body the nutrients and water it needs, blocks to healing need to be removed. Cure depends on an immune system and bodily organs that are intact and functioning normally. Under the principle of "vitalism" or "vital force," humans have an innate energy that promotes life and encourages homeostasis (balance). Treatments that are effective over the long term stimulate this life force. Treatments that block the life force may effectively suppress symptoms, but they are counterproductive for long-term recovery. Life-force-suppressing treatments include cancer chemotherapy and radiation, painkillers, drugs that suppress fever (a natural healing reaction that "cooks out" germs), steroids (which suppress the immune system), and antibiotics (which kill germs, but do it without stimulating the body's own immune system).

Antibiotics and steroids (including, hydrocortisone cream) are two popular drug categories that are particularly insidious. In critical situations, they can be "wonder drugs;" but they are used far too frivolously. The development of resistant strains from overuse has led to predictions that antibiotics will be obsolete in a few years. (See "Infection, Immunity.")

Besides current drug use, other factors that act to suppress the body's natural healing ability include previous surgeries, missing organs, a previous history of drug-taking (legal or illegal), smoking, poor nutrition, stress, hereditary conditions including birth defects and obstructions, and dental fillings of nonbiocompatible materials. If these obstructions can be removed, they should be, since if a patient is deprived of vital life force by any means, he will be less responsive to natural methods of healing intended to stimulate the life force. But even if obstructions can't be removed, results may be obtained by natural remedies to the extent that they are able to spark whatever life force remains.[13]

CHAPTER 3

VIBRATIONAL MEDICINE

Stimulating the Life Force

The principle of "vitalism" comes from homeopathy, another body-supporting therapeutic approach that is rapidly growing in popularity. Sales of homeopathic remedies are increasing by about 20 percent a year. Experience shows that the right homeopathic remedy can be uncannily effective. Yet the theory behind this approach is entirely foreign to Western medicine, so foreign that a chapter is warranted just to explain it. Unlike conventional medicine, which works chemically, homeopathic remedies are said to work on an energetic level to stimulate the body's own healing energy—rather like a tuning fork that sets disharmonious chords back on track.

Homeopathy involves inducing a mild reaction in the body by simulating the larger reaction that constitutes the disease. Where "allopaths" (conventional doctors) suppress symptoms, homeopaths encourage them, on the theory that they represent the body's attempt to flush out toxins. Homeopathic remedies consist of minute doses of natural substances—mineral, plant, or animal—that if given to healthy people in larger doses would cause the symptoms the patient is experiencing. The principle is the same as pharmaceutical vaccination. The difference is that vaccines are macromolecules that can induce unwanted side effects. High dose homeopathics are without side effects because the remedies are so diluted that no molecule of the original substance is likely to be left in solution.

Homeopathic medicines are made by preparing a mother tincture from the symptom-provoking substance. The mother tincture has a potency of 1x. The tincture is "potentized," or increased in potency, by diluting and succussing (shaking vigorously in a particular way). To raise the potency from 1x to 2x, one part of the 1x solution is mixed with nine parts of alcohol and succussed. To raise 2x to 3x, one part of the 2x solution is diluted with nine parts of alcohol and succussed. The process is repeated until the desired potency is reached. Anomalously, the highest and strongest potencies are the most dilute. The succussion is said to transmit the energy pattern of the original substance to the neutral matter in which it was diluted (usually water and alcohol).

Popularization of the homeopathic concept dates back to the German physician Samuel Hahnemann in the 1790s. Homeopathy has been widely accepted and practiced in Europe ever since and is now the leading alternative therapy used there. It was also quite popular in the United States in the nineteenth century; but it lost ground at the turn of the twentieth century to allopathic medicine, which was more lucrative, afforded its practitioners greater political leverage, and seemed to make more sense scientifically. Homeopathy's current renaissance in the United States is due in part to a series of studies that has finally brought scientific credence to its rather unlikely premises. On September 29, 1997, the British medical journal *Lancet* reported the results of a meta-analysis (a systematic review of a body of research) of 89 blinded, randomized, placebo-controlled clinical trials of homeopathy. It found that the homeopathic medicines used in those studies had an average effect that was 2.45 times greater than placebos.[14]

Also eliminating the possibility of the placebo effect are studies on animals. One noteworthy laboratory study involved tadpoles. When a glass bottle containing a homeopathic remedy (Thyroxine 30x) was suspended in the tadpoles' water, development of the tadpoles into frogs was slowed—although there was no interaction between the remedy and the water. Somehow, the remedy was radiating its effects through the glass.[15]

In another provocative laboratory study, researchers gave rats crude doses of arsenic, bismuth, cadmium, mercury chloride, or lead. Animals pretreated with homeopathic doses of these substances before and after exposure to the crude substances excreted more of the toxic crude substances through urine, feces, and sweat than did animals pretreated with a placebo.[16]

THE FINE ART OF SELECTING A REMEDY

Constitutional homeopaths can make deep, profound changes in health with single, high-potency doses of homeopathic remedies given over long periods of time. Many cases are on record in which serious or even fatal illnesses have been reversed and lab values have returned to normal in a few months, results that in Western medical practice would have been considered impossible. But constitutional homeopathy is an art, and results are uncertain. True constitutional homeopathy is a slow, progressive uncovering of the patient's real nature. In some cases the course of treatment can last ten years or more. The constitutional homeopath is concerned not so much with the symptoms as with understanding the individual who has them. Treatment is individualized and largely dependent on the practitioner's experience in selecting the correct remedy. Skilled constitutional homeopaths are not only difficult to locate but usually expensive. A visit can cost from $200 to $3,000.

SELECTING A REMEDY THROUGH ELECTRODERMAL SCREENING

To increase the accuracy of the remedy selection process, machines to help locate energy imbalances in the body are becoming increasingly popular with practitioners. Called electrodermal-screening devices, they date back to Reinhard Voll, M.D., a German researcher who developed EAV or "Electro-Acupuncture According to Voll" in the fifties. Like the EEG, ECG, and EMG, electro-dermal screening is based on measurements of electrical skin resistance. According to Richard Gerber, M.D., in his paradigm-shattering book *Vibrational Medicine*, the devices can also tell the type and degree of dysfunction in particular organs, as well as their actual causes and potential cures. How they do this is a function of biological resonance, the same principle underlying the later imaging systems of MRI and EMR scanning.[17]

Proponents contend that the accuracy of electrodermal screening is equal to or better than that of the various orthodox tests of Western medicine, without their risk of dangerous side effects. Electrodermal screening can establish an immediate case report without a prior patient history, based entirely on measurement readings. The machines can also tell what remedies will resonate harmonically to correct electromagnetic imbalances in the body.

CHOOSING YOUR OWN REMEDIES

Electrodermal screening takes some of the guesswork out of homeopathy, but the devices still require training, and the services of homeopaths who use them are often expensive. Even if initial fees are low, the cost of multiple remedies and repeat visits adds up. The first visit can be $150 to $800 and repeat visits $50 to $400.

An increasingly popular alternative is for the patient to educate her-self and select her own homeopathic remedies, an approach that for many conditions is safe and effective. One proviso is that it's much easier for a practitioner to treat a problem at the onset. If time is lost in self-treatment with the wrong remedies, the homeopath will have a much harder time of it. Another proviso is that homeopathic remedies given incorrectly in high potencies over a period of time can suppress the disease and finally make the case incurable. Those provisos aside, single remedies *in low potency,* and combination homeopathic remedies for minor ailments, are quite safe and effective. Combination remedies take a shotgun approach, including a range of likely homeopathic possibilities that helps take the guesswork out of the selection process.

General Considerations When Using Homeopathic Remedies

1. WHEN CHOOSING YOUR OWN REMEDIES without the advice of a practitioner, take only 3x to 30x potencies, nothing higher.

2. TAKE THE REMEDIES away from food and drink—a min-imum of 15 minutes before or after eating or drinking (except water). Your mouth should be clean and free of food, drink, tobacco, alcohol, tooth-paste, gum, and the like.

3. AVOID coffee and products containing camphor, mint, menthol, or eucalyptus (internal and external, such as gums, lozenges, Tiger Balm, Vick's VapoRub, white-flower oil, Noxzema creams, and BenGay), which can antidote the remedies or render them ineffective. (That's the rule, but for people who absolutely can't give up coffee, experience indicates that the remedies may still be effective if taken well away from it.) Homeopathic medicine should never be used along with steroid drugs, which work by an opposing mechanism. Homeopathic remedies encour-age the body to regain its original vitality, while steroids suppress the immune system's own efforts.

4. AVOID TOUCHING HOMEOPATHIC REMEDIES WITH THE HANDS.
For pellets: Shake them into the cap of the bottle, then drop them into the mouth. Keep them under the tongue until they dissolve.

For liquid: Let the drops fall from the dropper or bottle into the mouth, taking care not to touch the dropper to the tongue or lips; or put the drops in a little water. Try to hold the liquid in your mouth for 30 seconds before swallowing. Wait at least 30 seconds before taking another remedy.

For homeopathic vials: The vials are different potencies, which need to be taken in order. If one is broken, it should be replaced before going on to the next. Do not take the vials if you have a cold or flu. Wait until your symptoms have cleared, then resume your regular schedule.

5. TAKE STAUFEN HOMEOPATHIC VIALS FROM RIGHT TO LEFT. German remedies by Staufen, which are among the most effective of homeopathic remedies, are frequently mentioned in this book. The manufacturer advises taking the vials from left to right (lowest to highest potency) at the rate of one a week. But Dr. Bruce Waller, under whom Dr. Walker studied, advised a different approach. Dr. Waller acquired his experience from working with a small group of German homeopaths including Reinhard Voll, M.D., the homeopathic pioneer who developed EAV. These researchers concluded after studying the issue that the body had the greatest opportunity to heal if the remedies are given from right to left (highest to lowest potency). This approach causes greater "healing crises" but gives more dramatic results. Dr. Walker also advises taking the remedies at the rate of one every three days instead of once a week.

6. STORE THE REMEDIES in a dark place away from perfumes, medications, foods, herbs, and all strong smelling substances. The bathroom cabinet is not a good place. *Do not leave them in a hot car, as temperatures above 150 degrees can ruin them.* Don't store them on electronic equipment such as a TV, microwave, or radio set, as the remedies work vibrationally and can be damaged by competing radiation.

7. WHEN YOU FLY, don't let the remedies by X-rayed. Don't put them in your checked luggage, which is often X-rayed. Carry them separately in a little bag and put them on the key tray when you walk through the doorway at the security check. Pick them up on the other side. (If they accidentally go through the machine, they can still be used; they just may be less effective.)

8. BE PREPARED FOR A HOMEOPATHIC AGGRAVATION. A slight aggravation of your symptoms can sometimes take place before you feel better. This is not only normal but desirable: It indicates

the remedy is the correct one, and that healing is beginning to occur. If you feel worse, you may stop the remedy and simply observe the symptoms. You'll feel better in a few hours, or at most a few days; then you can continue taking the remedy. Some people are more sensitive than others. Find your own comfort level.

9. STOP WHEN YOU SEE AN IMPROVEMENT IN SYMPTOMS. Homeopathic remedies exert subtle influences on the system. Their purpose is to encourage the body on its health-building path. When the body is healthy, it no longer needs the remedy. Prolonged use beyond that time may result in nontoxic aggravation, producing the very symptoms the remedy was being taken to eliminate. (If that happens, don't worry; the symptoms will disappear when you stop taking the remedy.) If your symptoms return after discontinuing the remedy, try a few more drops. If you are seeing a practitioner, it's best to return within two to three weeks to determine whether you still need the remedy.

10. NUTRITIONAL RECOMMENDATIONS while taking homeopathic remedies include a diet centered around fresh, whole grains and fruits and vegetables, with low amounts of sugar and no added preservatives. Warm, cooked foods are encouraged; raw and cold foods are discouraged. It's best to avoid processed or preserved foods and dairy products (including milk, cheese, butter, and yogurt).

BACH FLOWER REMEDIES

Bach Flower Remedies are vibrational remedies that balance the emotions. Derived from flowers, they are entirely safe and nontoxic. Dr. Bach, a British physician, categorized 38 flowers, all of which work on different emotions of the body. "Walnut," for example, helps during stressful life changes such as moving or starting a new job; "Pine" helps with feelings of guilt; "Star of Bethlehem" helps with shock. Bach flowers are a great way to treat children for emotional trauma such as the first day of school, death of a pet, and so on. They can be taken in many ways: Put four drops directly under the tongue, up to five times daily; or place a dropperful in water and sip throughout the day; or put a dropperful in a spray bottle with water and spray in the room to calm fighting children as they inhale it.

CHAPTER 4

Nature's Medicine Chest

Getting Started

Here are some popular herbal and homeopathic remedies that are good to have on hand for emergency first aid and to treat ailments such as upset stomachs and congestion:

- *Tea Tree Oil*—this remedy has a wealth of uses. It can be used as an antifungal for athlete's foot, fungus in the mouth, fingernail or toenail fungus; a scalp cleanser for problems such as dandruff and lice; a gargle for sinus congestion, sore throat and sore gums; a topical remedy for canker sores, cold sores, acne, minor cuts, abrasions, insect bites, rashes, after shaving or waxing, or for minor burns.

- *Rescue Remedy*—by far the most popular Bach flower essence combination, Rescue Remedy is excellent for relieving stress and irritability. It can calm an upset child, an irritable teen, a stressed-out mother, even traumatized pets. It's completely safe, even for babies and pregnant women.

- *Biting Insects* by Molecular Biologicals—this is a great remedy to prevent insect bites or stop pain and itch after being bitten. It is safe and effective for children and easy to use. Take ten drops three times daily.

- *Peppermint oil*—a couple of drops in a glass of warm water will heal a stomach ache. For headaches, peppermint oil applied directly to the forehead stimulates prostaglandins to relieve pain.

- *Black Ointment*—this is a drawing salve that can pull out slivers of glass or splinters that can't otherwise be removed. It has been used successfully, for example, to draw out cactus needles in the foot. The day after its topical application, the needles become red and encapsulated and pop out when touched. Apply twice daily to the problem area.

- *Arnica homeopathic 6x or 30x tablets*—take orally to stop trauma to the body and to soothe sore muscles, aches, and sprains. Arnica can also be taken immediately before exercise to prevent sore muscles (two tablets under the tongue). After trauma, take two pills, four times daily as needed for aches and pain. This is the remedy you need when you stub your toe, slam your fingers in the door, or drop something on your foot; or after a car accident, when there might be injury or whiplash. It should be taken as soon as possible after trauma—two pills every 15 minutes for the first hour following a severe trauma, then four times daily as needed.

- *Trauma ointment or Traumeel ointment*—a homeopathic combination used topically to relieve aches and pains. Massaged into sore muscles or sprains, it helps eliminate pain. The product also comes as oral drops, which can be taken along with topical application at the rate of ten drops every 15 minutes the first hour, then ten drops four times daily.

- *Calendula tincture*—for wound cleaning and healing. Put two droppersful in one pint of water to soak or wash a cut or wound. Then wrap the wound with a calendula-soaked dressing. Healing time can be dramatically reduced with this treatment.

- *Nux Vomica homeopathic 6x or 30x*—will take care of a hangover. It's also excellent for an upset stomach from over-eating or -drinking, and can be used in the relief of hemorrhoids.

- *Calendula and Hypericum ointment*—can be a miracle cure on certain types of cold sores or cuts. Used topically, the ointment can heal cold sores in a single day.

- *Gunpowder 6x* is good for any type of minor infection, from that of a pierced ear to an abscessed tooth. The remedy pushes out the infection, aiding healing. Take three pills three to four times daily.

- *Bacticin drops*—these homeopathic drops stimulate your body to fight bacteria. Take ten drops three to five times daily for strep throat, acne, red inflamed infections, infections with an odor, and deeper infections causing pus formation and drainage.

- *ABC drops*—a combination of aconite, belladonna, and chamomilla homeopathics, this remedy is quite popular in Europe for colds and earaches. Take at the onset of symptoms.

- *Cold and Flu Solution Plus* (by Dolisos)—taken at the onset of cold symptoms, one every 15 minutes for the first hour, then one pill four times daily, this remedy has been known to knock out a cold in a single day.

- *Elderberry pills* (with vitamin C)—two pills taken three times daily at the onset of a cold help relieve symptoms.

- *Yunnan Paiyao*—this Chinese patent remedy, applied directly to a wound, will rapidly stop bleeding.

- *Ignatia 30x*—for unexpected grief: when the family dog dies, the boyfriend of your teenage daughter breaks up with her, and so forth.

- *Cantharis 6x*—this remedy will take the pain and sting out of a burn. Take two pills every 15 minutes as needed for pain, then three to four times daily to promote healing. Cantharis is also a great remedy for a bladder infection: take two every 15 minutes for one hour, then two every hour to relieve discomfort. (Also drink plenty of water. If the problem hasn't improved in six to eight hours, seek medical advice.)

- *Skullcap and Oats*—an herbal combination remedy for insomnia, anxiety, and stress.

Section

II

AN A-TO-Z GUIDE TO COMMON AILMENTS AND THEIR BEST TREATMENTS

The following guide presents a wide selection of common ailments in handy reference form, along with an analysis of their currently popular drug treatments and the natural alternatives available from various disciplines—homeopathy, herbalism, nutrition, flower essences, aromatherapy, and so on. The focus is on remedies actually reported by consumers to work.

*A*bscesses, Boils, Carbuncles, Skin Infections, Skin Aggravations from Body Piercing

An abscess is a collection of pus caused by an infection. The *ordinary (or pyogenic) abscess* may be found in any tissue of the body—in the center of bone, in the appendix, in the lymph glands, in infected gum tissue around the teeth, and so forth. For all pyogenic abscesses located near the surface of the body, the symptoms are the same: pain, tenderness, and a mass with a red, firm surface and soft center. The temperature and white blood count are usually elevated.

A *cold abscess* is a nontender swelling without fever.

Folliculitis is the presence of pustules in the hair follicles.

Boils and *carbuncles* are quite painful localized abscesses that form in the skin and underlying tissues, usually as a result of infection that has gained entry by traveling down into the hair follicles.

Other minor infections are caused by surface wounds to the body. One modern source is the increasingly popular body piercing.

For dental abscesses, see "Toothache."

CONVENTIONAL TREATMENT

Pyogenic abscesses containing pus are opened and drained, usually under general anesthesia. Carbuncles and boils are also opened when the presence of pus is demonstrated, but cold abscesses are aspirated (removed by suction), since there is a danger of secondary infection if they are opened. To rout out infection, antibiotics are usually prescribed.

Herbal Treatment

Herbs can help prevent folliculitis. Everyone has bacteria on the skin; but as with acne, not everyone gets folliculitis. Herbalists say the problem is caused by a reaction between the bacteria and toxins in the blood. Herbs can clear these toxins, preventing them from coming out in the hair follicles. *Burdock* taken internally cleans the blood and acts as a blood purifier. Other useful herbs are *dandelion, echinacea,* and *slippery elm.*

    Tea tree oil applied topically also helps clear folliculitis. For men with recurring folliculitis from shaving, tea tree oil shave lotion is available.

    For infection from splinters or cactus burrs, herbal *Black Ointment* by Nature's Way helps draw the infection out.

Homeopathic Treatment

Boils and carbuncles treated with antibiotics can often recur, and they can take months for resolution. Folliculitis also tends to recur when treated with antibiotics and can lead to abscess formation. Homeopathic remedies can resolve these conditions permanently. The best single remedies are:

- *Hepar Sulph 30x*, for the pus-forming abscess that is tender to the slightest touch, producing stabbing pain and irritability.
- *Silicea 6x*, for the slow-forming abscess that is deep and will not go away or come to a head.
- *Pyrogenium 6c*, for the deep infection with pus; for "rotting flesh."
- *Belladonna 30x*, for the early-stage abscess that is red, hot, inflamed and tender.
- *Gunpowder*, for folliculitis.

    The best combination homeopathic remedy for abscesses is *Bacticin* by CompliMed. This is a general remedy for any type of infection. People who have used it in place of antibiotics have typically found that prescription drugs weren't needed. Take ten drops every two hours for the first day, then four times daily until cleared.

    For infection resulting from body piercing, wash with homeopathic *Calendula* mother tincture to clear up the infected area and promote healing. Infection can also be inhibited in its early stages with homeopathic *Gunpowder 6x*. Take the recommended dosage every two hours on the first day, then four times daily. For most people, the infection should clear in two days. Inflammation may also be caused by an allergic reaction to the base metal in jewelry. Switching to solid gold and silver should help.

Boil Spontaneously Eliminated

A woman with a huge boil at the top of her left shoulder said she was reluctant to let her doctor lance it. She had had a previous boil lanced and it had taken months to heal. But this boil was becoming increasingly uncomfortable and she knew she had to do something for it. Homeopathic *Silicea* was recommended, to be taken four times a day. The day after she started taking the remedy, her boil opened spontaneously and drained. In less than a week, it was completely healed and had disappeared.

Acne

Acne is the most common skin disorder in the United States and the bane of more than 16 million American teenagers. Pimples result when sebaceous glands at the base of hair follicles get clogged with oil, causing inflammation and attracting bacteria. Bacteria can turn blackheads and whiteheads into red, inflamed pimples. White blood cells rush to the scene, causing swelling as they fight the infection. Hormones can aggravate the condition, leaving teenagers, women about to have their periods, and women on oral contraceptives particularly susceptible. Other aggravating factors include stress, food allergies, and poor diet.

Cystic acne is a serious form of the disease that can result in permanent pits and scars. Heredity is a factor in cystic acne as well as in a tendency to have oily skin.

The inherited tendency may actually be an allergy to certain foods. Milk products are common culprits. Blemish problems may also be traced to certain drugs. In fact drug eruptions are among the most common skin disorders encountered by dermatologists. Even over-the-counter drugs can be responsible. An article in the medical journal *Dermatologica* reported the case of a woman whose skin eruptions were traced to a daily aspirin habit. Another woman's complexion problems were traced to the fluoride in her city's water. The connection was established when her complexion cleared after she switched to bottled water and unfluoridated tooth products.[18]

ANTIBIOTIC TREATMENT

Antibiotics have been a mainstay of treatment, even for mild outbreaks of acne. But these drugs have been so overused that they are no longer producing the results they once did. Several recent studies have shown that the bacteria that cause acne have developed strains that are resistant to both oral and topical antibiotics. *Tetracycline, erythromycin, clindamycin,* and *doxycycline* are all losing their effectiveness. Dermatologists have therefore turned to a stronger and more expensive antibiotic called *minocycline,* the current market favorite. A semi-synthetic form of tetracycline, it is sold under the name Minocin. Its side effects are even greater than for its forerunners, however, and signs of resistance to it too have been cropping up.[19] Erythromycin can cause upset stomach, and tetracycline can cause photosensitivity that results in severe sunburn; but these inconveniences pale beside those recently reported for minocycline: severe liver disease resulting in death, hepatitis, severe arthritis, and the autoimmune disease lupus, all apparently caused by the body's immune system turning on itself. Minocycline can also cause dizziness, discoloration of the teeth, and inflamed and aching joints and shortness of breath.[20] On top of that, all antibiotics can lead to *candida* yeast infections, which may, ironically, provoke skin eruptions.[21] (See "Candidiasis.")

Resistance to antibiotics can develop from very long courses of the drugs, or from the use of two or more of them together or in quick succession. It can also result because patients don't finish the entire dose, allowing stronger bacteria to survive. To avoid bacterial resistance, dermatologists now recommend using the stronger drugs only when absolutely necessary. In milder cases, topical remedies are recommended first.

TOPICAL REMEDIES

Over-the-counter topical remedies have proliferated, including a variety of creams and gels based on drying agents such as *benzoyl peroxide.* But while there are now more choices (at higher prices), the products remain only marginally effective. They take four to six weeks to work, if they work at all; and when you stop using them, the acne comes back. They are also quite drying to the skin. Medicated cleansers are generally a waste of money, because the medication washes off. Granular facial scrubs work no better than a washcloth, and facial saunas can actually aggravate acne.

In 1996, the first new prescription topical drug for mild to moderate acne was introduced. Called *Azelex*, it is a cream containing azelaic acid, a naturally occurring substance found in wheat that helps remove the redness from pimples. Like other topicals, however, it takes a couple of months to work.

RETINOIDS: ACCUTANE AND RETIN-A

Accutane (isotretinoin), on the other hand, works quickly and effectively. One of a class of vitamin A derivatives called retinoids that have revolutionized dermatology, Accutane is nearly always successful in treating serious cases of acne. Called "the greatest single advance thus far" in the treatment of acne, the drug has now been used by more than a million patients. It can produce dramatic clearing of lesions in severe, recalcitrant, cystic acne that is unresponsive to conventional therapy.[22]

Unfortunately, the usefulness of this "wonder drug" is severely limited by its high risk of side effects and birth defects. In a study of 154 women who took the drug while pregnant, their odds of having a child with major malformations turned out to be about 50:50. Among those in the study for whom contraceptive information was available, a third of the women who bore malformed infants conceived despite using contraception. Spontaneous abortions were also common.[23] Nearly everyone receiving therapeutic doses of Accutane experiences drying and inflammation of the lips, and chapping, itching, inflammation, and dryness of the skin are frequent. Some patients experience dryness in the eyes and an increased sensitivity to sunlight, symptoms that may not go away after the drug course is completed. Some patients also suffer vague aches and pains in the muscles and bones. Some lose a portion of their hair. Some find that their skin problems get worse, especially if they are taking tetracycline antibiotics at the same time. Headaches, depression, irritability, and fatigue can also result. Liver function can become altered and cholesterol and triglyceride levels elevated, necessitating careful monitoring in patients with a history of coronary artery disease, hepatitis, or inflammation of the pancreas.[24] Specialists now recommend that Accutane be used only on patients with deeply-seated cystic or pustular acne that is unresponsive to any other form of treatment who have been carefully screened for contraindications by physicians who are thoroughly familiar with the drug.[25]

Mild acne can be treated with the topical cream *Retin-A (tretinoin)*, a milder retinoid that is subject to side effects similar to Accutane's but in lighter form. *Retin-A is likely to cause sun sensitivity, so its prescription should always come with warnings to use sunscreens.*

Birth-Control Pills

Hormones have long been known to have a strong influence on the skin. Acne rages during the raging hormone years of the teens, and flare-ups tend to be worse for women the week before their menstrual periods. Dermatologists are therefore investigating treatments that alter these underlying hormonal changes. The birth-control pill is thought to ameliorate acne because estrogen suppresses the sebaceous glands' production of oil.[26] In January of 1997, the FDA approved a birth-control pill called *Tri-Cyclen* for the treatment of acne. Approval was limited, however, to females over fifteen who want contraception, have no contraindications to pill use, and have tried other topical acne treatments to no avail.

The Pill has been used as an acne treatment since the sixties, when it contained quite high levels of estrogen. When doses were later lowered to safer levels, improvements in the complexions of Pill-takers became much less common. Many women also noticed a worsening of acne when they stopped taking it. The Pill has other side effects as well—and acne can again be one of them.[27]

Tracking the Cause

Accutane, antibiotics, and other drug treatments address the symptoms of acne, but a lasting cure needs to rout out the cause. Likely suspects include dietary offenders, environmental toxins, and certain drugs.

To find out if food allergies are the problem in your case, try going on an elimination diet, then systematically adding suspect foods back in.[28] If a food is definitely implicated by the return of symptoms, eliminate it from the diet for at least three months. It can then be tried cautiously. If no reaction occurs, it can be eaten in moderation.

Teenagers in underdeveloped countries whose diets are based on vegetables and grains are substantially less prone to complexion problems than Americans are. For people willing to undergo a radical dietary overhaul, macrobiotic fare (whole grains, no milk, none or few animal products) has been reported to work miracles on blemishes.[29] There is no scientific proof that chocolate, nuts, or colas trigger outbreaks, but anecdotal evidence suggests that they do. Since these foods have no redeeming dietary virtues, cutting them out can't hurt. Eating less fat and more fruits and vegetables can also make your skin less oily. Fresh-squeezed fruit and vegetable juices—particularly carrot and cucumber juices—help oxygenate the blood and the skin it feeds.

HOMEOPATHIC AND CHINESE PATENT REMEDIES

Homeopathic doctors view the skin as an important organ of elimination. If its eruptions are suppressed, the toxins the skin is trying to eliminate will be driven further into the body, manifesting later as more serious diseases such as cancer. Another problem with the suppression of eruptions by drugs is that the drugs must be used continually, since when you stop using them, the problem comes right back. Oriental herbs and homeopathic remedies can eliminate the problem for good, by encouraging the body's elimination of underlying toxins.

A very effective Chinese patent remedy that works on this principle is one called *Margarite Acne Pills*. Chinese doctors believe that toxins build up in the blood and come out through the skin. Another combination herbal remedy with quite satisfied users is a product called *Herpacine*. (Give it about three weeks to work.) Effective homeopathic acne products currently on the market include *Clear AC* by Hyland's (which comes both as an oral tablet and a topical cream) and *Nelson Acne Gel*.

Recurring Acne Cleared

Nineteen-year-old Kelley was enormously self-conscious about her complexion, which was severely stricken with acne. She was thrilled when her complexion began to clear two weeks after she started taking the Margarite Acne Pills. In three weeks, it looked great.

NUTRIENT SUPPORT

Acne around the mouth can indicate digestive problems. For this, *digestive enzymes* can help, along with general nutritional support. *Colostrum* (the first mammary secretions of lactating cows) is now available in pill form and can help reduce infection. A good mail-order source is Pacific

Research Laboratories, 1010 Crenshaw Boulevard, Suite 170, Torrance, CA 90501 (tel. 310-320-1132).

HOME REMEDIES

Some simple home measures can also help keep symptoms under control:

1. Wash with ordinary soap and water. *Dr. Bronner's pure castile soap* is good. Once or twice a day is sufficient, since washing your skin too much can actually worsen acne.

2. Resist the urge to pick at blemishes, a habit that increases the risk of pits and scars.

3. Use either no cosmetics or the water-based kind. Avoid greasy hair dressings, and wear your hair away from your face.

4. For a facial scrub, try *oatmeal.* Make a paste of rolled oats and water, let it dry on your face, then wash it off.

5. For a natural steam sauna, use *red clover, lavender,* and *strawberry leaves.*

6. For a natural facial mask and moisturizer, peel and core an apple, put it in the blender with a little lemon or apple juice, smooth it on your face, leave it for about 15 minutes, then wash it off. *Lemon juice* may also be used as a natural astringent. A slice of *raw tomato* wiped on the face is good for oily skin. *Cucumber* works as a refining lotion to tighten pores.

7. If you feel you need a commercial product, use natural formulations. *Aloe* is one that can give quick skin relief.

8. If you can, spend a week at the beach. *Sunshine* brings oil to the surface of the skin, and *saltwater* acts as an astringent and cleans out the skin. A good natural oil applied as an aftersun lotion will feed the skin.

9. To draw oil out, try applying *healing clay* or a paste of *baking soda* and water to blemishes. Other possibilities are a dab of *toothpaste* or *tea tree oil.*[30]

Cystic Acne Cleared with Bentonite

A 37-year-old builder who worked in the sun and sweated a great deal had cystic acne all over his back. He was advised to brush his skin before showering, then apply bentonite clay to his back every night. The remedy drew the toxins from his acne and cleared it up. (For skin brushing, see "Environmental Illness.")

Acne Rosacea

Acne rosacea is an acne condition in older people. It usually begins as flushing or redness that follows a pattern of flare-ups and remissions. It can be aggravated by cold weather, stress, alcohol and spicy foods. Genetics is also a factor. Over time, it may become more pronounced and persistent, leaving pimples, visible blood vessels, and sometimes an enlarged nose (the W. C. Fields look).

CONVENTIONAL TREATMENT

The standard treatment is *MetroGel* applied to the skin twice daily, and the antibiotic *minocycline* taken orally (see "Acne"). MetroGel contains *metronidazole*, the same strong antibiotic found in Flagyl, a parasite remedy. The drug is marked with the FDA warning, "Metronidazole is carcinogenic in rodents. Avoid unnecessary use." Minocycline, a type of tetracycline, also comes with warnings, including skin sensitivities, pigmentation of the skin, and severe phototoxic reactions (reactions to the sun). Hazards are compounded by the fact that these strong medications are being put on damaged and sensitive skin. The drug combination costs between $125 and $150 a month, and when you stop using it, your skin returns to the state it was in before starting on the medications.[31]

ALTERNATIVE TREATMENT

Safe and effective natural alternatives include *vitamin K cream* and oral antioxidants containing *oligomeric proanthocyanids (OPCs)*, for example *pycnogenol*. A device called a *Bioptron* machine is also very effectively eliminates the symptoms of acne rosacea. The device is a rapidly blinking light that stimulates the skin to heal. (See "Skin Problems.")

Avoid aggravating factors: stress, alcohol, spicy foods. Bundle up in cold weather and stay well-ventilated in hot weather. Eat right and exercise. Use a natural moisturizer.

Aging, Memory Loss, Longevity

Aging is attributed to cellular degeneration caused by reactive oxygen compounds called free radicals. Cell colonies can be kept alive and well in Petri dishes indefinitely. What seems to cause aging and cell death in the body is the buildup of toxins, starving the cells for oxygen. If toxins could be eliminated as fast as they accumulated, the body, too, might live indefinitely.

"If DNA can manage to make perfect arteries for five hundred centuries, each one containing millions of perfectly operating cells," writes Deepak Chopra, M.D., "there is no intrinsic reason why *your* DNA should botch the job after sixty years." According to the Indian Ayurvedic philosophy Dr. Chopra espouses, aging is a mistake of thinking. He observes that in 1978, a team of researchers made the remarkable discovery that transcendental meditation could retard or even reverse the aging process.[32]

Other researchers are discovering that this process can be reversed with certain natural substances, including antioxidants to neutralize free radicals, and hormones and hormone precursors to replace the hormones that decline with age.

Other remedies help reverse the memory loss that is a normal part of aging. The natural remedies discussed under "Alzheimer's Disease" are also good for normal memory loss.

DRUG TREATMENT

Hormone replacement with prescription forms of *estrogen* and *progesterone* has been popular for women since the sixties. The problem with the best-selling forms of these hormones, which are either synthetic or animal derivatives, is that they don't exactly match the body's own hormones. Since they don't quite "fit" in the lock they are designed to turn, they can produce side effects and fail to perform all the functions of the normal hormone. (See Brown & Walker, *Menopause and Estrogen*, 1996.)

Attempts are now being made to replace the waning hormones not only of women but of men. Although substantial clinical evidence is lacking, users maintain that supplemental *testosterone* (by prescription-only patch, pill, or injection) can boost energy and libido and build muscle. Excitement was also generated by a 1990 study in which *human growth hormone* (HGh) increased muscle mass and strength in a small sample of men over the age of 60, while reducing their body fat and cholesterol levels. But more recent studies have failed to confirm these results; and injecting HGh can have serious side effects, including joint pain, fluid retention, and exacerbation of diabetes. The treatment can also cost a prohibitive $300 to $1,000 per month.[33]

NATURAL HORMONE ALTERNATIVES

Natural plant forms of estrogen and progesterone are now on the market that afford the benefits of hormone replacement without the side effects of drugs. (See "Menopause.") These products are available without a prescription. So are their natural precursors, which the bodies of both men and women can convert to other hormones as needed.

Hormone precursors include:

* *DHEA:* The DHEA produced by the adrenal glands is converted into estrogen or testosterone as needed. In rats, studies confirm that DHEA extends life. This hasn't yet been shown in humans, but DHEA has been found to promote feelings of well-being, increase production of some types of immune cells, and enhance sexual response. Start with 5 milligrams daily and work up, not to exceed 50 milligrams a day. Side effects have been reported, but this may have been because much of the DHEA on the market is synthetic. Natural sources are safer bets. A good mail-order source of pure, all-natural supplements is Pacific Research Laboratories (310-320-1132).

* *Pregnenolone:* This hormone precursor hasn't yet been well researched, but it has been shown to boost memory in rats and to help in some types of arthritis; and users report an enhanced sense of well being.[34] In women, pregnenolone is recommended along with DHEA, since taking DHEA alone can throw off hormone levels. Pregnenolone helps keep hormone levels in balance.

- *L-arginine:* This amino acid is a precursor to growth hormone and has been shown to stimulate its release. Arginine aids in the healing of wounds and immunity from disease; decreases cholesterol levels and atherogenesis (degenerative changes in the arteries), in both animals and humans; increases the weight of the thymus, a gland essential for immunity; and stimulates wound healing actually better than an injection of growth hormone.[35]

- *Melatonin:* A hormone manufactured by the pineal gland, melatonin gradually falls off after reaching peak levels during the twenties. When the pineal glands of adolescent mice have been transplanted into old rodents, their average life span has increased by a third. Melatonin is also a potent antioxidant, and it kills some cancer cells. CAUTION: Regular melatonin use isn't recommended for people under 40, since there is evidence that it *reduces* longevity in young rats. For younger people with insomnia, *homeopathic melatonin*, which stimulates the body to make its own hormone, is recommended instead. (See "Insomnia.")

ANTIOXIDANTS

Antioxidants neutralize free radicals. Rodents and insects fed large amounts of them have been found to live longer than control animals; and a diet heavy in fruits and vegetables, which are rich in antioxidants, has been shown to be protective against heart disease and cancer in humans. But animals given extra antioxidants also tend to eat less, so part of their increased longevity may be due to their low-calorie diets. (See the following.) And taken alone, some antioxidants can actually create free radicals, so you should take a range of them. The most researched are *vitamins A, C, E,* and *selenium;* but there are others with more antioxidant power. *Pycnogenol,* from *pine bark extract,* contains antioxidant flavonoids called OPCs (oligomeric proanthocyanids). Pycnogenol is several hundred times stronger as an antioxidant than are vitamins C and E and is used by millions of people daily in Europe. *Grapeseed extract* is another excellent source of OPCs. A third very powerful antioxidant that helps slow the aging process is *alpha lipoic acid* (ALA). Other antioxidants include *coenzyme Q10, cysteine, glutathione, superoxide dismutase,* and *zinc.*

Ginkgo biloba is an herb used for hundreds of years in Europe and Japan to increase mental function and help memory loss. Research at the University of California has shown that the herb is a strong antioxidant, which increases blood circulation to the brain. Studies at the University of Berlin have demonstrated that 50 mg of gingko biloba extract taken three times daily can improve mental functioning within six weeks.

Another popular youth-preserving herb is ginseng. The two main species of this plant are the Chinese or Oriental (Panax ginseng) and American (Panax quinquefolium) forms. Clinical and laboratory studies have shown that ginseng stimulates, regulates, and normalizes the central nervous system; stimulates and strengthens the heart; normalizes the blood pressure; regulates blood sugar; stimulates and regulates the pituitary, thyroid, and adrenal glands; combats stress and shock; and enhances the body's resistance to cancer.[36] *Siberian ginseng* (Eleutherococcus senticosus root) is not a true ginseng but is grouped with it because of similar active chemicals and physiological effects. It is used to increase longevity and decrease weakness and fatigue. Ginseng, a "yang" herb, is better for men than for women.

Other herbs with anti-aging benefits are *bilberry* and *green tea*.

Cancer Relieved with Common Herb

A woman customer said she had been diagnosed with inoperable lung cancer and had been given only two to three months to live. Then she had read about green tea and started using it, and noticed feeling dramatically better. Two months later, she went back to her doctor, who confirmed her remarkable improvement. Six months after that, she called to order more green tea. Three months after she was supposed to be dead, she said she felt great.

CALORIE RESTRICTION

When mice, fish, spiders, or fruit flies are fed a third less than they would eat if given a choice, they live up to twice as long as when eating *ad libitum* (at will). Calorie-deprived rats also learn to run mazes faster than well-fed rats.[37] In animals, longevity has been increased by calorie restriction either by reducing the total daily food intake or by alternating normal periods of intake with periods of abstinence.

Enthusiasts have long considered *fasting* to be the road to youth and health. When the body no longer needs to use its energy in digestion, it turns to housecleaning, burning up old toxins in place of food. Fasts have been engaged in for thousands of years for religious reasons, to clear the mind and as a form of denial that strengthens the spirit. For therapeutic purposes, modified fasts that include juice, tea, and broth are popular in health spas, particularly in Europe. (Edgar Cayce advocated an apple fast that also permitted coffee.) When therapeutic fasts were popularized a century ago, water-only fasts of one or two months were reported to cure many otherwise incurable chronic degenerative diseases. Dr. Paavo Airola, writing in the 1970s, explained that after the first three days of a fast, your body lives on itself, burning and digesting its own tissues, but it eliminates the dispensable ones first. That means that diseased, aging, or dead cells; morbid accumulations; tumors; abcesses; damaged tissues; and fat deposits are the first to go. During this time, the individual loses his craving for food.[38]

Then in the 1980s, reports of deaths from drastic fasting caused doctors to label the practice hazardous. It seems that our environment has become so polluted and our bodies so laden with drugs, pesticides, and industrial wastes that long-term, stringent fasting can cause an onslaught of toxins to be released into the bloodstream that overwhelms the body. But fasting has again become popular in the 1990s—in moderation. A three-day fast is advocated in Pamela Serure's *The 3-Day Energy Fast: Cleanse Your Body, Clear Your Mind, Claim Your Spirit*. Dr. Joel Fuhrman, in *Fasting—and Eating—for Health*, states that he has successfully treated ills ranging from asthma to heart disease with a one- or two-week water-only fast followed by a low-fat, plant-based diet.

Dr. Airola recommended modified fasts on vegetable and fruit juices, and that not for more than seven to ten days unless under medical supervision. He also felt that daily enemas were essential to speed the elimination of toxins. The V. E. Irons fast promoted by Dr. Bernard Jensen in his classic book *Tissue Cleansing for Bowel Management* adds supplements (chlorophyll, beet, and the like), psyllium (plant fiber), and bentonite (a natural colloidal adsorbing solution). The prescribed regimen is a seven-day fast once every seven weeks for seven weeks. Consult Dr. Jensen's or another reference book for detailed guidance.

The *Sambu Cleanse Kit* by Flora is a complete kit for a three- or ten-day fast that cleans the colon, bladder and kidney, boosts the immune system, and clears the body of toxins. It comes with elderberry syrup that is drunk every couple of hours.

Youthful Old Age Attributed to Frugal Diet and Lifestyle

Luigi Cornaro, a fifteenth-century centenarian, maintained that the secret to living not only long but well to the end was a "regular" life—simple, free of stress, and involving extremely frugal eating habits. He limited his daily intake to 12 ounces of food and 14 ounces of drink. He wrote at the age of 95, "though at this great age, I am hearty and content, eating with a good appetite, and sleeping soundly. Moreover, all my senses are as good as ever . . . How different from the life of most old men, full of aches and pains, and forebodings, whilst mine is a life of real pleasure."[39]

NATURAL MEMORY BOOSTERS

Herbs and supplements specifically recommended to slow memory loss include *ginkgo biloba, gotu kola, phosphatidyl serine (PS), omega–3 fatty acids, choline* and other *B vitamins, amino acids* (especially *L-glutamine* and *L-phenylalanine*), *acetyl-L-carnitine (ALC), antioxidants* (especially *co-enzyme Q10*), *dimethylaminoethanol (DMAE), pregnenolone, Bacopa Monniera* (an Ayurvedic herb), and *nicotinamide adenine dinucleotide (NADH).*[40] See also "Alzheimer's Disease."

AIDS

AIDS (Acquired Immune Deficiency Syndrome) is a fatal immune deficiency disorder for which neither the cause nor the cure is certainly known. The disease seriously impairs immunity, leaving patients highly vulnerable to attack from opportunistic organisms, particularly *P. carinii* pneumonia (PCP); and to such malignancies as lymphoma and Kaposi's sarcoma, a once-rare form of cancer that attacks the endothelial cells lining the blood vessels.

AIDS is steeped in controversy. The cause is conventionally considered to be the HIV retrovirus; but Dr. Peter Duesberg, of the University of California at Berkeley, heads a growing number of scientists and physicians who question the theory. Dr. Duesberg, who helped pioneer the field of retroviruses, argues that HIV is too inactive, infects too few cells, and is too difficult to find in AIDS patients to be responsible for the immune damage that results. He observes that there are nearly 5,000 documented AIDS cases worldwide where HIV is not present, a discrepancy that has been covered up by reclassifying them as idiopathic CD-4 lymphocytopenia (ICL), although their symptoms and opportunistic infections are the same as for AIDS.[41] Alternative explanations for the immune deficiencies of AIDS patients include chronic consumption of drugs such as cocaine, amyl nitrates ("poppers"), AZT, and other immunosuppressive drugs; multiple, repeated venereal diseases leading to immune-system collapse; radiation exposure; and other viral and parasitic pathogens. Even the toxic benzene lubricants used by homosexual men have been proposed as culprits.[42]

Other researchers accept the viral theory but dispute the popular African green-monkey theory of its origins. Dr. Leonard Horowitz, a Harvard public-health researcher, traces the AIDS virus to National Cancer Institute laboratories, where researchers in the 1960s deliberately mixed viral genes from different animals to produce leukemia, sarcoma, general wasting, and death, producing the "cancer models" used to begin human vaccine trials.[43] Still other researchers blame the spread of AIDS on contaminated vaccines; for example, those given in Africa for smallpox. Such contamination hasn't yet been proven for a human vaccine, but contamination of a fowlpox vaccine with a retrovirus was reported in the *Economist* in November of 1997. The discovery confirmed that retroviruses are able to reproduce by inserting their genes not only into an animal host but into another virus.[44]

DRUG TREATMENT

The first prescription medicine approved for the treatment of AIDS was the antiviral drug *zidovudine ("AZT")*. Originally developed for treating cancer, AZT slows replication of HIV but doesn't specifically target the virus, doesn't cure active AIDS, and can't restore an AIDS patient's immune system once destroyed. It also has many unwanted side effects, including nausea, insomnia, severe headaches, muscle pain, and reduction in white blood cells. Suppression of the growth of bone-marrow cells results in a lack of red blood cells, producing anemia, and in a lack of white blood cells, increasing susceptibility to infection. Liver damage has also been documented. As many as half of all AIDS patients can't take AZT because of these side effects; and cost of the drug is prohibitive, running around $7,000 or $8,000 per patient per year.

AZT has also been used preventatively, since it seems to delay the development of AIDS in people who have the virus but have no symptoms—a category believed to include several hundred thousand Americans. The problem with using the drug preventatively is that HIV progressively develops a resistance to it. If people who are well take it for several years, it may be of no use to them once they begin to get ill; and they will have had to undergo AZT's side effects and risks in the meantime.[45] Risks include cancer; high doses of AZT have been linked to vaginal cancer in rats. For people who already have AIDS, this may be of small consequence, since their life expectancy is typically only a year or two after their first hospitalization. But for people who are infected with the virus but are asymptomatic, the ill effects of the disease may not be felt for years. Cancer could affect them before AIDS does.[46] And under Dr. Duesberg's theory, they might never even develop the disease.

In December of 1995, the FDA approved Hoffman-LaRoche's *Saquinavir,* the first of a new category of AIDS drug known as *protease inhibitors.* In March of 1996, two more protease inhibitors were approved, Merck's *Indinavir* and Abbott's *Ritonavir.* Protease inhibitors are reported to stop HIV from replicating and, in some cases, to substantially reduce the total viral load. But these drugs, too, can have serious side effects, although Indinavir seems to have the least; and the cumulative price tag is estimated at more than $40,000 for the drugs and another $20,000 to $40,000 for lab and doctor fees.[47] In 1997, researchers reported that the drugs weren't as effective as had been hoped, and that the AIDS virus seems to be becoming resistant to them.[48]

A range of other drugs that kill HIV is also used to treat AIDS, including *DDI (didanosine), pentamidine, ddC, d4T,* and *3TC;* but these drugs too can have serious side effects. Other drugs are used by AIDS patients to treat the opportunistic infections and malignancies resulting from their immune deficiency.

There is no vaccine effective against HIV and no drug that specifically targets it. Development of an effective AIDS vaccine, if possible at all, is thought to be more than a decade away.[49]

THE ALTERNATIVE APPROACH

AIDS is still a terminal disease, but people stricken with it are living longer than ever before. AIDS patients are an organized, cohesive group who share information and have developed a tremendous support system. Many AIDS patients and activists have concluded, like Dr. Duesberg, that antiretroviral medications do more to cause immune deficiency than to relieve it. These patients are opting for natural therapies that build up the immune system and improve the quality of life; or they are using a combination of therapies, conventional and alternative.[50]

Reversal of AIDS Symptoms by Detoxification Program

Roger Cobb, co-chairman of the consumer caucus for the Commission on AIDS Care, Service and Treatment for the Philadelphia area, admits to using crack, cocaine, and many other drugs for more than 21 years, until he learned he was HIV-positive. He took AZT for about 14 months, but decided it wasn't for him. Instead, he set out to detoxify his body of the legal and illegal drugs he credited with the destruction of his immune defenses. He used colon cleansers, herbs, wheatgrass juice, distilled water, juicing, dietary reform, and meditation. He now reports having more energy, feeling more rested and less stressed, and looking better than when he was taking drugs, legal or illegal.[51]

Promising Natural Treatments

Many natural therapies are being used to treat AIDS worldwide. A Chinese practitioner in Melbourne, Australia, reports the elimination of active symptoms in pre-AIDS cases with the use of *acupuncture*.[52]

An Ayurvedic practitioner in India, T. A. Majeed, claims high success with an AIDS compound consisting of 25 *Ayurverdic herbs* that build up the immune system. He says he has worked with more than 300 AIDS patients, and that except in serious cases, his compound has worked quickly for most of them. Few patients in India are willing to discuss their cases, but one exception was a woman named Chitra, who contracted HIV from her husband in 1991. Amazingly, she says, 43 days after starting on Majeed's Ayurvedic medicine, she turned HIV-negative. One concern was that in the United States, immune suppression from AZT and other drugs would counteract the immune-stimulating effects of Ayurvedic medicine; but about 40 U.S. patients have been treated with the Ayurvedic compound, and all have reportedly shown significant improvement.[53]

Another promising treatment is *boxwood extract*. An informal six-month U.S. trial organized by AIDS patients showed that the extract helped reduce the level of HIV in the blood of most participants, and it had no toxic side effects. The extract is manufactured under the name SPV-30 and costs about $800 a year in the United States, less than one fifth that of the newest AIDS drugs.[54]

Ozone therapy is also widely used in Europe with reportedly good results. See "Immunity."

For the latest in other new treatments and support, see the Internet. There are several Web sites devoted to AIDS, including **http://www. thebody.com; www.aidsquilt.org/;** and **www.unaids.org.** For Hoffman-LaRoche's presentation of the latest pharmaceutical approaches to AIDS, see **www.roche-hiv.com.**

Alcohol Abuse

Ten million Americans are alcoholics. In 1988, the Supreme Court stopped short of ruling that alcoholism is a disease, saying only that the Veterans Administration didn't have to treat it as one for disability purposes. But the medical trend is to reclassify the condition as a disease and to search for genetic errors and neurochemical imbalances. Besides physiological factors, there are obviously emotional ones: Alcohol is used to escape personal problems, anxieties, and stress.

CONVENTIONAL TREATMENT

The standard treatment is a drug called *Anabuse*. It works as a deterrent by making you violently ill if you ingest alcohol in any form. One downside is that you can have a severe reaction if you accidently drink alcohol, for example, in cough syrup.

NATURAL ALTERNATIVES

An herbal remedy called *kudzu* (an American vine) and a homeopathic remedy called *Nux vomica* work remarkably well in quelling alcoholic tendencies without side effects.

The "Liver Cleanse Diet" is another very useful aid. (See "Liver Disease.")

For a complete program, including vitamins and amino acids, claimed by many people to be effective, see *Seven Weeks to Sobriety; The Proven Program to Fight Alcoholism Through Nutrition*, by Joan Larson (Fawcett Books, 1994).

Marriage Saved with Herbs and Homeopathy

A woman sought help for her husband, who was drinking nightly and getting progressively more abusive and aggressive. She said he had tried to stop but seemed just to be getting worse. She went home with kudzu and Nux vomica. A month later, her husband returned and bought more. The following month, the woman came back to confirm the remarkable change in her husband. He hadn't had a drink in two months, he was happy, and their marriage was going well. Nearly a year after he began taking the remedies, she reports he still hasn't had a drink. He took the remedies consistently for about four months. Now she keeps them on hand just for occasional use—whenever he becomes cranky and irritable, perhaps once a month.

Allergies, Hay Fever

Allergies plague an estimated 20 percent of Americans. They are responsible for one in five visits to the pediatrician and are the leading reason for hospitalization in children. *Hay fever*, or *allergic rhinitis*—an inflammation of the nasal passages caused by an irritant—is by far the most common allergy, striking some six million children annually. The increased incidence of allergies in industrialized countries has been linked to an increase in pollutants, chemicals, pesticides, and other allergy-provoking foreign substances.

Several studies reported in 1997 also linked both allergies and diabetes (two auto-immune diseases) to immunization and a decreased incidence of childhood infections. When nearly 300 children in Guinea-Bissau were tested for allergic reactions to airborne allergens, allergies (asthma, eczema, hay fever, and so forth) were found to be significantly more common in children who had never had measles. Vaccination against the disease, it seems, didn't give the same protection as actually getting it. In two other recent studies conducted in Italy, allergies were found to be less common among the poor and among people who grew up in big families or unsanitary surroundings. Exposure to hepatitis A and tuberculosis was shown in other studies to afford immunity to allergies. The suggested explanation is that the evolving immune system needs to keep busy. If it has no invaders to cope with, it turns its defenses on otherwise-harmless stimuli.[55]

DRUG TREATMENT

Standard allergy treatment includes drugs similar to those for colds. In fact the *antihistamines* familiar in treating colds are actually more helpful in treating allergies, since allergies result from the *inappropriate* release of histamine into the blood stream.

Antihistamines have been available since the 1940s, but the older versions (*Benadryl, Allerest, Chlor-Trimeton*) produce drowsiness, making driving a car or operating machinery unsafe and work difficult. A later-model antihistamine called *terfenadine (Seldane)*, which overcame this defect, shot to number one on the prescription drug charts the year it came out (1985). But enthusiasm for it was tempered when a rash of deaths was attributed to its use in conjunction with certain other drugs, and in 1997 the FDA withdrew Seldane from the market.

Other drugs of this type, however, are still available. *Claritin* is the current market leader among nonsedating antihistamines. Other options include *Histmanal* and *Zyrtec*. (Histmanal has the same heart risks as Seldane, and 14 percent of users on Zyrtec report drowsiness.) Seldane's makers have also produced *Allegra,* an allergy drug touted as having the same benefits as Seldane with fewer risks.[56] But the chemical structures of these drugs are all similar to Seldane's, making them all potentially risky.

Other allergy medicines that are new to the over-the-counter market include *cromolyn sodium* products that come either as a nasal spray (*Nasalcrom*) or eyedrops (*Opticrom*). Unlike antihistamines, which reach histamine only after the allergic response is in full swing, these drugs are said to prevent the response at its outset by preventing white blood cells from releasing histamine and other immune-system chemicals. Their drawbacks are that they need to be used three to six times a day all through hay fever season, and they can have side effects, including headaches, sneezing, nosebleeds, and stinging in the nose.

There are also *steroid-containing nasal sprays* for the treatment of hay fever (*Vancenase, Flonase,* and others). Although steroids taken by mouth have serious systemic effects, the sprays are thought to reduce these effects since they hit only the nose, not the whole body. But their safety, too, remains to be established. The new steroid inhalers for asthma, which were also thought to be safer than steroids taken by mouth, have now been found to have some of the same side effects as the oral drugs. (See "Asthma.") The sprays also take two to four days to work and can irritate the nose. The hazards of steroids in general are discussed under "Infection, Immunity."

WARNING: For the treatment of hay fever, decongestants or decongestant/antihistamine combinations should be avoided. They can cause a rebound effect and are potentially addicting if used for more than a few days; and hay fever tends to last more than a few days.

ALLERGY SHOTS

Allergy desensitization injections are generally reserved for people with severe allergies, since they're a long and expensive commitment with an uncertain outcome. A typical course can take three to five years, and it may be a full year before you see any improvement. The required once- or twice-weekly office visits have been called annuities for allergists. Whether the shots actually reduce or eliminate allergies has never been proven, since many young people outgrow their allergies even without treatment. A study reported in the *New England Journal of Medicine* in January of 1997 found that most children with asthma don't benefit from allergy shots.[57]

NATURAL ALTERNATIVES: HOMEOPATHIC REMEDIES

Effective homeopathic remedies are available that help desensitize the body to specific allergens. A number of companies also make good combination allergen remedies. (See Appendix.)

THE WATER CURE

F. Batmanghelidj, M.D., in *Your Body's Many Cries for Water*, asserts that asthma and allergies are diseases of water dehydration. He states he has seen many cases cured simply by increasing the patient's intake of pure water to half the body weight in ounces per day—for example, 64 ounces, or 8 glasses, for a body weight of 128 pounds.[58] (See Chapter 2 for other details of this therapy.)

AVOIDING THE CAUSE

Avoiding the known offenders, such as cats or down pillows, is another obvious precaution. For allergies to airborne substances, an air conditioner or air filter on your heating system can help. So can a humidifier or vaporizer, but it can also aggravate some allergies by producing a moist environment that encourages the growth of allergy-producing molds.

Food allergies account for many less obvious childhood symptoms, including eczema (skin rash), chronic coughs and bronchitis, diarrhea, migraine headaches, colitis, and even otitis media.[59] Again, substantial improvement may result from avoiding the common offenders—eggs, milk, nuts, soy, wheat, and the nightshades (tomatoes, potatoes, green peppers, eggplant, tobacco). This can require substantial effort by the parent, but it is liable to be worth the trouble, since children often outgrow their allergies. If the food isn't avoided, the allergy is more likely to remain.[60] The desensitization process can even be started before the child is born. If one parent has allergies, the chances are one in three that the child will too; and if both parents have them, the chances are two in three. Mothers who suspect food allergies can start by passing up allergy-causing foods while they're pregnant and nursing. Eggs, milk products, nuts, and peanut butter are leading suspects to be avoided.[61]

Allergies can also be precipitated by parasites.

Allergies Traced to Parasites and Eliminated

David's fourteen-year history of symptoms included persistent nausea, gas, bloating, intestinal upset, and severe fatigue; and allergies had plagued him for years. He had tried all the conventional remedies to no avail. A six-week course of *Para-A* to treat his parasites had the remarkable effect of eliminating his allergies as well, although he was never treated specifically for that condition. (See "Chronic Fatigue Syndrome," "Parasites.")

NATURAL DECONGESTANTS

For congestion, try hot tea made with natural decongestants, such as *fenugreek, anise* and *sage. Garlic, onions*, and *hot and spicy foods* can also thin out mucus.

Another trick is the nasal douche: washing out your nose with saltwater. This can be done with a nose dropper, or with an Indian device called a *neti pot.*

Exercise is a natural adrenalin stimulant that can produce direct nervous stimulation to the nose.[62]

For other suggestions, see "Asthma."

Alzheimer's Disease

Alzheimer's disease is a mental deterioration in the elderly that can't be explained by normal aging. Discovered in 1906, it was once erroneously thought to result from hardening of the arteries but is now known to involve degeneration of nerve cells. It is characterized by twisted, tangled nerves and hardened deposits of chemical plaque in the brain. Alzheimer's disease has recently become an epidemic, afflicting over a million Americans—up to half of the elderly who are over 75, and half of those with senile dementia. Nearly 20 times as many deaths were reported from Alzheimer's disease in 1993 as in 1979.[63] It is now the fourth leading cause of American deaths, and accounts for 30 percent of nursing-home admissions. Symptoms include gradual memory loss, disorientation, loss of language ability, and personality changes that can extend over a number of years, devastating not only the patient but his family.

THE CONVENTIONAL APPROACH

Conventional medicine has no cure for Alzheimer's disease. The only available treatment, a drug called *tacrine (Cognex)*, can slow deterioration somewhat, but it can also cause uncomfortable and dangerous side effects, and it is expensive and hard to administer ($260 a month for the drug and weekly blood monitoring).[64] Other drugs can ease pain, agitation, and paranoia. But conventional treatment for the most part consists simply of helping the patient and his or her family cope with the disease.

Concerning prevention, women who take *hormone replacement therapy* have been found to have a lower risk of Alzheimer's disease. For the natural approach to hormone replacement, see "Menopause."

As for the cause, conventional research has focused on genetics; but the cause of Alzheimer's remains elusive.

A NOVEL NATURAL APPROACH: ELIMINATING HEAVY METALS

Even people with a genetic predisposition to a disease may not develop it unless they are pushed over the edge by toxic environmental factors. Among those factors, mounting evidence points to accumulation in the brain of heavy metals, including mercury, aluminum, and lead. The blood/brain barrier is intended to keep toxins out of the brain, but those that do get in are prevented by it from getting back out. They continue to build up over the years, progressively blocking brain and nerve function.[65]

The link with aluminum has been demonstrated by accumulations of the metal found in the brains of patients who have died of Alzheimer's disease. Pathological changes similar to those seen in Alzheimer's have also been observed after exposure to aluminum.[66] Earlier observations linking the metal to the disease were confirmed in a study of 88 county districts in England and Wales, which found a definite connection between the incidence of Alzheimer's and average aluminum levels in the water supply.[67] The use of aluminum-containing antiperspirants is also associated with a higher risk of Alzheimer's dementia.[68]

Research links Alzheimer's disease not only to aluminum but to mercury. Cats fed fish containing methyl mercury show Alzheimer's-like brain lesions, and humans who eat mercury-laden fish exhibit neurological symptoms including memory loss, tremors, irritability, insomnia, numbness, and visual disturbances.[69] The greatest human exposure to mercury, however, seems to be the standard silver/mercury amalgam dental filling. A 1990 *New England Journal of Medicine* editorial called mercury fillings "possibly the chief source of exposure [to mercury] of a large segment of the U.S. population."[70] Recent research has established that mercury from fillings is released into the body with chewing, and that it accumulates in the tissues of the brain.[71]

In 1990, University of Kentucky researchers found significant elevations of mercury in the brains of 180 Kentucky residents who were autopsied after dying of Alzheimer's disease. When concentrations of trace elements were analyzed, the most important imbalance found was an elevation in mercury.[72] These findings meshed with earlier studies demonstrating a direct correlation between the amount of mercury in the brain and the amount in mercury dental fillings. In studies of the cadavers of accident victims, those with a mere five amalgams had three times the amount of mercury in their brain tissues as cadavers without amalgams.[73] A later autopsy study done by the Mayo Heavy Metals Lab on an 82-year-old decedent with confirmed Alzheimer's disease found 53 times the normal level of mercury in the woman's brain. The "neurofibrillary tangle" characteristic of Alzheimer's disease was also found. The woman had multiple amalgams in her teeth. Other research shows that people with mercury fillings have higher levels of mercury not only in their brains but in their urine and blood.[74]

Alzheimer's Disease Reversed

Tom Warren, in a book called *Beating Alzheimer's,* attests that his own diagnosed case of Alzheimer's disease was reversed after he had all of his teeth pulled and replaced with dentures. (His teeth contained 28 mercury amalgam fillings.) He also had chelation treatments and took homeopathic remedies to remove heavy metals from his tissues, changed his diet, took heavy doses of nutritional supplements, and eliminated environmental toxins and allergens from his surroundings. He maintains that his is the first case on record in which Alzheimer's, a disease conventionally considered incurable, has been reversed. Other cases he cites include that of a physician who recovered from the disease in a stunning two hours, with the removal of 13 teeth containing root canals.[75]

CHELATION

Getting heavy metals out of the teeth is only half the battle. Metals also must be eliminated from brain tissues, a much trickier proposition. Tom Warren used intravenous and homeopathic chelation for this purpose. The chelation process and other available chelators are described in detail under "Heavy Metal Poisoning."

A placebo-controlled trial of *desferrioxamine,* which removes aluminum from the body by binding with it, found that the drug significantly reduced the rate of decline in the ability of a group of people with Alzheimer's dementia to care for themselves.[76]

OTHER NATURAL REMEDIES

In April of 1997, the *New England Journal of Medicine* reported on a remedy compared to which "no treatment for Alzheimer's disease has shown similar benefits." The remedy was easy to administer, inexpensive, and had no unwanted side effects. It was ordinary *vitamin E,*—at an extraordinary dosage of 2,000 IU.[77]

The herb *ginkgo biloba* has been shown in more than a dozen double-blind studies to reduce mental decline. One was in the *Journal of the American Medical Association* in October of 1997. Ginkgo, the world's oldest species of tree, is considered in traditional Chinese medicine to benefit the brain. It seems to increase blood flow to the brain, improving the supply of oxygen and glucose.

Another natural substance found to help Alzheimer's patients is *nicotinamide adenine dinucleotide (NADH)*. NADH is present in all living things and plays a central role in cellular energy production. Patients given 10 mg of this nutrient half an hour before breakfast for 8 to 12 weeks showed significant improvement on a mental-state examination.[78]

An Italian study found *acetyl-L-carnitine* to be effective in slowing the progression of Alzheimer's.[79]

Alzheimer's patients given *zinc* (90 mg), *selenium* (2 mg), and *evening primrose oil* (6 grams) scored better than a placebo group in another study on a battery of mental-function tests.[80]

Alzheimer's patients tend to be low in *vitamin B12*, even when dietary intake is adequate. Apparently they have a problem absorbing the vitamin. For this, B12 shots can help.[81]

Improvements have been documented in Alzheimer's patients given *coenzyme Q10, iron*, and *vitamin B6*. Other studies have found improvements with various protocols using *DMSO*.[82]

A Chinese herbal tea also has reported benefits. For centuries, traditional Chinese healers have claimed that a tea made from a plant called *club moss (Shen Jin Cao)* improves memory and failing mental capacity. A drug now undergoing testing for Alzheimer's called *Hyperzine A* is a derivative of club moss. The tea version is currently available in the Chinatowns of large American cities.[83]

F. Batmanghelidj, M.D., documented a case in which a patient's Alzheimer's symptoms were reversed simply by increasing his *water* intake to eight glasses a day. (See Chapter 2 for protocol.)

Anemia

Anemia is a condition in which body tissues get insufficient oxygen, either because there aren't enough red blood cells in circulation or because the blood is low in hemoglobin, an essential protein. Anemia can result from blood loss or from something that destroys blood cells or interferes with their production in the body. Chronic blood loss can result from stomach ulcers or hemorrhoids. Iron-deficiency anemia occurs when the body lacks iron, a necessary constituent of hemoglobin. It can be the result of heavy menstrual bleeding or a lack of iron in the diet. Anemia may also result from a lack of other nutrients, including folic acid and vitamin B12. Other types (for example, sickle-cell anemia) are hereditary.

Drugs and alcohol can also cause anemia. One cause of iron-deficiency anemia is the daily loss of imperceptible amounts of blood in the stool from habitual aspirin use, as by arthritis victims. This effect is particularly insidious because it produces no symptoms. It can be a serious threat to older people who don't get enough iron and to women who have heavy periods. Besides iron, aspirin also increases your need for certain vitamins, notably C, B1, and folic acid.

Conventional Treatment

Anemia is usually treated with supplemental iron, but iron supplements aren't very effective in rebuilding the blood. They take a long time to be absorbed, can be constipating, and are highly toxic in overdose. Enteric-coated supplements can't be effectively absorbed and should be avoided. There is also research linking high levels of iron in the blood to an increased risk of heart attacks in men. It has been hypothesized that the lower risk of heart attacks in premenopausal women may be due, not to their higher estrogen levels (as has been thought), but to menstruation, which lowers their total iron levels.[84] *Don't take iron supplements unless you need them.* If you do need them, *ferrous gluconate* is the most absorbable form.

Anemia may also be treated conventionally with supplements of *folic acid* or other nutrients in which the patient's blood levels are low. Serious types of anemia, for example those caused by bleeding of the digestive tract, are conventionally corrected by surgery.

The Oriental Approach

In Chinese medicine, diagnosis of anemia is made from a pale tongue or the faintness of the lines on the palm of the hand. The condition is referred to as "blood deficiency." Chinese doctors say there is not enough blood in these cases to "nourish the heart," so the *Shen* (spirit), which resides in the heart, is disturbed. The patient can't sleep, has nightmares, experiences heart palpitations, becomes pale, loses her hair. The Chinese formula for correcting this condition in women is called *Women's Precious Pills* by K'am Herbs. Take 2–3 pills 3x daily.

Normal, healthy women can become anemic just from menstruating. Normal, healthy men, on the other hand generally don't become anemic. If they do have this problem, and if it's not from a known source of blood loss like an injury, they probably aren't manufacturing blood properly. Professional help should be sought to determine the cause, so the underlying problem can be treated.

NUTRITIONAL AND HERBAL REMEDIES

Chlorophyll, the "blood" of plants, can help rebuild the blood of humans. However, eating sufficient amounts of green vegetables to accomplish this result is difficult. The easier alternative is to take supplemental *chlorophyll* (two ounces in water two to three times daily), or green pills: *spirulina, chlorella* or *The Ultimate Green* by Nature's Secret.

Angina Pectoris

Angina pectoris, or chest pain on exertion, may be the first symptom of an impending heart attack. Chest pain results when the supply of blood fails to meet demand, preventing the heart muscle cells from getting enough oxygen to pump at required levels. Insufficient oxygen delivery usually results from the buildup of a calcified fatty plaque in the arteries that diminishes blood flow. The process by which hardening of the arteries impairs heart function is discussed under "Atherosclerosis."

DRUG TREATMENT

Drug treatment for angina generally involves *beta-blockers, calcium channel blockers, nitrates,* or some combination of them. Beta-blockers reduce angina pain by preventing the nervous system from stimulating the heart to work harder. Calcium-channel blockers do it by dilating the blood vessels, making more room for blood to flow through. Both can have side effects, ranging from annoying to life-threatening. (See "Hypertension.") A combination of low doses of these two drug types has become popular in angina treatment on the theory that the combination will cover more bases with fewer side effects. But recent data suggest that in most patients, combination therapy actually increases side effects, without increasing benefits.[85]

Nitrates include nitroglycerin, isosorbide dinitrate, and pentaerythritol tetranitrate. They work by dilating the blood vessels in the heart. They don't affect peripheral blood vessels but do dilate blood vessels in the head, leading to their most troublesome side effect, painful headaches. Up to 50 percent of users suffer from headaches at one time or another.

Nitroglycerin tablets that can be dissolved under the tongue are used either to relieve angina attacks that are in progress or to prevent anticipated attacks from exertion. They work for about 30 minutes.

A newer drug-delivery system is the *transdermal patch*, a device that lets controlled doses of the drug enter the bloodstream continuously through the skin. The patch can't be used for acute attacks, since maximum concentrations don't reach the blood until an hour or two after application. But for maintenance therapy, it has several advantages over pills, including convenience and constant bioavailability. The major drawback of the transdermal nitroglycerin patch is that continuous doses can cause the body to develop a tolerance to the drug. That means not only that it won't work but that serious problems can result on withdrawal. One study concluded that in most patients with stable angina, side effects of the patch outweigh its benefits.[86]

NATURAL REMEDIES

Good natural heart regulators are available that avoid these adverse effects.

In the herbal line, *hawthorn berry (Crataegus Oxycantha)* is an excellent tonic for the heart. Studies have shown that it increases coronary blood flow and allows the heart to function with less oxygen. Hawthorn berry increases not only oxygen use by the heart but enzyme metabolism in the heart muscle, making the heart pump more efficiently. It also dilates the peripheral blood vessels (blood vessels distant from the heart), lowering blood pressure and reducing the heart's burden in pumping blood. Hawthorn berry helps overcome cardiac weakness and is particularly useful for people with angina, high blood pressure, or a history of heart attack. It has also been used to lower serum cholesterol.[87]

Nutritional supplements can also help. Injections of *magnesium sulfate* have brought about dramatic clinical improvement in patients with angina and coronary thrombosis. *Co-enzyme Q10* is another nutrient with documented effectiveness in strengthening the heart and the body in general.[88]

In the homeopathic line, *Glonoine* is a useful remedy for heart problems. Glonoine is appropriate for the heart patient with chest pain, confusion, dizziness, sensations of pulsing throughout the body, heart flutterings and palpitations. *Cactus Comp* formula is another homeopathic remedy that can do wonders for the heart.

Angina Symptoms Relieved

Extremely weak and barely able to walk, Mrs. Hicks had been given no hope of survival by her doctor. But her husband Irl, an old-time Idaho farmer, was a firm believer in alternative medicine. He owned a homeopathic book and had read it through many times. When he sought help in choosing a remedy, he was advised to try Cactus Comp. In a matter of weeks, his wife was out of bed, walking around, and full of life. Her doctor couldn't believe it. She remains alive and well two years later.

For another interesting case in which Cactus reversed heart symptoms, see the discussion under "Nail Health" of a patient whose spoon-shaped nails indicated heart problems.

LIFESTYLE MODIFICATION

Exercise can help prevent angina from developing. An Israeli study of more than 10,000 middle-aged men and women found that the risk of developing angina was more than twice as great for men with sedentary lifestyles as for those who were more active; and for sedentary women, it was more than three times as great.

Exercise has also been shown to reduce angina pain. A regular exercise routine lowers the pulse rate, which means the heart doesn't have to work so hard or use so much oxygen. In a study reported in the medical journal *Mayo Clinic Proceedings*, eight men with mild angina were put on an exercise program involving 45-minute sessions three times a week. Five were completely symptom-free after one year, and three experienced significant reductions in angina pain.[89]

A strict vegetarian diet can be even more effective. In a British study, four out of four patients with severe angina who had not responded to medication became symptom-free after five to six months on a "vegan" diet that entirely excluded animal products. They were able to engage in strenuous activities without pain. One patient was followed for a full ten years, during which his pain did not return even when mountain-climbing.[90] In an earlier study, when six angina patients were put on a diet consisting of rice, fruits, vegetables, and a specially prepared mixture of amino acids, their angina pain decreased, their ability to exercise increased, and their serum cholesterol levels dropped nearly 40 percent. Again, prior drug treatment had failed to improve their conditions.[91]

THE DENTAL FACTOR

Toxins from bacterial abscesses or heavy metals in the teeth have also been linked to angina. For a full discussion of recommended protocols for removal, see Ellen Brown, Richard Hansen, D.M.D., *The Key to Ultimate Health* (La Mirada, California: Advanced Health Research Publishing, 1998).

Angina Pain Eliminated

A 74-year-old man complained of chest pains, arm pains, and an irregular heartbeat. He was on nitroglycerin for angina and Verapamil for high blood pressure. He had spent two days in the hospital undergoing tests, but the medication he was given for his irregular heartbeat only made his symptoms worse. Dental examination revealed an extremely infected tooth. The man waited too long to get it fixed, however, and it had to be extracted. When it was, his heart symptoms disappeared. He got off his heart medications and onto a nutritional maintenance program, and said he had never felt stronger.

Anxiety

Approximately 50 million U.S. adults suffer from anxiety, a mental state that can induce not only psychological symptoms (tension, fear, difficulty concentrating, apprehension) but physical symptoms including tachycardia (rapid heart beat), increased blood pressure, hyperventilation, palpitations (irregular or strong heart beats), tremors, headache, and sweating. Less obvious effects can include weakened immunity, nervousness, indigestion, problems concentrating, sleeplessness, and chronic fatigue.

General anxiety disorder, characterized by disabling apprehension, worry, irritability, and vigilance, initially manifests around age 20 to 35 and is slightly more predominant in women. When anxiety progresses to full-blown panic disorder (unpredictable episodes of intense anxiety), physiological responses can result, including rapid heartbeat, dizziness, trembling, and choking.[92] Other distressing signs and symptoms are dyspnea (shortness of breath), palpitations, headache, a sense of smothering, nausea, bloating, and a feeling of impending doom. Recurrent sleep panic attacks (not nightmares) occur in about 30 percent of people with panic disorder. The condition tends to be familial, with onset under age 25, and affects 3 to 5 percent of the population. The premenstrual period is a time of heightened vulnerability.

Other anxiety disorders include phobias—claustrophobia, agoraphobia (fear of open spaces) acrophobia (fear of going out or leaving home); obsessions (obsessive/compulsive disorder, compulsive handwashing, counting rituals, mechanical impulses like turning a light switch off and on); hair pulling, nail biting, hypochondria, Tourette's syndrome, and eating disorders.

CONVENTIONAL TREATMENT

In the fifties, the drugs of choice for anxiety were a class of prescription sedative/hypnotics called *barbiturates (phenobarbital, amobarbital, butabarbital),* which produced an intoxication similar to alcohol. Only moderate overdoses could be fatal, making them favorite drugs among the suicidal. They were the drugs that killed Marilyn Monroe, Judy Garland, and Elvis Presley. At heavy intake levels, withdrawal can also be fatal, and the barbiturates can produce a host of other side effects.

The *benzodiazepines,* or "minor" tranquilizers, were considered a major advance over the barbiturates. *Librium (chlordiazepoxide hydroxide)* was the first of these drugs, and *Valium (diazepam)* was the market leader for many years. In 1980, Valium was among the top five drugs prescribed in the United States, while *Dalmane (flurazepam)* was the benzodiazepine most often prescribed as a sleep remedy.

Originally thought to represent an improvement over the barbiturates in not having addiction potential, Valium now heads the list of drugs that cause dependence. By the time the fallacy of this presumption became apparent, unfortunately, thousands of people were already hooked on it. By 1988, when its side effects and addiction potential were well known, Valium had dropped to twenty-seventh among brand-named prescription drugs.

Meanwhile, the newer benzodiazepines *Xanax (alprazolam)* and *Halcion (triazolam)* had climbed to third and sixteenth.[93] Halcion became the world's best-selling sleeping pill. But charges against these newer benzodiazepines, too, are mounting. Halcion has been linked to violent behavior and to seizures, amnesia, hallucinations, personality disorders, and other side effects.[94] And some researchers assert that Xanax is potentially one of the most dangerous drugs on the market. It can cause powerful withdrawal symptoms, including severe convulsions. It and other benzodiazepines have also been linked to casualties ranging from highway fatalities to hip fractures caused when elderly patients tripped or fell out of bed.[95]

The newer benzodiazepines have shorter half-lives (an indication of the amount of time they stay in the body). Longer-acting drugs such as Valium are typically used to treat daytime anxiety, while the shorter-acting drugs are typically used for insomnia. (Insomniacs want the effect to have worn off by morning.) The main problem with the drugs with shorter half-lives is that they can have more serious side effects when you try to break the habit. Since Valium stays in your system longer, withdrawal is more gradual. On shorter-acting benzodiazepines, rebound insomnia and anxiety can occur after only short periods and at only low daily doses. That means you can have *more* trouble sleeping and feel *more* anxious than before you started on the drugs. This syndrome can cause you to keep taking them when you'd rather quit.[96] Studies also suggest that over the long term, patients who take Xanax for panic attacks can wind up more anxious than they were to start with.[97]

Prozac and its corollaries (*Zoloft, Paxil,* etc.) are current drug favorites for anxiety, depression, and a host of other ills, including premature ejaculation and even depression in pets. Prozac obliterates anxiety and depression because it numbs the whole system, but that means it also kills the desire for sex and the ability to perform. Other common side effects are sleeplessness, nervousness, nausea, and anxiety. Some 3.5 percent of patients who weren't suicidal before treatment get that way on the drug, and homicides have been blamed on it, generating a spate of lawsuits. (For a fuller discussion, see "Depression.")

NATURAL ALTERNATIVES

Fortunately, there are excellent natural remedies for treating anxiety. Research shows that herbs can be as effective as prescription drugs without their dangerous side effects.

One option is the South Pacific plant *kava*. In one study, it reduced symptoms as well as the benzodiazepine *oxazepam (Serax)* without being addictive or producing the side effects of the drug (which included drowsiness, dizziness, headaches, and vertigo).[98] In another study comparing these two remedies, the drug impaired the quality and time of response to a word recognition test, while the plant extract did not.[99] Kava can be made into a relaxing drink or taken in pill form. Recommended daily kava dosage is 70 to 200 mg of kavalactones (the pharmacologically active constituents).

Other herbs that are effective for treating anxiety include *skullcap, oats (aveno sativa)*, and *kava kava*. Also very useful for anxiety are *Stress X* by Trace Minerals Research, *Kalm-Asure* by Nature's Plus, *Rescue Remedy*, and cherry plums, a Bach flower remedy.

For "anticipatory anxiety"—nervousness before a speech or an exam—the homeopathic remedy *Gelsenium 30x* helps calm the nerves. Take three tablets as needed, up to four times a day.

St. John's wort is an herbal substitute for Prozac that many people find to be effective at a much reduced cost. See "Depression." For people with depression and anxiety, a combination herbal product called "*Nutrizac,*" containing St. John's wort and other herbs, is quite popular and effective.

For phobias and to bring out and eliminate the underlying cause of anxieties, constitutional homeopathic treatment from a qualified practitioner is often effective.

CAUTION: If you are on prescription antianxiety or insomnia drugs, switching remedies should be done only under professional supervision.[100]

Rescued from Panic Attacks

Karen, a dog trainer, had been depressed and experiencing panic attacks for about a year. She had been on Prozac since her symptoms first appeared and said she was much better with the drug than without it; but she still had symptoms and wanted to be drug-free. She telephoned in an acute state of panic after trying to stop the Prozac herself.

Karen was 42 years old with no previous history of anxiety or depression. A review of her symptoms indicated that her underlying problem was simply menopause. She was given "Rescue Remedy" and "Skullcap and Oats" (by Eclectic Institute), to be taken as needed for support while her underlying problem was treated. Within two days she called to say how much better she felt. A week later she stopped by to say she no longer needed the "Skullcap and Oats:" she felt terrific. Two months later, Karen reported that she had lost weight and felt better than she had for years. She had no depression or anxiety. She was convinced that she had never needed the Prozac and that her real problem was hormonal changes induced by menopause.

RELAXATION, MEDITATION, AND OTHER CALMING THERAPIES

In some circumstances, simple relaxation can be as effective as drugs in alleviating anxiety. In a study of patients about to undergo surgery, *acupressure* (a form of massage) and relaxation/meditation tapes were found to work as well as or better than Valium. *EMG biofeedback* relaxation methods have also been proven effective in relieving both anxiety and insomnia.[101] *Music therapy* and *color therapy* are other possibilities. Blue light is calming. Dietary habits may also play a role. Anxiety may be triggered by hypoglycemia or food allergies. Stimulants such as caffeine, ma huang (herba ephedra, ephedrine), and alcohol can also induce symptoms.

Arthritis

About one in seven Americans suffers from arthritis, and most are senior citizens. *Osteoarthritis*, the most common form of the disease among the elderly, is a chronic degenerative condition that comes from wear and tear on the joints. It afflicts 16 million Americans but is poorly understood, and there is no effective conventional treatment. *Rheumatoid arthritis* is the most intractable and painful form of the disease. The evidence is inconclusive, but many researchers feel it's caused by a virus or bacterium. *Bursitis* is a painful inflammation of the bursae, the fluid-filled sacs that cushion the bones, tendons and ligaments where they move against each other. *Ankylosing spondylitis* is an inflammation of the spine and hip joints. Many other conditions also involve an element of inflammatory arthritis, including *lupus, ulcerative colitis,* and *gout* or *gouty arthritis*. (See "Gout.")

CONVENTIONAL TREATMENT

Standard treatments recommended for osteoarthritis include exercise, weight loss for overweight people to ease stress on the joints, and pain relievers including *acetaminophen* and nonsteroidal anti-inflammatory drugs such as *Motrin* or *Naprosin*. The drugs, however, don't cure the disease but only relieve pain; and they do it by suppressing natural bodily processes. The result can be side effects ranging from gastrointestinal bleeding and ulcers to kidney problems. Drugs given to slow progression of the disease aren't very effective and can have even worse side effects.

ASPIRIN, ACETAMINOPHEN, AND NONASPIRIN NSAIDS. *Aspirin* has long been the preferred pain reliever for arthritis. *Acetaminophen* is easier on the stomach, but it doesn't reduce inflammation, which is involved in most forms of arthritis. Even many rheumatoid arthritis patients find that aspirin works as well as prescription medications with fewer side effects; and it's much cheaper.

The drugs that are giving aspirin a run for its money are the newer non-steroidal anti-inflammatory drugs (NSAIDs), including *ibuprofen* (Advil, Motrin, Medipren), *naproxen* (Naprosyn), *piroxicam* (Feldene), *sulindac* (Clinoril) and *indomethacin* (Indocin). The newer NSAIDs are said to have the advantages over aspirin of better tolerance, less gastrointestinal distress, once-daily dosing (piroxicam), general variety of choices, and that they cause merely reversible blood problems, as opposed to salicylates, which can cause irreversible problems. But the FDA asserts that the safety of one NSAID can't be clearly distinguished from another;[102] and in some cases, the newer NSAIDs are actually less safe than aspirin. The *Medical Letter* warns that all NSAIDs (including aspirin) inhibit the synthesis of prostaglandins that are necessary to regulate kidney blood flow, filtration, and sodium and water excretion. In patients with kidney disease, heart failure, or cirrhosis, kidney toxicity can occur after only a few days of therapy, and the result can be fatal. This can also happen in patients taking diuretics to treat high blood pressure. *For this reason, patients regularly taking any NSAIDs are advised to have periodic checkups to determine their white blood-cell counts and other blood factors.*[103]

Concerning the claim that the nonaspirin NSAIDs are easier on the stomach than aspirin, a 1986 British study found that people over 60 who took these drugs were three times as likely as nonusers to be hospitalized with bleeding gastric and duodenal ulcers.[104] Concerns about these side effects led the FDA to require new labels for all NSAIDs, which now must state in part:

> Serious gastrointestinal toxicity such as bleeding, ulceration, and perforation can occur at any time, with or without warning symptoms, in patients treated chronically with NSAID therapy.

WARNING: For lupus and ulcerative colitis, sufferers should avoid both aspirin and other NSAIDs, due to the higher risk of kidney or intestinal damage for these patients.

STEROIDS. For severe rheumatoid arthritis and other arthritic pains for which none of the foregoing works, *steroid drugs* such as *hydrocortisone, prednisone,* or *dexamethasone* may be given. The steroids are powerful anti-inflammatories, but again they don't cure arthritis. Joint destruction continues although pain is relieved. And steroids can have quite serious side effects, including ulcers. Ideally, they should be given only in small doses on alternate days for only one or two months at a time; but symptoms can become worse when the drugs are stopped than before the patient started on them, so he is liable to wind up on them indefinitely. As a result of this problem, steroids are now recommended only short term for emergencies.

"DISEASE-MODIFYING" DRUGS. Some arthritis specialists believe the progression of rheumatoid arthritis can be slowed if large doses of certain drugs called disease-modifying antirheumatic drugs are given early in the disease. These drugs include *gold*, given either by mouth or injection; *hydroxychloroquine* (Plaquenil), an antimalarial drug; and *chemotherapeutic drugs* that suppress the immune response, for example *cyclophosphamide* (Cytoxan), *methotrexate,* and *azathioprine* (Imuran). However, there is little evidence to support the claims that these drugs actually slow arthritis progression.[105] And the drugs' side effects can rival the disease. Gold can cause skin rashes, blood disorders, kidney and liver damage, and acute attacks of arthritis. Chloroquine must be taken in high doses to be effective, and these doses can cause irreversible damage to the eyes, resulting in blindness. Immune-suppressing drugs cause damage to the bone marrow (resulting in blood disorders) and deterioration of the muscles.

A preferable drug in the disease-modifying category is *colchicine*. Side effects have been attributed to it, but it's a derivative of a natural plant—*saffron*—and many users swear by it.

Another drug often given for severe rheumatoid arthritis is *D-penicillamine*. It, too, has side effects, and how it works isn't certain. However, D-penicillamine is a chelating agent; and rheumatoid arthritis patients have been found to have abnormally high levels of copper, lead, and mercury. Chelators are chemicals that pull heavy metals from the blood. Some authorities feel arthritis pain is the result of heavy metal accumulation in the joints. The drug evidently works by eliminating this toxic buildup. Side effects may have resulted because, not understanding the mechanism, doctors have given the drug for too long a time. Only enough chelation is necessary to remove toxic metal accumulation. Beyond that, it can do harm.

ELIMINATING THE CAUSE: HEAVY-METAL TOXICITY

Not only oral chelation (as with D-penicillamine) but intravenous chelation has proven remarkably effective in reversing arthritis symptoms. Ray Evers, M.D., a pioneer of chelation therapy for heart and arthritic conditions, analyzed the heavy-metal levels in his arthritis patients and found elevated levels of lead in nearly all of them. Mercury and other heavy metals were also high. The link was confirmed when chelation successfully relieved the symptoms of these patients.[106]

A. Hoffer, M.D., reports dramatic results in arthritis victims given vitamin regimens including high doses of *niacin* (2,000 to 3,000 mg per day).[107] Niacin, like chemical chelators, eliminates heavy metals from the tissues. Again these results suggest that at least one cause of arthritis can be an accumulation of heavy metals in the joints. For protocols for chelation and the Niacin Flush, see "Heavy-Metal Poisoning."

A series of French studies found that autoimmune diseases including chronic polyarthritis can be triggered by heavy metal accumulations from silver/mercury amalgam dental fillings.[108] Arthritis symptoms have been relieved both by removing these fillings and by removing or redoing infected root canals.[109]

ELIMINATING THE CAUSE: THE FOOD FACTOR

For many arthritics, symptoms are also brought on by certain foods. About 10 percent of arthritis patients, says Dr. Hoffer, are allergic to the solanine family of plants (potatoes, tomatoes, peppers).

The idea that diet could either cause or cure arthritis was long considered quackery. Then in the 1980s, several studies linked rheumatoid arthritis to food intolerances. In April of 1987, a study published in the *Annals of Internal Medicine* showed that about 5 to 10 percent of all cases of the disease were due to them.

In another double-blind study, patients with rheumatoid arthritis were first fed a two-week washout diet of foods unlikely to cause allergic reactions. Then they were challenged with capsules of either placebos or known food allergens—dairy products, wheat, corn, citrus, coffee, and chocolate. The effect of different foods was a very individual one, but about 15 percent improved dramatically and 70 percent showed varying degrees of improvement without their particular offending foods.[110]

Another study linked rheumatoid arthritis to *dietary fat.* Complete remissions resulted when the six subjects changed to a fat-free diet. Symptoms returned within three days of ingesting fat, whether in the form of animal fat or vegetable oils. The researchers concluded that dietary fats in amounts normally eaten can cause the inflammatory joint changes seen in rheumatoid arthritis.[111]

Dietary links then began appearing for osteoarthritis. A study published in the September 1, 1996, *Annals of Internal Medicine* showed that the disease may respond to a component of *vitamin D.* The researchers looked at the records of people in the Framingham Heart Study with X-ray evidence of osteoarthritis in the knees. They found that people with diets and blood levels high in vitamin D were least likely to have further degeneration later in life. The recommended daily allowance (RDA) of vitamin D is only 200 international units, but the best results were shown among people who were taking between two and eight times that amount. The researchers suggested that the vitamin's contribution is linked to its beneficial effect on the surrounding bone. The same researchers also found that a diet high in *vitamin C* slows the progression of osteoarthritis. These results are preliminary but provocative.[112]

The latest in nutritional supplements for relieving arthritis pain is a blend of fatty acid esters called *Cetyl Myristoleate.* In a large double-blind placebo-controlled study, 63 to 87 percent effectiveness was reported for this product ("CM Plus").

SUN THERAPY

The subjects in the vitamin D studies were taking it orally, but our principal source of the vitamin remains the sun. The use of sunlight for treating arthritis actually dates back for centuries. In Russia, a significant reduction in arthritis has been found in miners given routine sunlight treatments. In another study, one group of children with severe arthritis was given cortisone while another group was given sunlight treatments. In the sunlight group, relief came more slowly than in the cortisone group, but it did come; and unlike with cortisone, there were no unwanted side effects. Resistance to infection also increased.[113]

CHLOROPHYLL

Julian Whitaker, M.D., recommends another type of solar therapy for arthritis: *chlorophyll*. Deep-green plants are constantly exposed to the high-energy rays of the sun, which they transform into chlorophyll. Chlorophyll protects plants from oxidative damage, is an excellent cleanser, and it has anti-inflammatory properties. Chlorophyll can be taken as a supplement or in green food drinks including *Green Magma, Barley Green, Kyo-Green,* and *Green Radiance.*[114]

Prednisone Avoided with Greens

Dr. Whitaker cites the case of a patient who had had severe rheumatoid arthritis for about four years. She was taking the toxic drug Plaquenil, and Prednisone had been recommended next; but she had declined. Instead, Dr. Whitaker started her on large doses of a green drink called *GREENS+*, along with antioxidants, glucosamine sulfate, fish-oil supplements, and flax-seed oil. The patient gradually reduced her dosage of Plaquenil. After two weeks her symptoms had significantly lessened and the movement in her hands had significantly increased.

REBUILDING CARTILAGE: GLUCOSAMINE AND CSA

Jason Theodosakis, M.D., maintains that a combination of two nutritional supplements sold in health-food stores—*glucosamine* and *chondroitin sulfate (CSA)*—can relieve the pain of osteoarthritis and even regenerate deteriorating cartilage in joints. These nutrients, he says, are the building blocks for joint cartilage. They pass through blood to the joints, where they stimulate the production of new cartilage cells and reduce the action of enzymes that harm cartilage. In his book *The Arthritis Cure*, he cites 15 studies in Europe and Asia showing that patients reported less pain when taking the nutrients, which are found naturally in foods but in very small quantities. Dr. Theodosakis' book generated enormous interest, selling 100,000 copies in its first five days on the shelves in January of 1997.[115]

Other authorities dispute whether glucosamine and CSA represent a "cure." But they agree that this nutrient combination does relieves pain, and unlike aspirin and other NSAIDs (which don't cure arthritis either), the nutrients have no known side effects. Dr. Theodosakis observes that they have been given in dosages up to ten times those he recommends with no signs of toxicity.[116]

The two popular glucosamine forms are *glucosamine sulfate* and *N-Acetyl-Glucosamine (NAG)*. Glucosamine and chondroiton are both derived from cartilage. You can also buy cartilage itself, as *shark cartilage* or *cow cartilage*. Another cheap and readily available option is plain *gelatin*. Mix the powder in juice and drink.

Trace Minerals Research in Ogden, Utah, makes a good combination nutritional supplement for arthritis called *Arth-X Plus*, containing glucosamine sulfate and trace minerals among a long list of other nutrients and herbs.

Knee Surgery Avoided

A prominent Massachusetts businessman sought advice while vacationing in Sun Valley, after his doctor recommended surgery to replace both knees. He was an avid golfer, but he was having problems walking. He was given "Arth-X Plus," along with some acupuncture to open his energy fields. Two days later, he was back on the golf course. He still calls periodically from Massachusetts and reports that he continues to play golf and to do remarkably well without surgery—so well that his business associates thought he had had the surgery. He says they were very surprised that he would try alternative healing methods, but his results spoke for themselves, and many of his friends have stopped by to ask questions and purchase herbs for their own ailments.

HERBAL AND NUTRITIONAL SUPPLEMENTS

A Chinese herbal remedy called *Tin Tzat* is quite effective in alleviating arthritis pain in the hands and wrist. Liberal doses of *garlic* can also help.

Crippled Hands Restored

The hands of a 42-year-old team roper were so crippled with arthritis that he could no longer rope cattle. He had tried many remedies, but none was satisfactory. He was using Feldene on the days he knew he was going to rope, even though it ripped his stomach up terribly, because he couldn't rope without it. He sought a nontoxic remedy and went home with Tin Tzat. When he came back, he bought a whole case of it. He was so impressed with how well it worked that he continues to send other arthritis sufferers in for it.

THE pH FACTOR

Some authorities maintain that arthritis results from too much acid in the body. A product called *Alkazone* changes the body's pH.

HORSE TRAINER'S ARTHRITIS RELIEVED

Joan, a 57-year-old horse trainer, was so stiff with arthritis that she could hardly move. Riding was so painful that she dreaded going to work. The first week after trying Alkazone, her pain disappeared. More than a year later, she says it's her best friend. Her cupboard is fully stocked with it, since the thought of going back to being crippled with arthritis terrifies her.

TOPICAL REMEDIES

Natural topical creams are available that can temporarily alleviate arthritis pain. *Natural progesterone cream* rubbed into painful joints is also effective over a period of time.

OTHER NATURAL THERAPIES

Other nondrug therapies useful in the treatment of arthritis are physical and occupational therapy, including warm-water swimming and other exercise, heat treatments, acupuncture, homeopathic remedies, and rest. Total bed rest, however, is no longer recommended, since it causes loss of muscle tone. Correcting anatomical problems such as unequal leg lengths or abnormal foot positions can also relieve symptoms, and so can exercise that puts the joints through their full range of motion.

Many arthritis patients swear by *copper bracelets*. Why they work is uncertain, but an Australian study found that they actually relieve symptoms.[117] Good copper bracelets are available from Sergio Lub Copper Bracelets, P. O. Box 3400, Walnut Creek, CA 94598; (510) 932-6085.

Asthma, Emphysema, Lung Disease

Asthma is a disorder of breathing characterized by wheezing, difficulty exhaling, and often coughing. It afflicts an estimated 14 million Americans, including 4.8 million children—one in four children in industrialized countries—and is responsible for more admissions to the hospital than any other childhood condition. Once considered nonfatal, asthma now has a death toll that reached 5,167 in 1993—nearly twice what it was in 1979—and is on the rise. Asthma medications have become the second largest category of prescriptions written by doctors.[118]

Asthma can precipitate emphysema, a more serious lung disease characterized by chronic coughing and loss of elasticity in the lungs. The most common cause of emphysema, however, is heavy smoking.

Asthma can be triggered by many things, including food allergens, exercise, cold weather, and environmental irritants such as dust mites, mold, animal dander, and chemical odors. Cockroaches are a major trigger in inner-city children, and a cluster of infant deaths from lung disease has been linked to a toxic fungus found in the home.[119] The high level of airborne pollutants in industrialized countries is a leading suspect in the growing incidence of asthma.

Drugs are also a factor. Childhood asthma can develop in babies given *cortisone* for a skin rash. *Aspirin* can also trigger a reaction. Other drug suspects are early childhood *immunizations*. Asthma is rare in parts of the world, in parts of town, and in families where childhood diseases are allowed to run their course, giving the immune system something to "cut its teeth" on.[120] (See "Allergies.")

The surge in asthma deaths is also attributed in part to the drugs used to treat the disease.

DRUG TREATMENT

In the sixties, an epidemic of asthma deaths in England, Wales, and New Zealand hit at about the time metered-dose inhalers became the treatment of choice among asthma patients. The epidemic was attributed to the increased sale and use of a high-dose aerosol containing the drug isoproteneronol, on which patients were relying for self-treatment rather than seeking medical care. Today, this drug is no longer available without a perscription and is infrequently used; but the huge increase in availability and use of other aerosol preparations in metered-dose inhalers for dilating the bronchial tubes may be having the same effect. The products afford a false sense of security in the face of a dangerous condition. All anti-asthma medications can produce life-threatening reactions, and the likelihood of these reactions is multiplied by the increased use of the medications. Increasing use of over-the-counter asthma inhalers was shown in studies presented to the FDA in 1995 to be a factor contributing to the alarming increase in ashthma deaths. The death of a teenage girl the same year was linked to over-the-counter "Primatene Mist." The tragedy was thought to have been caused, not directly by the drug, but because she had relied on it in the throes of an acute attack. The drug opens the air tubes, but only temporarily. She evidently needed something more long-lasting.[121]

Drugs for the treatment of asthma include "relievers" (used for acute attacks) and "controllers" (used for maintenance therapy). The drugs fall into several main types:

1. *Sympathomimetic drugs* stimulate the muscles that open the bronchial tubes. Ephedrine, contained in "Bronkotabs," "Mudrane," "Quadrinal," "Quibron" and "Tedral," is used for acute attacks. It can cause the heart to pound and can have other distressing side effects, including nausea, high blood pressure, dizziness and sleepless nights. Aerosol inhalers containing adrenalin in the form of *epinephrine* ("Primatene Mist," "Bronkaid") or *isoproterenol* ("Isuprel," "Mucomyst," Medihaler-Iso", "Duo-Medihaler," "Norisodrine") can cause some of the same side effects as ephedrine. The sympathomimetic drugs used in the newer aerosol bronchodilators, including *albuterol* ("Ventolin," "Proventil"), *terbutaline* ("Brethine"), and *metaproterenol sulfate* ("Alupent"), are less likely to have distressing side effects, but overuse can cause them to lose their effectiveness and can cause a rebound effect that actually makes the condition worse. For children, a popular option is "Alupent" bronchodilator elixir or syrup. It can have side effects, including tachycardia (increased heart rate), irritability, hyperactivity, and insomnia; but because the drug is specific to the lungs and has limited effects on the body, it represents an advance over the systemic steroids for asthmatic children.[122]

2. *Corticosteroids (steroids)* are pharmaceutical copies of the steroid hormones produced by the adrenal glands. Steroids reduce inflammation, opening the airways of the chest; and they suppress much of the immune

system's response to allergens. For asthma emergencies, systemic steroids like *methylprednisolone* (the injectable form) or *prednisone* (the oral form) can be very effective. But these drugs should not be used long-term and should be used only when all other treatments fail. In children, they can't be used for asthma attacks more than about four times a year without significant adverse effects. The drugs don't cure the problem but act mainly by inhibiting the body's reaction to it; and when you take extra steroids, your adrenals quit making their own. As a result, when you need the natural steroids to cope with stressful emergencies, they're no longer available. What can go wrong was illustrated in the case reported in 1997 in which a child died from chicken pox while taking prednisolone. The drug was thought to have suppressed his immune system so that he couldn't fight the disease. Other adverse side effects of steroids include cataracts, bone loss, diabetes, weight gain, easy bruising, and emotional and growth problems in children. The drugs shouldn't be taken by people with ulcers, tuberculosis or ocular herpes, and should be used only with caution by children, pregnant women and nursing mothers.[123]

The newer *steroid inhalers* ("Asmacort," "AeroBid," "Beclovent," "Vanceril") are safer than oral steroids, because they're sprayed directly into the lungs and a much lower dose is required to get an effect. They aren't effective if reserved merely for acute attacks but must be used regularly to be effective. Because they're inhaled and are poorly absorbed, they have been considered safe enough for daily use even by children, since the potential for adrenal suppression has been thought to be minimal. But research reported in July 1997 cast doubt on the safety even of these drugs. The link with cataracts found with oral steroids was found with the inhalers as well, and the inhalers were associated with a higher risk of glaucoma. Steroid inhalers can also contribute to the development of fungal mouth infections. For this reason, use of a mouthwash is advised after each dose. The problem is that antiseptic mouthwashes, like antibiotics, can wipe out friendly flora along with unfriendly ones, leading to other ailments and imbalances.[124]

3. *Cromolyn sodium,* an alternative anti-inflammatory in the "controller" category, is contained in an asthma inhaler called "Intal." A longtime favorite in Europe, it is less effective but safer than steroids, making it a popular choice for children. Unlike antihistamines, which generally battle histamine only after it has already been released, cromolyn prevents histamine release.

4. *Xanthine bronchodilators* are traditional mainstays for daily maintenance treatment. *Theophylline* has been used for nearly 150 years to clear obstructed air passages. Theophylline is found in the prescription drugs "Theo-Dur," "SloPhyllin" and "Quibrin," and in non-prescription "Bronkaid" and "Primatene" tablets. Oral bronchodilators are frequently prescribed for people who can't tolerate inhalers or who have chronic asthma. Theophylline can have side effects, including nausea, vomiting, abdominal pain, loss of appetite, headache, nervousness, anxiety, increased heart rate, heart palpitations, behavioral changes and short-term memory loss. It isn't recommended for children whose symptoms are only intermittent, whose behavior changes on the drug, or who do better on other drugs; or for pregnant women or nursing mothers. It should be used only with caution by people with liver disease or uncontrolled hyperthyroidism. It can aggravate ulcers, fibrocystic breast disease, and heart disorders.[125]

5. *Salmeterol* ("Serevent Inhaler") is another popular bronchodilator in the "controller" category. A long-term, twice-daily inhaler, it won't help an acute attack but works only slowly over time. This feature has proven fatal in several cases, in which deaths resulted when patients with acute broncospasm evidently tried to use it to stop their acute attacks. Its other adverse effects are similar to other bronchodilators, but its effects on the heart and blood vessels aren't as pronounced.[126]

WARNING: If you have a serious asthmatic condition, it is particularly important that you be under the regular care of a physician specializing in the field. Asthma attacks can be life-threatening. Appropriate medication is necessary during an acute attack. A peak flow meter should be used to monitor breathing.

NUTRITIONAL BRONCHODILATORS

The foregoing provisos aside, natural substances are available that can open constricted bronchial tubes without side effects. There are also natural therapies and other measures that can be taken to reduce the need for medication and the likelihood of an acute attack.

Researchers have known for half a century that *magnesium sulfate* acts as a natural bronchodilator that opens constricted bronchial tubes without adverse effects. Richard Firshein, D.O., director of the Firshein Center for Comprehensive Medicine in New York City, which specializes in the treatment of asthma through natural and alternative therapies, recommends 500 milligrams of magnesium aspartate daily. He observes that magnesium alone won't cure a severe attack, but intravenous magnesium sulfate can be given by a trained practitioner along with drugs to relax smooth muscle and rapidly open the bronchial tubes. Oral magnesium supplements are used for long-term maintenance. Dr. Fishman adds that the only accurate test of magnesium levels is an RBC or red-blood-cell magnesium test. His holistic asthma treatment protocol also includes *licorice, gingko biloba, fish oil or flaxseed oil, organic foods, breathing exercises,* and *mind-body techniques.*[127]

Another nutritional supplement that opens the lungs for easier breathing is *black currant seed oil.* This remedy is very useful not only for asthma but for any type of breathing problem (emphysema, and the like). It eases breathing by reducing inflammation in the lungs. Recommended dosage is two pills every morning. To relieve exercise-induced asthma, take two pills before workouts.

Inhalers Avoided with Black Currant Seed Oil

Chloe, 19, had a long history of asthma and recurring colds and chest infections. She wanted to attend college without constant illness and the need to rely on inhalers. She used a combination of homeopathic products and herbs over approximately a year to clear her problems. She continues to take the black currant seed oil daily, increasing the dosage to two pills three to four times daily if she feels her lungs are getting "tight." She is now off inhalers and doing well, and reports that she has not had a cold or lung problem in the last two years.

Exercise-induced Asthma Relieved

Sheila, 45, complained that she was gaining weight after her daily workouts had to be curtailed due to exercise-induced asthma. Then she began taking two black currant seed oil capsules daily before working out. She says she has had no asthma problems since.

HERBAL AND HOMEOPATHIC REMEDIES

Asthma drugs have natural counterparts. Theophylline is found naturally in tea. It belongs to a group of drugs called *xanthines* that also includes caffeine (found in coffee) and theobromine (found in cocoa). *Ephedrine,* too, has natural counterparts. In these more natural forms it has been used to treat asthma for thousands of years. Even cromolyn is new only to Western medicine. In the form of *ammi seeds*, it has been part of Bedouin folk medicine for centuries.[128]

The herb *elecampane* can help build up the lungs. *Lung Complex* by Enzymatic Therapy is an herbal formula to support the lungs.

Asthma by BHI is a homeopathic remedy that supports the lungs. A German homeopathic remedy by Staufen called *Asthma* is also quite effective. For allergic asthma caused by cockroaches, the appropriate homeopathic remedy is *Blatta 6x or 30x* taken three times daily.

The lungs of *emphysema* victims are unable to open appropriately to take in oxygen. A homeopathic remedy called *Lung RegenRx* by Futurplex can help regenerate the lung and improve cellular oxygenation.

Hockey Player's Asthma Alleviated

A hockey player in his early thirties suffered from severe asthma when he was on the ice. He was also prone to contracting pneumonia once or twice a year. He wound up resorting to progressively more inhalers, steroids, and antibiotics. He took the Staufen homeopathic remedies for asthma and pneumonia, then began taking two black currant seed oil capsules before a hockey match. He reports being well ever since. He can breathe on the ice now without wheezing, and his game is much better.

TREATING THE EMOTIONAL FACTOR

A common cause of asthma, say Chinese doctors, is "cold in the lungs." That would account for the hockey player's asthma. Another cause can be emotional: suppressed anger or grief. The typical case is the older woman who suddenly becomes a widow. She is so busy with the funeral and arrangements, she has no time to grieve. Within a year of her husband's death, she begins to have lung problems: coughing, congestion in the morning, frequent colds and flu, perhaps turning into pneumonia or bronchitis. Homeopathic remedies like *Ignatia 200x* can help release this "grief trapped in the lungs."

Chronic Lung Condition Relieved with Herbal and Homeopathic Remedies

Barbara's husband died suddenly of a heart attack when she was 62. It was so unexpected, no arrangements had been made. She did not know about their financial matters. Her husband always handled them. With so many things to consider, along with her family coming from out of town for the funeral, she hardly had time to grieve. Her relatives wouldn't let her grieve even if she had had time. Whenever Barbara started to cry, someone found something to keep her busy or talked to her to "cheer her up."

Months later, Barbara was hard at work with her new job. Her new life wasn't going well, but she kept plugging on. She never cried, but she found herself staying up all night "thinking." Meanwhile, she had developed a chronic cough and was coming down with colds every three weeks or so. When her cold went into pneumonia, she sought advice. The recommended remedies were the herb elecampane to build up her lungs and homeopathic Ignatia 200x to release her grief. After a course of these remedies, her cough went away and she was fine—but only after she had had a good cry.

OTHER NON-DRUG ALTERNATIVES

Acupuncture can help alleviate asthma. A Chinese study published in 1989 reported a disappearance or decreased frequency of asthma attacks in 88.9 percent of cases treated by a particular acupuncture method. *EMG biofeedback* techniques have also shown success in treating asthma.[129]

Exercise is a natural adrenalin stimulant, which can produce direct nervous stimulation to the nose.[130] Learning to *breathe properly* from the diaphragm and to empty the lungs completely on exhalation is also very important.[131]

F. Batmanghelidj, M.D., reports some remarkable asthma cures with *water therapy*. (See Chapter 2.)

For other natural remedial and preventive approaches, see "Allergies."

Atherosclerosis, Coronary Heart Disease

Atherosclerosis, or hardening of the arteries, results from an accumulation of calcified fatty plaque in the blood vessels. Atherosclerosis has been called a "silent killer." For one out of four victims, the first sign of trouble is sudden death. Lesions in which function has been impaired by atherosclerotic growths develop in Western man at an average age of 20. These lesions spread so that they cover about 2 percent more of the surface of the coronary arteries every year. By the time 60 percent of this surface has been covered with coronary lesions, the opening through which blood passes is narrowed enough to set the stage for trouble. Until they reach this critical threshold, however, these lesions cause no symptoms. Then they can take only minutes to manifest as a fatal *heart attack*.[132] Besides heart attacks, atherosclerosis is the chief cause of *coronary heart disease (CHD)* and *strokes* it is a major cause of *high blood pressure* and contributes to *circulatory disorders*, including *Raynaud's disease.*

Heart disease was rare at the turn of the century, accounting for only 8 percent of U.S. deaths. Today, it has shot up to the number-one killer, accounting for 45 percent of all deaths. Dietary cholesterol is commonly blamed for the epidemic, based on the Framingham Heart Study, in which 5,209 adults living in Framingham, Massachusetts, were followed for 18 years beginning in 1949. People with lower blood pressure and serum cholesterol levels were found to live significantly longer than people with higher levels. Long-term studies of people on low-fat, high-fiber vegetarian diets have also consistently shown a reduction in serum-cholesterol and blood-pressure levels, as well as an actual increase in life expectancy.[133]

One snag in the cholesterol theory is that since 1990, dietary cholesterol has steadily gone *down*, not up. The consumption of other suspect foods, however, has increased. Foods on the increase that have been linked to increased heart disease risk include *vegetable (not animal) fats*, *sugar*, and *heated* milk protein. The latter has been shown to increase the formation of blood clots, or thrombosis.

Problems with the cholesterol theory have prompted some researchers to revive the theory that heart disease results, not from dietary cholesterol, but from the toxins from which it is protecting the arteries. (See "Heart Attacks.") The body itself produces cholesterol, which accumulates in the form of plaque in the arteries as a protective mechanism. Cholesterol is necessary to repair injuries and protect against irritation to the arterial wall. Cholesterol is also the stuff of which hormones are made. Without enough of it, your body will be hormone-deficient. Dietary cholesterol can be dangerous, but research has shown that the dangerous form is the cholesterol that has been oxidized by high temperatures and exposure to air.[134] *Antioxidants* can help protect against this form of damage.

THE CONVENTIONAL APPROACH

The conventional approach to preventing heart disease is to use drugs to reduce its major risk factors: high blood pressure and high cholesterol levels. The problem is that the long-lived people in the studies pinpointing these targets didn't get their low blood pressure and cholesterol levels from drugs. They got them from their lifestyles or their genes. In most studies in which these risk factors have been lowered with drugs, long-term benefits have been disappointing.[135] Recent studies have actually linked the drugs used as mainstays to lower blood pressure—beta blockers and calcium channel blockers—to an *increased* risk of death from heart disease. For a detailed discussion of studies of their long-term effects, see "Hypertension," "Cholesterol, High."

Pharmaceutical *estrogen* is another drug that has been promoted as lowering heart disease risk. On January 18, 1995, *JAMA* reported the results of the Postmenopausal Estrogen/Progestin Interventions (PEPI) Trial, the first randomized, double-blind, placebo-controlled prospective study of the effects of estrogen on cholesterol and triglyceride levels. It found that estrogen significantly increased levels of high-density lipoprotein cholesterol (HDL-C, the "good" cholesterol). HDL-C is thought to be the best predictor of heart disease risk in women: the higher the HDL-C, the lower the risk.

Confounding the issue was the fact that triglycerides also went up in women on estrogen, suggesting an *increase* in heart-disease risk. And taking synthetic progestins with the estrogen (the hormone-replacement protocol popular in the United States) reduced the HDL-C benefit by a full 75 percent. Meanwhile, a second PEPI report, issued in the *Journal of the American Medical Association* (*JAMA*) on February 7, 1996, strongly advised women who still had their uteruses not to take estrogen alone, due to a substantially increased risk of endometrial cancer.

Still to be proven is that the effects of estrogen on HDL-C translate into an actual increase in survival. In 1997, researchers reported in the *Annals of Internal Medicine* that neither the current nor the long-term use of estrogen, either alone or with synthetic progesterone, significantly affects the risk of myocardial infarction (heart attack) in postmenopausal women.[136] Offsetting the lack of a heart-protective effect for estrogen is an increased risk of breast cancer, another growing epidemic. Researchers writing in the British medical journal *Lancet* in 1997 reported that breast cancer risk is increased after only one year of estrogen use, and that it increases thereafter by almost 2.3 percent per year. These findings were based on a review of about 90 percent of the worldwide epidemiological evidence, including 51 different studies.[137]

In short, the drug approach merely delays death from heart disease; and whether it does even that has yet to be unequivocally established.

THE DIETARY APPROACH

In 1988, the notion that heart disease might actually be reversible was a revolutionary one. That was the year that Dr. Dean Ornish, a San Francisco cardiologist, proved that the fatty-plaque deposits blocking the coronary arteries of advanced heart patients could be made to shrink using natural therapies alone. The therapies used in his study were a strict low-cholesterol diet, meditation, and yoga. The official position of conventional medicine before that was that heart disease progressed inexorably to the patient's death, no matter what he ate, did, or believed.[138]

Half the patients in Dr. Ornish's study were counseled (but not required) to lower cholesterol and blood pressure and to quit smoking. The other half were required to quit smoking, to walk one hour three times a week, to reduce stress by daily yoga and meditation, and to eat a low-fat vegetarian diet. The only animal products allowed were nonfat milk and yogurt. Only 8 to 10 percent of their total calories came from fat—about a quarter of the usual American intake. After a year, arterial blockage was significantly reduced in 10 of 12 patients in the vegetarian group. By comparison, 11 of 17 patients in the control group got worse. Cholesterol levels also dropped markedly in the vegetarian group, while decreasing only modestly in the other group.[139]

In a second study, sponsored by the National Heart, Lung and Blood Institute, the formation of *new* lesions was prevented simply by cutting fat to about 27 percent of total calories (compared to 36 to 37 percent in the normal diet).[140]

Fish or *fish-oil capsules* can also protect the heart. Taking their cue from the heart-hardy Eskimos, British researchers found a 29 percent lower death rate from heart attacks in men who ate *omega-3 fatty acids* (especially EPA, or eicosapenentaenoic acid) in the form of fatty fish or fish oil capsules. Omega-3s thin the blood, reducing the risk of blood clots. Omega-3s also reduce blood triglycerides, and they may lower blood pressure and reduce cardiac arrhythmias.

NUTRITIONAL SUPPLEMENTS

Other nutritional supplements can also lower cholesterol and the risk of heart disease. One is *niacin*. (See the "Niacin Flush" under "Heavy Metal Detox.") Another is *vitamin E*. In two studies reported in 1992 involving more than 130,000 people, women who took at least 100 IU per day of vitamin E for two or more years reduced their risk of heart disease by 26 percent, and men on the same regimen reduced their risk by 46 percent. People who took megadoses of vitamin E had no greater reduction in risk than those who took 100 IU daily.[141]

Vitamin E is an antioxidant that evidently reduces the oxidation of cholesterol, preventing damage to the heart and arteries. Other antioxidants may also accomplish this result. Matthias Rath, M.D., a German researcher, attributes heart disease to a deficiency of vitamin C, another antioxidant. The simple cure, he says, is to take more vitamin C. Red wine, thought to be responsible for the French Paradox (low blood cholesterol despite a high-cholesterol diet), contains potent antioxidants called *OPCs*, also found in *grapeseed extract.*

The herb *hawthorn berry (Crataegus berry)* also contains OPCs. Hawthorn berry has been shown in clinical studies to have cardiovascular benefits in the treatment of coronary-artery disease, high blood pressure, mild congestive heart failure, angina, and cardiac arrhythmias.[142]

Another powerful antioxidant, traditionally found in foods but new as a nutritional supplement, is *alpha-lipoic acid (ALA)*. ALA prevents cell damage, slows aging, regulates blood sugar, and chelates toxic metals out of the blood. It has the advantage that it is both water- and fat-soluble, so it can permeate all the body's cells. Besides in supplements, it is found in foods including *spinach, kidney, heart, skeletal muscle (beef), and broccoli.*[143]

Arginine, an amino acid, has been shown to decrease blood-platelet stickiness in people with very high cholesterol levels. Platelet stickiness is associated with heart failure and stroke. The dosage studied—8.4 grams a day—was well tolerated and without side effects. The effect of a two-week course of the amino acid lasted 16 weeks.[144]

Garlic also has natural blood-thinning, cholesterol-reducing, and blood-pressure-lowering properties.

Scientists at London's National Heart and Lung Institute have concluded that *natural progesterone* has a direct impact on reducing platelet aggregation. In 1997, researchers at Oregon Regional Primate Research Center showed that natural—but not synthetic—progesterone may help prevent heart attacks.[145]

Evening primrose oil, a traditional North American Indian remedy, has been shown to lower blood pressure and serum cholesterol. It also decreases the amount of insulin required by diabetics and aids in weight loss by increasing fat metabolism. Cofactors that should accompany its intake are zinc and vitamins C, B3, and B6.[146] Evening primrose oil and *black-currant oil* both contain gamma-linolenic acid (GLA), which is converted in the body to a prostaglandin called PGE1. PGE1 prevents the blood-platelet aggregation that causes heart attacks and strokes, opens up blood vessels and improves circulation, helps the kidneys remove fluid from the body, and slows down cholesterol production. PGE1 also controls arthritis, improves nerve function, gives a sense of well-being, regulates calcium metabolism, aids the immune system, and seems to inhibit cancer development.

Tufts University researchers reported in 1997 that foods rich in *B vitamins*, particularly *folic acid*, are essential to a healthy heart. The reason, however, involved a new culprit besides cholesterol: homocysteine. This essential amino acid was linked to an increased risk of heart attack and stroke when it accumulated in the blood, perhaps because it damaged the lining of the blood vessels. Folic acid helps keep blood homocysteine levels from going too high. Leafy greens such as spinach, fruits, and beans are good food sources.[147]

The mineral magnesium, when given intravenously to patients with suspected heart attacks, has reduced cardiovascular mortality by a remarkable 25 percent.[148]

The herb *mistletoe* works like oral chelation to remove plaque from the arteries. (Concerning chelation, see "Heavy Metal Poisoning.")

For cases in which simple natural remedies have brought dramatic improvement for specific heart conditions, see "Cholesterol, High," "Heart Attacks," "Hypertension," "Strokes."

CHELATION

Antioxidants help neutralize oxidized fats, but fats aren't the only toxins that can injure artery walls and cause heart disease. Others include toxic chemicals, pesticides, and heavy metals. Chelation to eliminate heavy metals from the arteries has effected some remarkable recoveries from heart disease. It and other detox protocols are discussed under "Heavy Metal Poisoning."

HELP FOR CIRCULATORY DISORDERS

Acupuncture is particularly helpful in circulatory disorders such as Raynaud's syndrome.[149] Herbal tinctures good for circulatory disorders include *Aesculus*, *Polygonum*, and *Solidago* by Nestmann.[149]

Helpful herbs to increase circulation are *butcher's broom, cayenne (capsicum)*, and garlic.

Attention Deficit Disorder, Hyperactivity

Attention deficit hyperactivity disorder (ADD), also called "minimal brain dysfunction," is a childhood condition considered to be a form of brain damage. The main problem is diagnosis. Studies have been unable to find consistent, objective evidence of the condition, and it is not defined by a consistent cluster of symptoms. According to the American Psychiatric Association, a child is considered to have attention-deficit-hyperactivity disorder who shows eight of the following symptoms for at least six months, beginning before his or her seventh birthday:

1. Often fidgets his hands or feet or squirms in his seat

2. Has trouble staying in his seat when required

3. Is easily distracted

4. Has trouble waiting his turn

5. Often blurts out answers before the question is completed

6. Has trouble doing chores or otherwise following through with instructions

7. Has trouble sustaining attention to work or play activities

8. Often shifts from one unfinished task to another

9. Has trouble playing quietly

10. Often talks too much

11. Often interrupts others or butts into other children's games

12. Doesn't seem to listen to what's being said

13. Often loses things (toys, pencils, books, assignments)

14. Does dangerous things without considering the consequences, such as running into the street without looking.[150]

The vagueness of these criteria has led to obvious problems in categorization, since most children display some of these symptoms.

DRUG TREATMENT

Vagueness in diagnosis, in turn, has led to serious problems with treatment. Thousands of children may now be on narcotics unnecessarily. The prescribed regimen, an amphetamine called *Ritalin (methylphenidate)*, is used to treat more than a million American children.[151] Other amphetamines used for this purpose are *dextroamphetamine (Dexedrine, Dexampex, Ferndex)*, and *pemoline (Cylert)*. Where the only alternative is to institutionalize the child, these drugs are obviously the best choice of treatment. But like other amphetamines, they have unwanted side effects; and they are often given to children whose problems can be corrected by other means.

Although amphetamines are stimulants, they have the paradoxical property of calming down hyperactive children. In this their effects are said to differ from those of amphetamines on adults, but in fact they are similar. In both age groups, stimulants increase the ability to concentrate on a task. Like the adult with his cup of coffee, the child sits still and gets down to work. Children on Ritalin perform better on certain types of tests, especially those requiring attention and motivation. In one study, two thirds of the hyperactive children tested did better academically, socially, or both on the drug.[152] Amphetamines are notorious for their illicit use by college students to get through exams. One problem with Ritalin is that high-school students are peddling it to their friends for the same purpose. A more fundamental problem is that, as with studying on "speed," a significant amount of information learned on the drug is forgotten when the child is taken off it. Most reviewers have concluded that Ritalin has neither short-term nor long-term beneficial effects on academic performance.[153]

The drug's side effects are like those of other amphetamines: sleeplessness, loss of appetite, irritability, headaches, fatigue, withdrawal, crying for no apparent reason, and a sensitivity to criticism. There may also be a stunting of growth. The most serious potential side effect is the development of tics—involuntary, darting, purposeless motor movements of the face or arms. The tics can progress to "Tourette's syndrome," a condition characterized by generalized jerking movements in any part of the body, accompanied by a tendency to use foul language and repeat words.[154] These side effects have led to a spate of lawsuits on behalf of children allegedly harmed by inappropriate use of the drug.

NON-DRUG ALTERNATIVES

Ritalin masks the problem without addressing the cause. When the child is taken off the drug, the problem returns, often with greater force than before. The first step in a holistic approach to ADD is to determine the cause. Possibilities include reading or other learning disabilities, problems at home, problems at school (ineffective teaching or boring subject matter), nutritional deficiencies, low blood sugar, food allergies, hay fever, buried emotional trauma, toxic chemical poisoning, and parasites. The second step is to treat this underlying problem. Research has shown combinations of fatty acids can play an important role in the development of vision, learning ability, and coordination. Fatty acids are found in fish oil, evening primrose oil, vitamin E, and thyme oil.

ADD Traced to Parasites and Eliminated

A mother who had been treated for parasites and had gotten dramatic relief mentioned that her ten-year-old daughter was having problems at school. The girl slept a lot, wasn't very active, and had little going for her. Within two weeks of taking remedies for parasites, the girl "came alive" again. (See "Parasites.") She soon began getting straight As, had more friends, felt much better, and was much more active. Both mother and daughter, it turned out, had toxoplasmosis, a parasitic infection acquired from cats. The mother may have had it while pregnant. It had evidently settled in the child's brain so she couldn't think clearly.

THE ALLERGY FACTOR

Hyperactivity has also been traced to *food allergies*. In a study of over 100 children reported by pediatrician and allergist William Crook, hyperactivity was traced to this cause in about three fourths of them. In a study conducted at London's Institute of Child Health and Hospital for Sick Children, 28 hyperactive children were fed one of two selected foods, each for one week. The "suspect" food was one that had been associated with symptoms in the child. The "control" food was one that hadn't. When the children's behavior was rated by a psychologist, a pediatric neurologist, and the parents, dramatic improvement was noted during the week the control food was eaten.

The late Ben Feingold, M.D., chief of the allergy clinics of the Kaiser Foundation in California, linked hyperactivity not only to foods but to food additives and chemicals, including those in Ritalin itself. Other likely ingested allergens are sugar, cow's milk, citrus fruits or juices, wheat, corn, chocolate, eggs, nuts, fish, and berries. If you suspect a food allergy in your child, try eliminating possible offenders, then adding them back into the diet one by one. If a food is definitely implicated by the return of symptoms, eliminate it from the diet for at least three months. It can then be tried cautiously. If no reaction occurs, it can be eaten in moderation.[155]

Hay fever can also cause irritability, mood swings and insomnia; and the drugs used to treat it can make victims drowsy and slow. The result can be a short attention span, difficulty learning, and disruptive behavior in school.[156]

Hidden sensitivities to *toxic chemicals and metals* are another possible cause of ADD. Childhood autism, which is conventionally considered irreversible, has been reversed in several cases by chelation to remove heavy metals. See "Heavy-Metal Poisoning."

ADD Traced to Pesticide Poisoning and Eliminated

A nine-year-old Boise boy with ADD was on major antidepressants and antipsychotic medications after he had gone through all the usual medicines including Ritalin without getting better. Investigation revealed that he lived in an area that had been heavily sprayed with paraquot, a highly toxic pesticide, in the sixties and seventies. He was given homeopathic remedies for detoxification, including a German formula specifically for paraquot poisoning, and products called *Addiclenz* and *Enviroclenz* by Deseret. (See "Environmental Illness.") The process was very difficult for the boy, and the detox had to be done slowly. He was started at one drop a day, working up to ten drops over a long period of time. When his system was finally cleared of the toxic chemical, however, his delighted mother reported dramatic improvement: he was much calmer, no longer got depressed, suicidal, or angry, and no longer picked on other kids.

MENTAL AND EMOTIONAL FACTORS

If the problem is mental or emotional, there are again better ways to deal with it than drugs. For specific learning disabilities, tutoring or remedial reading classes are available. If the problem is social or psychological, counseling is recommended. For emotional trauma, homeopathic remedies can help.

Hyperactivity Traced to Childhood Trauma and Eliminated

A hyperactive adopted girl of seven would not go to sleep until her mother had stayed by her bed for several hours each night. If she woke up and her mother wasn't there, she screamed and became hysterical. Rescue Remedy and an antimiasmatic homeopathic remedy called *Multiple Miasm* by Deseret made a dramatic difference in her. The girl began telling her mother of dreams and memories of her early years with her natural parents, who had abused her. *Multiple Miasm* is said to revive old memories, bringing them to consciousness so they can be cleared and are no longer suppressed in (and suppressing) the system. The mother was thrilled with the changes in the girl, who seemed to have matured by four or five years in six months, would finally sleep alone, and fell immediately to sleep.

Back Pain, Sciatica

Afflicting four fifths of Americans at some time in their lives, back pain is the leading cause of disability for people under 45. Acute back pain comes on quickly and is typically the result of a sudden motion or injury. Chronic back pain comes on slowly and can last for months or years. The cause of chronic pain may be hard to trace. It can be the result of a dysfunction in the body somewhere other than where the pain is actually felt.[157]

Sciatica results from compression of the sciatic nerve at the base of the spine. It is characterized by pain radiating through the buttock down the back of the thigh and leg, sometimes to the foot.

CONVENTIONAL TREATMENT

Where X-ray reveals a surgically correctable problem such as a herniated disk, surgery is done. For other back pains, conventional treatment is generally limited to symptomatic relief with pain-relieving drugs.

THE ORIENTAL APPROACH

Acupuncture can strengthen the low back to prevent pain. A Chinese patent remedy that effectively helps relieve back pain is one called *Sciatica Pills.* Another that is good for strengthening the low back is *Specific Lumbaglin.* Take two capsules three times daily for one week, then one capsule three times daily for maintenance.

Out of the Wheelchair and Walking

A woman sought a remedy for her husband, who suffered from back problems so severe he was unable to walk. He had been in a wheelchair for the past four years. The woman left with a box of Sciatica Pills. A few days later, she returned and bought an entire case. Remarkably, she said, her husband was out of the wheelchair and walking for the first time in years. He was also sleeping better than he had for a long time.

HOMEOPATHIC REMEDIES

Homeopathic remedies can also help relieve back pain. A good combination product is *Sciatica* by BHI. Take one pill every fifteen minutes as needed for acute pain, then three times daily for maintenance. *Sciataide* by B&T is another good homeopathic remedy. For upper back pain, try *Spinaflex* by CompliMed or *Back and Neck Aide* by B&T.

PHYSICAL AND MANIPULATIVE THERAPIES

Studies have shown that *chiropractic* is more effective than conventional medicine for relieving back pain. Other effective physical therapies are *massage, acupressure,* and *body work.*

Exercises are important for maintaining low-back strength. A good resource is *The Healthy Back Book* by Elizabeth Sharp.

Losing weight is also recommended. A sizable belly can pull the back out by the "fulcrum effect."

A *dental overhaul* may also help. TMJ (temporomandibular joint) dysfunction has been linked to some cases of back pain, and so have infected root canals. See E. Brown, R. Hansen, *The Key to Ultimate Health.*

Scoliosis and Chronic Nasal Congestion Alleviated

A private investigator in his early forties suffered from scoliosis (curvature of the spine) and frequent colds, flu, and nasal congestion so bothersome he had trouble sleeping. He had been to many therapists without relief. Surprisingly, when a root canal in one of his front teeth was cleaned out, his upper spine, which had been bowed to the side, began straightening out. When a particularly large silver filling was subsequently replaced with a biocompatible material (low-fusing Degussa porcelain), his nasal congestion and insomnia also cleared.

Bell's Palsy

Bell's palsy is a paralysis of one side of the face resulting from a lesion on a particular nerve. Typically the eye on that side can't be closed, and speaking and eating are impaired. In about two weeks, the paralyzed muscles begin to atrophy. Some facial paralyses may clear up in a few months, while others are permanent. The triggering cause may be infection, trauma (particularly surgical), or weather exposure, but the underlying cause remains elusive. A recent study linked Bell's palsy to the same *herpes simplex* virus that causes cold sores.[158]

CONVENTIONAL TREATMENT

Western medical treatment consists of *salicylates, heat treatments, electrotherapy,* and *steroids.* Steroids are given to stop inflammation. However, they aren't very effective for this purpose, and they seriously impair the body's recovery, deadening the immune system and making natural methods aimed at stimulating it much less effective. (See "Infection, Immunity.")

THE ORIENTAL APPROACH

Oriental doctors attribute Bell's palsy to a condition called "wind in the channels." In the typical case, the victim has fallen asleep under a fan. If the condition is treated immediately with *acupuncture*, the paralyzed nerve can be stimulated back to health in a few days. But if the palsy has been treated with steroids that suppress the immune system, allowing the nerve to atrophy for several months, cure is much harder to effect.

Prompt Treatment Produces Prompt Cure

Jan, 46, sought health advice the day after she awoke with a crooked face after falling asleep under a fan on a hot day. Immediately treated with acupuncture needles, she immediately improved. After receiving three acupuncture treatments a day for the next three days, her symptoms completely resolved.

Another woman who had fallen asleep under a fan and developed Bell's palsy wasn't so fortunate. She had already had the condition for four or five months and had been treated with steroids before she sought relief from acupuncture. She couldn't smile or close her eye completely to sleep. Acupuncture treatments succeeded in stimulating the nerve enough that she could close her eye and smile, and she was therefore happy with the result.

HOMEOPATHIC TREATMENT

The appropriate homeopathic remedy for Bell's palsy is *aconite.* It needs to be taken, however, immediately on contracting the condition. Later in

the course of the disease, acupuncture is much more effective in reviving
deadened nerves.

Bladder Infection (Cystitis)

Bladder infections plague one in three women sometime in their lives.
They are the second leading cause of lost work days for women and are
responsible for millions of doctor visits annually. Symptoms include frequency, a sense of urgency, painful burning, and sometimes bleeding on
urination. Women are far more likely to get the condition than are men,
apparently because a woman's urethra is shorter than a man's and is close
to the anus and vagina.

Most bladder infections are caused by the bacteria *Escherichia coli*
normally found in the intestines. Improper wiping is a possible route of
infection, but lack of estrogen can affect internal flora and contribute to
bladder infections as well. The condition has also been linked to vigorous and frequent sexual activity, but the reason may not be the obvious
one.

About a decade ago, physicians began noticing high numbers of
urinary-tract infections among women using diaphragms for contraception. When refittings did not solve the problem, researchers finally
traced the link to a popular spermicide called *nonoxynol-9* that was being
applied to the contraceptive device. A 1996 study found that women
were more than three times as likely to get urinary tract infections if
they used condoms with nonoxynol-9 more often than once a week.[159]
The spermicide evidently kills not only sperm but the friendly bacteria
residing in the urinary tract, leaving it susceptible to invasion by
unfriendly bacteria.

Interstitial cystitis is an ailment that does not show up on bacterial
cultures. At one time, it was thought to be a merely psychosomatic condition of hysterical women. But the approximately 450,000 sufferers of
interstitial cystitis, who urinate dozens of times daily and experience lower
abdominal pain and other distressing symptoms, have succeeded in raising public awareness of the ailment enough that it is now a fast-growing
research area of the National Institutes of Health.[160]

Drug Treatment

Antibiotics are the usual treatment for cystitis. Before the drugs are given, however, a bacterial culture must be done; and for women with interstitial cystitis, the bacteria don't show up on culture. For another 20 percent of cystitis patients, antibiotics don't work; and for still another 25 percent, the drugs may work in the short term but the cystitis keeps coming back.

When antibiotics aren't effective, other medications may be prescribed. *Elmiron*, which is believed to create a protective coating over the bladder lining, helps about a third of patients. Soothing medicines may also be instilled in the bladder, including *anesthetics*, the anti-inflammatory *DMSO*, and *hydrocortisone*; but again only about a third of patients respond.[161] *Elavil*, an antidepressant, is often prescribed to relieve chronic pain.

A new painkiller called *Uristat* is also now being sold over the counter for relieving bladder-infection distress. Ironically, its manufacturer, Ortho Pharmaceuticals, is the same company that makes one of the popular contraceptive creams containing nonoxynol-9, the ingredient shown to cause chronic urinary-tract infections.

Homeopathic and Herbal Remedies

Homeopathic doctors maintain that antibiotics don't cure urinary tract infections but merely suppress their symptoms. Homeopathic remedies draw the problem to the surface and help the body eliminate it.

For bladder infections, homeopathic *Cantharis* is excellent. The recommended dosage for treating intense burning before, during and after urination is three pellets of Cantharis 6x or 30c four times daily.

Sarsaparilla 6c to 30c is also effective. Homeopathic authority Roger Morrison, M.D., calls it "one of our great specifics for the urinary tract . . . and . . . our best remedy for uncomplicated cystitis."[162] The dosage is three pellets four times daily.

These single homeopathic remedies work when taken at the onset of a bladder infection (on the first or second day). However, a combination of homeopathic and herbal remedies is more effective after the problem has gone on for several days. Take either *Bacticin* by Complimed or *Tao Chin Pien* (a Chinese herbal combination), along with *Bladder Irritation* by Natura-Bio or *Uri Control* by BHI, following these schedules:

- *Bacticin*: 10 drops every 15 minutes for the first hour, then once an hour for 4 hours, then 4 times daily until the infection is completely gone.
- *Bladder Irritation*: 10 drops every 15 minutes for the first hour, then once an hour for 4 hours, then 4 times daily until the infection is completely gone.
- *Uri Control*: 1 tablet every hour for the first 4 hours, then 1 tablet 4 times daily.
- *Tao Chin Pien*: 4 pills twice daily for 5 to 10 days.

Bladder Infection Cycle Broken

Peggy's bladder infections had been recurring for years, despite repeated courses of antibiotics. The problem resolved only when she discovered the homeopathic remedy Cantharis. She has had no recurrences now for several years.

NUTRITIONAL REMEDIES

Cranberry juice, an old wive's remedy for bladder infections, has been shown in clinical studies to actually reduce cystitis pain and recurrences. The juice not only acidifies the urine, inhibiting bacterial growth, but engulfs the infecting bacteria and prevents them from becoming attached to the cells lining the urinary tract. You need to use the pure juice, however. "Cocktails" can contain as little as 2 percent of it. The bitter cranberry taste can be alleviated with cold seltzer or sweeteners, or a teaspoon of pure juice can be added to a cup of tea. *Uva ursi*, a type of cranberry, can also be made into tea; or you can buy cranberry capsules.

A combination of *parsley and celery juices* (fresh-squeezed) acts as a natural diuretic that flushes the body. Avoid citrus juices, which can encourage bacterial growth.

An old home remedy for calming an inflamed bladder is to mix one-quarter teaspoon of baking soda with a half glass of water and drink it twice daily. A more modern alternative is a product called *Alkazone*, a patented, concentrated alkaline supplement that increases the pH of water, changing ordinary water into an alkaline solution.

If antibiotics are taken, follow them with *acidophilus* to replace friendly intestinal flora.

Most important, drink eight to ten glasses of water (preferably distilled) daily to flush out the bladder, dilute toxins, and prevent bacteria from going back up the urethra and infecting the kidneys.

OTHER HELPFUL TIPS

- Empty the bladder frequently. Holding the urine can increase bladder infections. Empty the bladder after intercourse.
- Avoid the use of spermicidal jellies or diaphragms. Even diaphragms used without spermicides can bruise the neck of the bladder and increase susceptibility to infection.
- Wear underwear with cotton crotches.
- Wipe from front to rear.
- Avoid hot tubs.
- Change sanitary napkins frequently (and tampons if you use them, but they're best avoided).

Bone Loss (Osteoporosis)

Osteoporosis, or age-related bone loss, causes an estimated 1.3 million fractures annually in the United States, at a national cost approaching $10 billion. The most damaging consequences are hip fractures, particularly for elderly women, who are seven times as likely to suffer from them as elderly men. Each year, 60,000 women die within six months of their fractures, and the numbers are going up. For the survivors, hip fractures can mean a nursing home.[163] Among other risk factors are a low vitamin-D and calcium intake, a family history of osteoporosis (fractures or rounding of the upper back), an early menopause or hysterectomy/oophorectomy, and low hormone levels.

DRUG TREATMENT

Until recently, the only FDA-approved drug treatment for osteoporosis was *estrogen* therapy. Bone loss takes a dramatic jump when hormone secretion falls off at menopause, and adding estrogen seems to slow it down. The package insert for Premarin (the most popular prescription estrogen) concedes, however, that "[t]here is no evidence that estrogen replacement therapy restores bone mass to premenopausal levels." It merely slows down bone loss. The dose necessary to do this is higher than you need to control other postmenopausal symptoms, increasing the breast cancer risk accompanying synthetic hormone replacement;[164] and to keep receiving estrogen's benefits, you have to keep taking it for life. Researchers have found that within four years of discontinuing ERT, there is no detectable difference in bone mineral content between women who have never taken the drug and those who began treatment but gave it up.[165] And even if you keep taking estrogen, it may not keep preventing bone loss. A review in the *American Journal of Medicine* concluded that "administration of this hormone six years or more after menopause may no longer be effective."[166] Another limitation of estrogen as a bone loss remedy is that it isn't appropriate for men.

Two other drugs have now been approved by the FDA for treating osteoporosis: *alendronate (Fosamex)*, a nonhormonal product; and a *salmon calcitonin nasal spray (Miacalcin)*. But these pharmaceutical options, like estrogen, aren't very effective; and they are quite expensive. In one review of osteoporosis-treatment trials, bone density of the hip increased by less than 1 percent when patients underwent ERT. With nasal-spray calcitonin, Bone density in the lumbar spine *decreased* by 0.2 percent. Adding calcium supplements improved these results, but only moderately: bone density increased on ERT by as much as 2.7 percent, and on calcitonin by 1.15 percent.[167] Alendronate has been found to increase bone mineral density by 7 to 8 percent over a three-year period—better, but still not dramatic enough to justify the cost. Alendronate and calcitonin are more than five times as expensive as Premarin, which already costs up to $30 per month.[170] And the drugs have unwanted side effects.

Provera (synthetic progesterone) has also been shown to modestly increase bone mass, but it too comes with a long list of side effects. Natural progesterone is a much better alternative. (See "Menopause.")

NATURAL HORMONE THERAPY

While the increased bone loss of elderly women is generally attributed to loss of estrogen after menopause, new research suggests that progesterone, which is also produced by the ovaries, may actually be the missing catalyst. An eight-year study conducted by John R. Lee, M.D., reported in the *International Clinical Review* in 1990 and in *Medical Hypotheses* in 1991, showed that natural progesterone not only retards age-related bone loss but actually reverses it. Within a three-year period, bone density was brought back to safe levels in 100 percent of the patients treated, something not even estrogen would do.[169] The product used in this study was not the synthetic progesterone found in popular hormone-replacement-therapy regimes, however. It was a natural progesterone cream derived from Mexican yams. (*Pro-Gest* by Transitions for Health.) The women rubbed the cream on the skin at bedtime for 12 days out of the month (or the last two weeks of estrogen use, if estrogen was being used). One third to one half of a one-ounce jar of progesterone cream was used per month, applied to the softer skin under the arms or of the neck and face, alternating sites each night.

The women were also instructed to take the following measures known to counteract bone loss: They were to get sufficient *exercise, vitamins, calcium and other minerals*; eat a *low-protein diet high in calcium-rich leafy green vegetables and low-fat cheeses*; avoid cigarettes, excess phosphates (especially in soft drinks), excess protein, and certain drugs (excess thyroid hormone and corticosteroids); and limit alcohol intake. The following nutritional supplements were taken: vitamin D (350–400 IU), vitamin C (2,000 mg in divided doses), betacarotene (15 mg or 25,000 IU), and calcium (800–1000 mg by diet and/or supplements). In addition, a modest exercise routine was prescribed (20 minutes per day, or 30 minutes three times a week).

As a result of this program, bone pains were relieved, muscle and bone strength and mobility increased, osteoporotic fractures dropped to zero, and regular fractures healed unusually well. No unwanted side effects were reported.

Expected bone loss in the women over a three-year period was 4.5 percent. At best, estrogen would have slowed this loss down; but the natural progesterone regimen actually put bone back on. In the 63 tested patients, bone density over three years increased by an average of 15.4 percent—double the results of the best of the prescription osteoporosis drugs, and more than five times estrogen's bone-restoring effects. The women's bones typically got 10 percent thicker in the first 6 to 12 months and increased 3 to 5 percent per year thereafter. Several patients' bone densities jumped 20 to 25 percent during the first year. This increase occurred regardless of age. In fact the patients who started out the worst improved the most. Bone density also increased regardless of whether estrogen supplements accompanied the progesterone. In many of the women, bone density eventually stabilized at the levels of healthy 35 year olds; and in all of them, it stabilized at safe levels. The women also lost weight and had more energy, and many volunteered the observation that their lost libido (sex drive) had returned. Blood pressures dropped, and there were anticancer effects. Unlike in studies with synthetic progestins, cholesterol levels did not rise.[170] So far, says Dr. Lee, natural progesterone has reversed bone loss in every woman on whom he has tried it (beginning in 1982), so long as the other essential factors were included: proper diet and exercise, supplemental micronutrients, and so forth.[171]

DHEA is another hormone that declines with age. Research in this area is new, so there are no long-term studies establishing the effects of supplementation on bone density, but studies do show that blood levels of DHEA are significantly correlated with bone density. Very low blood levels are seen in patients with osteoporosis.[172] For women, the hormone precursor *pregnenolone* is recommended along with DHEA, to help keep hormone levels in balance.

Natural estrogen is also available in the form of a cream derived from plants (*OstaDerm*). These creams have yet to be thoroughly tested, but to date, unlike synthetic and animal-derived pharmaceutical estrogens, they have not demonstrated side effects.[173] (See "Menopause.")

NUTRITIONAL SUPPLEMENTATION

Calcium supplements can help reduce bone loss, but if you merely supplement with calcium, you'll still lose bone.[174] Only a few studies have shown any effect of calcium on bone density, and in those few, the calcium sources were particularly bioavailable (available for use by the body).[177] *Vitamin D* is also necessary to aid calcium absorption, and *magnesium* is necessary to help move calcium out of the bloodstream and into the skeleton. When magnesium is out of balance with calcium, the calcium you eat may never make it to your bones.

CALCIUM SUPPLEMENTS. *Calcium carbonate* is a cheap form of calcium contained in certain antacids, but it is an inorganic form that is only about 5 percent absorbed. Other forms that are inorganic and poorly absorbed include calcium from *oyster shells* and *dolomite* (a rock).[176]

A more bioavailable option is *calcium citrate*. Calcium absorption from calcium citrate is as much as four times as great as that from calcium carbonate. Absorption from a combination chelate called *calcium citrate-malate (CCM)* is better yet.[177]

Another bioavailable source is animal bone. The ideal *bone meal* is a cold-processed product that has not been heated above 125 degrees F. A downside of bone meal is that it may be contaminated with lead, but this problem is avoided in a highly bioavailable bone calcium called *microcrystalline hydroxyapatite compound (MCHC)*, the organic protein calcium matrix found in the raw young bones of cattle and sheep raised on insecticide- and pesticide-free pastures. It differs from bone meal in that it is not heated in the reduction process or washed with chemical solvents. In two recent studies comparing MCHC with calcium gluconate and a placebo in the treatment of osteoporosis (age-related bone loss), only the MCHC groups experienced a significant increase in cortical bone.[178]

The most assimilable way to get calcium and other minerals is in *ionized* form, the form in which it must be reduced to be absorbed by the body. (See Chapter 2.) A balanced ionic mineral source is the "coral water" drunk by certain Japanese islanders reported to have unusual longevity. Their drinking water has a high content of ionized minerals leached from the coral on which the island was built. The result is a highly alkalinized water that keeps the body alkaline and resistant to disease. Researchers have found that this "coral" water can actually neutralize waste products contained in it, including bacteria, heavy metals, fluoride, and chloroform. A balanced ionized mineral product made from this water is available by mail order from Pacific Research Laboratories (310-320-1132). The recommended daily dose is one-quarter teaspoon of *Coral Legend* mixed with one-quarter cup of *Aloe Balance,* an organic aloe-vera juice fortified with negative ions that improves the bioavailability of ionized minerals taken with it.

MAGNESIUM. Guy E. Abraham, M.D., a research gynecologist in Torrance, California, succeeded in increasing bone density in post-menopausal women by 11 percent in one year, by *decreasing* their calcium intakes to 500 mg per day and *increasing* their magnesium intakes to 600–1000 mg per day. These results were significantly better than in studies involving calcium alone. The dose of magnesium was based on bowel tolerance: diarrhea was the limiting factor.[179]

Magnesium is abundant in whole grains, beans, nuts, seeds, and vegetables; but fertilizers reduce its content in the soil, and sugar and alcohol increase its excretion through the urine. Although the RDA for magnesium is only 350 mg for women of all ages, Dr. Mildred Seelig, executive president of the American College of Nutrition, suggests that older people eating a good diet can benefit from magnesium supplements of 700–800 mg per day.[180]

VITAMIN D.   The typical recommendation for vitamin D is 400 IU per day; but neither foods nor vitamin supplements are actually ideal sources. Vitamin D is produced in the body only after sunlight striking the skin initiates a series of reactions there.[181] The vitamin D produced commercially, called vitamin D2 (ergocalciferol), is not the same as the vitamin D manufactured by the body (vitamin D3). Studies show that blood levels of the vitamin are only weakly correlated with dietary intake. A much stronger correlation has been shown with exposure to sunlight.[182] Fortunately, to satisfy your vitamin D requirement, you needn't stay out in the sun long enough to risk skin cancer. Researchers at Tufts University have shown that in the summer, minimum vitamin D requirements are met by exposure of just the hands, face, and arms for 10 to 15 minutes a day, three times a week. These recommendations were made specifically for the elderly.[183]

HOMEOPATHIC REMEDIES

Calcium Absorption by BioForce is a homeopathic remedy that aids the body in assimilating the calcium it takes in.

Frail Hip Bones Strengthened

A 45-year-old woman said she had been diagnosed with osteopeny, a rare bone condition in which the bones, and particularly the hip bones, can break very easily. She had her bone density tested by bone scan, then began using *Pro-Gest* cream, a calcium/mineral product called *BoneUp*, and *Calcium Absorption*. A year later, to her delight and the surprise of her doctor, another bone scan showed that her bone density had significantly increased.

DIETARY MODIFICATION

Women in some non-Western cultures manage to escape the increased rate of hip fractures experienced by Western women after menopause, although their calcium intakes are below those of American women.[184] The solid bones of non-Western women have been attributed to low intakes of protein, meat, and phosphorus; a high intake of potassium; and regular exercise. A too-high protein intake leaches calcium from the bones.[185] A too-low protein intake is also hazardous, on the other hand, because protein is necessary for the liver to detoxify estrogen.[186] The RDA for women is 44 grams.

Excess phosphorus has also been linked to bone loss. Each phosphorus atom in the bloodstream must be accompanied by a calcium atom. The calcium pulled out of the blood to pair up with this phosphorus is replaced with calcium from the bones. Phosphorus is also antagonistic to potassium, a mineral found in the unprocessed vegetables, fruits, and whole grains that are abundant in traditional non-Western diets. Calcium- and potassium-robbing phosphorus is supplied in the Western diet not only by meat but by a worse offender, the carbonated soft drink.

Exercise is another variable. Clinical studies show that weight-bearing exercise such as brisk walking, jogging, low impact aerobics, and trampoline jumping improves the density of your bones and prevents osteoporosis. It also forestalls cardiovascular disease and prevents or relieves obesity, muscle weakness, and depression.[187]

THINGS TO AVOID

Besides excess protein and phosphates, bone loss has been linked to fluoridated water and to mercury amalgam dental fillings.[188]

Drugs that cause dizziness, sedation, and fuzzy thinking can also be responsible for the falls that produce fractures. In one study, older people were found to be about twice as likely to suffer hip fractures if they were taking tranquilizers with long half-lives, such as *flurazepam (Dalmane);* tricyclic antidepressants, including *amitriptyline (Elavil), doxepin (Sinequan),* and *imipramine (Tofranil);* or antipsychotics, including *thioridazine (Mellaril), haloperidol (Haldol),* and *chlorpromazine (Thorazine).*[189] Diuretic drugs can also contribute to hip fractures, by prompting elderly women to get up to the bathroom in the middle of the night.

Other drugs linked to bone loss are *aluminum-containing antacids.* Aluminum displaces calcium from the bones, causing them to be brittle and to break easily, and antacids inhibit calcium absorption by neutralizing stomach acid, raising the pH of the stomach. Calcium can be absorbed only in its soluble ionized form, which requires a low pH.

Bone Demineralization Linked to Antacids

The Annals of Internal Medicine reported the cases of two 42-year-old women with liver failure requiring liver transplants. Both women had serious bone demineralization, which was linked on X-ray examination to heavy deposits of aluminum in their bones. Both also had long histories of taking aluminum hydroxide-containing antacids (Amphojel and Mylanta) for the prevention of peptic ulcer. In one woman, bone pain completely disappeared after the aluminum was removed by chelation therapy. (This treatment involves the injection of a solution that chelates, or binds, heavy metals, which are then excreted in the urine. See "Heavy Metal Poisoning.") The other woman died before a liver donor could be located. But bone staining at autopsy was strongly positive for aluminum.[191]

Bone Spurs

Bone spurs are abnormal growths on the ends of the bones, which can cause excruciating pain when they press on nerves and muscles during activity. They typically develop on the feet, spine, or neck. When they occur in the upper neck, the condition is called *cervical osteoarthritis*. Bone spurs result when vertebrae shrink with age: the bone compensates for the expanding spaces between vertebrae by growing bony protrusions.

CONVENTIONAL TREATMENT

Conventional treatment is with anti-inflammatory painkillers (aspirin, ibuprofen); devices to take pressure off the nerves (orthopedic collars, back braces, foam-rubber shoe pads); or surgery. But these aren't actually cures. Even surgery doesn't reach the underlying problem, since the spurs are liable to grow back.

NATURAL ALTERNATIVES

Bone spurs can be an indication that the body is either low in calcium or isn't using its calcium properly. *Urticalcin* by BioForce is a homeopathic remedy that aids calcium absorption. Supplemental calcium can also help. (See "Bone Loss.")

For bone spurs on the feet, effective homeopathic remedies are *Hekla Lava, Calc Flor* or *Calc Phos.* One of these three will usually eliminate bone spurs in a month or so. You can also try changing your shoes. Improperly fitting shoes are a common cause of bone spurs.

For stubborn bone spurs on the spine, Metagenics makes a combination protocol designed to be taken over approximately a six-month period. This remedy has worked when conventional treatment failed.

Bone Spurs on Neck Eliminated

Nancy was skeptical. A woman of about 60, she had bone spurs on her neck that were distressingly painful; but she couldn't believe that an herbal protocol would cure the condition. She came back five or six times to study the Metagenics literature before she finally made her purchase. She returned six weeks later pleased to report that the remedy had worked. Her neck was fine, and it still is as of this writing.

Cancer

Cancer cannot legally be treated by alternative practitioners and is beyond the scope of this book. See Ellen Brown, *Forbidden Medicine* (Murrieta California: Third Millenium Press, 1998.). Good comprehensive guides to natural, nontoxic cancer therapies include the *Alternative Medicine Definitive Guide to Cancer* (Tiburon, California: Future Medicine Publishing, Inc., 1997), by W. John Diamond, M.D., and W. Lee Cowden, M.D., in collaboration with Burton Goldberg and a long list of M.D. contributors; Dr. Ralph W. Moss's *Cancer Therapy: The Independent Consumer's Guide* (New York: Equinox Press, 1992); and Richard Walters' *Options: The Alternative Cancer Therapy Book* (New York: Avery Publishing Group, 1993).

Candidiasis, Thrush

Fungi are the most common parasites, led by the ubiquitous yeast *Candida albicans*. Candida organisms are natural residents of the body, but they're normally found in harmless proportions. The body's natural defense against fungus infection is its resident population of normal bacterial flora, which prevents invasion by foreigners. But yeasts are impervious to the antibiotics that wipe out bacteria. When friendly bacteria are wiped out along with unfriendly ones by these drugs, the field is left wide open for the yeasts to move in.

Thrush is a fungal infection typically appearing as a bright-red diaper rash that doesn't respond to the usual rash ointments. It can also appear as white patches in the mouth that leave red sores. Thrush can be acquired by the newborn when passing through the birth canal, or it may follow a course of antibiotics.

CONVENTIONAL TREATMENT

To treat fungal invasions resulting from antibiotic "overkill," the conventional approach is to prescribe another drug. For strictly local infections, *nystatin (Mycostatin)* is used topically or as a "swish" in the mouth. The drug is relatively safe, but it can produce nausea, vomiting, and diarrhea.

For vaginal yeast infections and topical use on diaper rash, *clotrimazole* is currently the most popular option. Brand names include *Lotrimin, Gyn-Lotrimin,* and *Lotrisone* (clotrimazole with a topical steroid). These drugs don't work, however, on more serious systemic (whole-body) fungal infections. For their treatment, the likely candidate until recently was *amphotericin B,* a toxic drug that can seriously damage the kidneys and has to be injected. The current favorite is *Diflucan (fluconazole),* which has fewer short-term side effects and can be taken orally. But the 1998 *Facts and Comparisons* indicates that it, too, can have insidious long-term side effects, including a remote but real risk of serious liver damage.

For mild systemic and local infections, another option is *ketoconazole.* Less toxic than amphotericin B, it can still cause nausea, liver damage, sexual dysfunction, impotence, and enlarged breasts in men. *Griseofulvin,* an antifungal used for infections of the hair and nails, can also be toxic. Side effects listed in the 1998 *Facts and Comparisons* include headaches, upset stomach, tiredness, insomnia, allergic reactions, blood disorders, and fungal superinfections.[191]

HERBAL AND NUTRITIONAL ALTERNATIVES

Garlic is known for its antifungal properties. In laboratory experiments, its antifungal activity has been shown to be greater than that of either nystatin or amphotericin B.[192] Health-food stores now sell deodorized garlic tablets that make this age-old remedy both easy to take and socially acceptable.

Other useful herbal and nutritional remedies include *barberry*, an antimicrobial herb; *pau d'arco*, a South American anti-infective herb; *caprylic acid*, a medium-chain fatty acid found naturally in the body that counters microorganism growth; *undecylenic acid*, another fat found naturally in the body, produced commercially from castor-bean oil; *oregano*, an herb with antifungal properties; and *citrus-seed extract*, a natural antimicrobial.

Excellent essential oils are *oil of oregano* and *oil of cilantro*.

Lactobacillus acidophilus, Bifidobacterium bifidum, and *Lactobacillus bulgaricus* are "good" bacteria that protect the digestive tract from invasion by unwanted microorganisms.[193]

Many alternative practitioners also recommend avoiding foods on which yeast thrive—those containing sugar, molds, or yeasts, mushrooms and aged or fermented foods, including breads made with yeast, aged cheeses, vinegar, and beer. For a thorough discussion of this subject, see *Candida* by Dr. Luc De Schepper.

For natural remedies for vaginal yeast infections, see "Vaginitis."

THE HOMEOPATHIC APPROACH

Homeopathic doctors believe there is a "maintaining cause" that has suppressed the immune system, allowing the fungus to grow. Treatment aimed at killing the fungus or controlling it through diet by eliminating sugar and fermented foods is an imperfect solution, since the fungus returns once sugar or fermented foods are eaten again. The homeopathic approach is to use remedies that boost the immune system so the body stops the fungus from multiplying. Good options are *Mycocan Combo* by PHI (ten drops three times daily) or *Candida Plus* by Deseret.

Candida Precipitated by Garment Industry Job Routed with Natural Remedies

Sherry's high-stress job in the garment district kept her at work 10 to 14 hours a day. She had chronic recurring vaginal yeast infections, craved sugar, and had trouble sleeping at night. She had been diagnosed with and treated for candida on several occasions, but the infection kept coming back. While on a candida diet, she was fine; but if she ate a piece of cake or drank a beer, the next day her yeast infection would return. Her "maintaining cause" was evidently her job, which kept her body run down. She was also exposed to toxic fumes, constantly breathing the formaldehydes in the fabrics. For her extreme case, the German homeopathic *Monilia Albicans* was suggested. She took it for a month. She also went on the Liver Cleanse Diet and a formaldehyde detox program. (See "Environmental Illness.") At the end of two months, her yeast infections were gone, and they have not returned.

OTHER HELPFUL TIPS

To control candida, try these measures:

1. Avoid antibiotics unless critically necessary. If you must use them, replace friendly flora with acidophilus and bifido products after completing the course of drugs.

2. Avoid toxic chemicals, tap water, fabric softeners on underwear, scented detergent.

3. Don't wear damp socks or wet clothing after perspiring.

4. Practice safe sex. If using oral contraceptives or a spermicide with nonoxynol-9, supplement with beneficial flora.

5. Avoid fermented foods—mushrooms, yeast, beer, wine, alcohol.

6. Eat pure, sugar-free foods. For creative alternatives, see *Get the Sugar Out* by Anne Louise Gittleman.

7. Get enough sunshine and exercise, and avoid stress.

Cardiac Arrhythmias, Disrhythmias, Fibrillations

Cardiac arrhythmias, or irregular heartbeats, are of concern mainly because they can warn of an impending heart attack. Arrhythmias may be caused not only by heart disease but by infections, hypertension, and emotional stress. They can also be caused by drugs, including nicotine, caffeine, diet pills, and other stimulants. They may be accompanied by symptoms such as weakness, fainting, or shortness of breath; but sometimes they're the only symptom.

Atrial fibrillation, or *disrhythmia* in the atrium of the heart, is considered a risk factor for stroke, since it occurs twelve times as often in stroke patients as in other adults.

Drug Treatment

Because cardiac arrhythmia is a known risk factor for subsequent sudden death in people who have already had a heart attack, patients with this symptom were treated with antiarrhythmic drugs, until an upsetting major study led researchers to conclude that routine medication with these drugs was unwarranted. The study found that the popular antiarrhythmics *flecainide (Tambocor)* and *encainide (Enkaid)* not only did not forestall a second attack in arrhythmia patients but actually doubled the chances of bringing one on.[194] Correcting the symptom, it seems, aggravated the underlying disease.

Paralleling the use of antiarrhythmic drugs to prevent heart attacks, anticoagulant drugs have routinely been prescribed for atrial fibrillation or disrhythmia to prevent strokes. However, a 1987 study reported in the *New England Journal of Medicine* found that atrial fibrillation unaccompanied by other symptoms is associated with a very low risk of stroke, at least in patients under 60. Again, the researchers concluded that routine medication is probably unwarranted.[195]

Natural Alternatives

A homeopathic formula called *Cactus* can effectively normalize nonlife-threatening cardiac arrhythmias, used in conjunction with *hawthorn berry*, an herb which supports the heart, and *co-enzyme Q10*, which strengthens the heart. *Magnesium* can also help since magnesium depletion can cause rapid or irregular heartbeat. For other natural remedies good for heart function, see "Atherosclerosis," "Heart Attacks."

Arrhythmias Cured with Simple Natural Remedy

A 35-year-old woman was concerned about her repeated bouts of palpitations. She would wake up short of breath, her heart beating too fast. Her doctor had put her on beta blockers, but the drugs had only made her tired without eliminating the frightening palpitations. She sought a natural remedy. She went home with Cactus and did not come back for a year and a half. When she did, she said she hadn't had a single episode of palpitations since she had begun taking the remedy and that she hadn't felt so well in years.

Maintenance Dose Keeps Heart Palpitations at Bay

A 60-year-old man was doing well after his heart surgery seven years ago and was exercising heavily every day, until one day while riding his bicycle up a hill, he experienced a very strong irregular heartbeat that wouldn't go away. He became quite concerned after his doctor tried him on several medications to no avail. He began taking *Cactus* by MarcoPharma, and within a day his heart was back to its normal rhythm. However, two and a half weeks after he stopped taking the remedy, the palpitations came back. He started taking the remedy again and they stopped. He is now on a regular maintenance dose of 20 drops daily and has had no further problems.

Carpal Tunnel Syndrome

Medical experts report that carpal tunnel syndrome, or repetitive stress injury, has grown to almost epidemic proportions worldwide, a phenomenon attributed largely to the explosion in computer use.[196] Carpal tunnel syndrome begins with tingling and numbness in the fingers and wrist joints, particularly at night, progressing to persistent pain and aching in the hands and arms. Pregnant, menopausal, and overweight women are particularly affected.

CONVENTIONAL TREATMENT

Wrist splints can relieve symptoms and are particularly useful while sleeping. Pain relievers are also often prescribed. In the extreme case, surgery may be performed. But none of these remedies addresses the underlying cause. Even surgery may need to be repeated every few years.

NATURAL ALTERNATIVES

Acupuncture, chiropractic, massage, ultrasound, and yoga can help relieve pain, not by masking it but by increasing circulation. Homeopathic remedies also help. Avoiding unnecessary repetitive stress is another obvious precautionary measure.

For many women, however, the underlying problem is a little-suspected one: hormones. Estrogen causes water retention in the tissues. The resulting edema (swelling) can impinge on the nerves. Women who have been afflicted with carpal tunnel syndrome for years have been cured in a matter of weeks simply by applying *natural progesterone cream (Pro-Gest)* to their wrists. Progesterone is estrogen's antagonist and works to normalize hormone levels.

Wrist Splints Abandoned after 17 Years

As an obsessive/compulsive, overachieving law student, one of the authors (Ellen) spent her days furiously scribbling notes. Then she noticed her writing hand going numb. When she got pregnant after graduating from law school, both hands went numb, especially at night. She had to get up once or twice to shake the blood into them before she could get back to sleep. She consulted several medical practitioners; but this was in the seventies, when carpal tunnel syndrome was an obscure condition. They didn't know what the problem was. Her neighbor finally diagnosed it and suggested wearing braces on my wrists. This simple home measure allowed me to sleep through the night; but she was a fairly new bride, and the remedy was unromantic. She consulted the appropriate medical specialist to see if anything more permanent could be done. The doctor confirmed her neighbor's diagnosis and suggested surgery, but he conceded that it would probably have to be repeated every few years. She respectfully declined and resigned herself to wearing the brace, something she did every night for the next 17 years.

Then when she hit 50, she was suddenly able to sleep without it. She concluded this was because her estrogen levels had dropped. Estrogen causes edema (water retention). But she had also been applying natural progesterone cream to her abdominal area every night for several years. (See "Menopause.") Dr. Walker subsequently confirmed that she has seen carpal tunnel syndrome reverse itself in about thirty women in a matter of weeks, with the regular nightly application of natural progesterone cream directly to their wrists.

Cataracts, Macular Degeneration

Cataracts and macular degeneration are the two leading causes of blindness in the elderly.

A *cataract* is a clouding of the lens that focuses light in the eye. Most cataracts are the result of natural aging, but oxidative stress seems to play a central role in their development, suggesting that diet can be a factor. An increase in cataracts has been blamed on exposure to ultraviolet light and the thinning ozone layer, but the use of sunglasses is controversial. Some authorities maintain that they cause the pupils to dilate and allow even more harmful rays to enter the eye.[197]

Macular degeneration is scarring on the "macula," a tiny spot at the center of the retina in the back of the eye where images are transmitted to the brain. Macular degeneration can be "dry" or "wet." The wet form involves a leaking of blood and requires immediate attention. Aspirin, which interferes with blood coagulation and increases bleeding, has been linked to macular hemorrhage (bleeding).[198]

CAUTION: If you are having chronic eye problems, you should see an ophthalmologist (an M.D. specializing in eye diseases).

CONVENTIONAL TREATMENT

The only treatment available for correcting a cataract that has already formed is surgery. Cataract surgery is one of the most successful of operations, improving vision in 95 percent of cases. "Wet" macular degeneration can also be successfully treated with laser surgery.

NATURAL THERAPIES FOR PREVENTION

Both cataracts and macular degeneration are thought to indicate an overall deficiency in *antioxidants*. Research shows that people with age-related macular degeneration have low levels of *glutathione*, an antioxidant enzyme. Chronic exposure to UV radiation and chemicals (e.g. in smog and chemicalized water), along with insufficient intake of vegetables and fruits, could lower glutathione and other antioxidants over time to the point where the macula, an oxidant-sensitive tissue, is completely destroyed.

Laboratory and population studies show that a higher intake of antioxidant *vitamins C and E* and *carotenoids* lowers cataract risk. In one study, women who used vitamin C supplements for more than ten years had a 75 percent lower prevalence of early clouding of the lens (cataract formation) than did other women.[199]

Other research has shown that dietary supplementation with *lutein* helps prevent cataracts and macular degeneration. Lutein is a carotenoid found in vegetables (especially corn, spinach, and carrots) and available in pill form. Eyes taken from autopsies of people with macular degeneration have about 30 percent less of the mixed carotenoids than do healthy eyes. In one study, supplementation with 30 mg per day of lutein increased lutein levels by a factor of ten in the two subjects of the study.[200]

For other natural remedies good for the eyes, see "Eye Problems."

Chlamydia

Chlamydia is now the leading sexually transmitted disease in the United States. Though the condition is little discussed, its cost in suffering may actually be higher than for AIDS. An estimated four million new cases occur each year, but most go unreported, largely because the disease can be without symptoms. This is also one reason for its spread, since it may be hard to detect in either your partner or yourself. When there are symptoms, they include difficult or painful urination and, in men, penile discharge; or in women, a yellowish vaginal discharge, bleeding between periods or after intercourse, and pain in the pelvic area during intercourse. Untreated chlamydia can lead to sterility in men and to pelvic inflammatory disease in women, resulting in infertility, ectopic pregnancy, and sometimes death.

Chlamydia bacteria can also be responsible for a chronic eye inflammation called *trachoma*, which is one of the world's leading causes of blindness.

DRUG TREATMENT

Penicillin won't work on chlamydia. Drug treatment is usually with tetracycline antibiotics. But even they may fail, often due to reinfection by an untreated sexual partner.[201]

HOMEOPATHIC TREATMENT

Staufen, a German company, makes an effective homeopathic treatment for this condition. Called *Chlamydia*, it is taken at the rate of one ampule every three days for a month. While undergoing treatment, the patient should use condoms to avoid spreading the infection.

Interstitial Cystitis Traced to Chlamydia and Cleared

A woman confided that she had been diagnosed with interstitial cystitis, a disease of the bladder in which the patient feels as if she has a bladder infection, constantly needs to urinate, and is in pain, but no bacteria can be found on a lab culture. The condition is typically misdiagnosed, and its victims may suffer for years without relief. (See "Cystitis.") This woman had suffered with it for about six months before she finally diagnosed herself, after reading about the condition on the Internet. Her doctor had then confirmed her self-diagnosis, but he had no cure for it.

A careful homeopathic history revealed that the woman had contracted chlamydia and had been treated with antibiotics for it ten years earlier. About three months after the first round of antibiotics, she had been told she had chlamydia again and another course of antibiotics had been prescribed. *Chlamydia* by Staufen completely cleared her condition. The homeopathic explanation is that the chlamydia hadn't been cured by the antibiotics but had merely been pushed deeper into the system, where it had manifested as bladder irritation.

PREVENTION

Condoms, diaphragms and spermicides containing nonoxynol-9 may help reduce the spread of chlamydia. However, nonoxynol-9 is a synthetic estrogen mimic that can have other side effects. (See "Bladder Infection," "Uterine Prolapse.") The safest course remains abstinence or careful selection of partners. The sexually active should get regular checkups by a physician.

Cholesterol, High

Elevated cholesterol levels are now considered an illness, based on studies finding that people with very high levels have an increased risk of heart disease.

The often quoted statement, "For each 1 percent reduction in cholesterol, we can expect a 2 percent reduction in CHD [coronary heart disease] events," was based on the Lipid Research Clinics Coronary Primary Prevention Trial (LRC), a $150 million project reported in the early 1980s. Based on the LRC, the government-sponsored Cholesterol Consensus Conference called for mass cholesterol screening. Anyone with cholesterol levels over 200 was considered at risk. Dietary recommendations included replacing saturated fat and cholesterol with vegetable fat (that is, butter with margarine). Estimates are that more than $60 billion is now spent annually in the United States on cholesterol screening and treatment.[202]

Yet independent researchers who tallied the LRC data found no difference in heart disease incidence in the drug and nondrug groups. Other researchers were troubled by the little-publicized finding of an increase in deaths from cancer, intestinal disease, stroke, violence, and suicide in the drug-taking group in the LRC.

Today, researchers are wondering whether we haven't gone too far in trying to eliminate cholesterol from our diets. Cholesterol is produced by the body itself, and it has many necessary functions.

One is to make hormones. Cholesterol is at the top of the hormone cascade. Insufficient dietary cholesterol can result in weak sexual organs, precipitating hysterectomies and other surgeries, and in problems handling stress. People lacking sufficient cholesterol to make the stress hormone cortisol are less able to cope with crises. Several studies have found a threefold increase in suicide, homicide, or other violent deaths among men taking cholesterol-lowering drugs. In a study reported in 1995, men in a psychiatric ward whose serum cholesterol levels were in the lowest twenty-fifth percentile were 2.2 times more likely to have tried to commit suicide than men in the upper seventy-fifth percentile for serum cholesterol.[203] Another of cholesterol's essential functions is to protect the arteries. This can, in fact, explain its abnormal accumulation in the arteries of patients with heart disease. The culprit may not be cholesterol itself but the toxins from which the cholesterol is protecting the arterial walls. (See "Atherosclerosis.")

CONVENTIONAL TREATMENT

The approach of conventional medicine is to lower serum cholesterol levels with drugs. In the 1980s, three major trials tested three different cholesterol-lowering drugs. In each of them, the incidence and death rate from heart disease were reduced. But these results were misleading, since *total* deaths remained the same or actually increased in the drug-taking groups. The first study, reported in 1980, was conducted by the World Health Organization and tested the drug *clofibrate*. The drug evidently killed more people than it saved. Deaths in the treated group were one third higher than in the controls (163 vs. 127).[204] The second study, the Lipid Research Clinics Coronary Primary Prevention Trial, was reported in 1984 and tested the drug cholestyramine (Questran). Nonfatal heart attacks were reduced by 20 percent, but total deaths in the treated and control groups weren't significantly different (68 vs. 71).[205] The third study, the Helsinki Heart Study, was reported in 1987 and tested the drug *gemfibrozil (Lopid)*. CHD was reduced by 34 percent, but again there were actually more deaths in the treated than in the untreated groups (45 vs. 42).[206]

Offsetting the reduction in heart-disease deaths in these studies was an increased fatality from accidents and violence. This finding could have been passed off to coincidence, except that it happened repeatedly. The drugs evidently induced mood changes, precipitating the accidental and violent deaths. People on cholesterol-lowering drugs were also more likely to develop gallstones, which in certain cases led to death, and they had a higher incidence of certain types of cancer and of bleeding in the brain.[207]

Until 1997, only one cholesterol-lowering remedy was found to actually increase overall survival. This was niacin.[208] Besides being more effective than the other remedies, it was only one tenth their cost. The reason? *Niacin isn't a drug.* It's an unpatentable vitamin, B3. It's discussed more fully on page 113–114.

Then in November of 1997, researchers studying *lovastatin (Mevacor)*, a leading cholesterol-lowering drug, reported a breakthrough. In their landmark study, taking Mevacor significantly reduced the risk of heart attack or sudden death even in people with only slightly elevated cholesterol levels (around 220). The researchers, whose study was financed by Mevacor's manufacturer, suggested that cholesterol-lowering medicines should be considered for an additional eight million Americans.[209]

Enthusiasm for this approach to high cholesterol levels was tempered, however, not only by the cost (about $100 per month per patient), but by another study announced the same month, which found that daily Mevacor use may somewhat dull the mind and worsen attention and dexterity.[210] The drug has also caused cataracts and birth defects in animals.[211]

The Mevacor study also contradicted the results of other studies. In 1994, Yale researchers reported in the *Journal of the American Medical Association* that high cholesterol levels hold no apparent risk, at least for the elderly. Tracking 997 Connecticut senior citizens for four years, they found that people with the worst cholesterol profiles had virtually the same rates of heart disease and death as those with the best profiles.[212]

Those concerns didn't stop *Zocor*, a newer cholesterol-lowering drug from Merck touted as being "even better" than Mevacor, from hitting number four on the U.S. prescription-drug charts in 1997. (Mevacor was only number nine in 1996 and had dropped out of the top ten by 1997.) Skeptics suggest that the hype about Zocor may be less about breakthrough advances in drug formulation than about the fact that Mevacor has reached the end of its patent-protected life. Zocor is the manufacturer's new patentable substitute.

DIETARY ALTERNATIVES

Cheaper and safer alternatives are available. Studies show that most people can lower their cholesterol levels without side effects of any sort, merely by changing their diets.[213] For details of Dr. Dean Ornish's landmark dietary program achieving this effect with a low-fat lacto-vegetarian diet, see "Atherosclerosis."

Another option is to fortify your diet with *soy products*. A study reported in the *New England Journal of Medicine* on August 3, 1995, found that eating 47 grams of soy protein daily (about the amount in three-quarters pound of firm tofu) lowered cholesterol by a full 20 percent in people whose levels were initially too high. Soy protein also significantly reduced LDL or "bad" cholesterol and triglycerides, both of which are primary heart-disease risk factors. The effect was attributed to the phytoestrogen compounds called *isoflavones.*[214]

Plant fiber is another natural cholesterol-lowering nutrient. The most effective type is the soluble fiber in fruits, vegetables, and oat bran. Unlike the insoluble fibers, which remain coarse and gritty in water, the soluble fibers dissolve to form a gel. All plant foods are rich in both types of fiber, but some contain more of one than the other. Insoluble fiber, the kind in wheat bran, increases stool bulk and promotes bowel function. *Soluble fiber*, the kind in *oat bran*, forms a gel that traps cholesterol-rich bile acids. These bile acids would otherwise be recycled. When they're trapped and eliminated, the body has to use other cholesterol to make more bile acids, and serum cholesterol is reduced.[215]

Soluble fiber is also the kind found in bulk laxatives, such as *Metamucil*, containing *psyllium*. In one study, volunteers with an average serum cholesterol level of 250 mg/dl were given a teaspoonful of Metamucil three times a day. After eight weeks, their cholesterol levels had dropped an average of 35 mg/dl, or 14 percent. This result was about as good as with the bile-acid resins Questran and Colestin. In fact, psyllium works in much the same way as these drugs. It binds bile acids in the intestines and prevents them from being reabsorbed. The advantages of psyllium are that it's easier to swallow and its side effects are limited to occasional mild stomach cramps and gas.[216]

Psyllium comes from the seed of a common weed that you probably wouldn't eat except in processed form. If you're into the truly natural, you can get its effects from common edible plant fibers, including the *pectin* found in apples and other fruits and vegetables. The mechanism is the same as with the bile-acid resins. In combination with calcium, pectin binds readily to bile acids, rendering them useless as digestive enzymes. The liver senses there is a shortage of bile acid and compensates by extracting cholesterol molecules from the blood. These molecules are then modified into bile molecules. The result is a drop in serum cholesterol.[217]

HERBAL AND NUTRITIONAL SUPPLEMENTS

Hawthorn berry (*Crataegus*) is an herb shown in clinical studies to have cardiovascular benefits. Indicated for the treatment of coronary-artery disease, high blood pressure, mild congestive heart failure, angina, and cardiac arrhythmias, it contains *OPCs*, which are powerful antioxidants.[218]

An herbal product called *Cholestin* contains yeast such as that eaten in quantity by the Chinese for thousands of years. In combination with diet and exercise, it is reported to reduce serum cholesterol by an average of 25 to 40 points, without side effects except for occasional mild indigestion.[219]

An Ayurvedic remedy called Guggulow is also remarkably effective at lowering serum cholesterol. We recommend Jarrow's version called *Opti-Guggul* or *Doctor's Best Ultra Guggulow*.

Dangerously High Cholesterol Stabilized with Ayurvedic Herb

Jim, 54, had cholesterol levels that were well over 300. He had tried Mevacor and Zocor without relief. After two weeks on Guggulow, his cholesterol had dropped to 280. It eventually stabilized at around 210.

THE DETOX APPROACH

Some people have high cholesterol levels although their diets are unimpeachable. In those cases, cholesterol may be high not because of something they ate but because their bodies are padding their arteries with cholesterol to protect them from toxic onslaughts. Potential artery aggressors include heavy metals, pesticides, and other poisonous chemicals. To reach the cause of this type of problem, you need to eliminate the aggressors.

That seems to be why niacin works so well in lowering cholesterol and increasing survival. The "niacin flush"—the red face and skin you get when you take sufficient quantities of the vitamin—indicate that your capillaries are ejecting toxins. Niacin opens the capillaries, increases circulation, and normalizes cholesterol. The first time you try it, 100 mg can give you a flush; but with repeated use, it is actually possible to get up to 5,000 mg without one. At that point, your capillaries are considered "clean." For protocols, see "Heavy Metal Poisoning."

The therapeutic dose given for high cholesterol levels is usually around 3,000 mg a day, but many people can't tolerate the "flush" and other side effects at that dosage. Time-released niacin has therefore been used clinically to try to reduce the impact of the sudden flush. But researchers concluded its risks outweighed its benefits, after signs of liver toxicity were reported from time-release niacin at that high dosage.

Regular niacin nevertheless remains quite valuable in not only lowering cholesterol but actually extending survival, at a very reasonable price. CAUTION: High doses of niacin should be taken only with professional supervision.

If the offending toxins are traced to heavy metals in the teeth, the first order of business should be dental overhaul to remove the metal. Then metal vapors that have settled in the tissues will need to be removed. This can be done with homeopathic remedies and with oral and intravenous chelation. Protocols are described under "Heavy Metal Poisoning."

Dangerously High Cholesterol and Thyroid Levels Normalized Naturally

Dan's cholesterol level was nearly 400—dangerously high. His blood pressure had shot up before that, but medication had brought it back to normal. The problem was that his cholesterol had then shot up. Cholesterol medication had dropped his cholesterol level to normal, but his thyroid levels had then shot up. His thyroid hormone level was so high that his doctor wanted to surgically remove Dan's thyroid. But an extensive patient history and careful examination revealed nothing to indicate that his thyroid was his real problem.

Dan's wife then revealed that her husband had had an enormous amount of trouble with his teeth. He'd had caps that had been filed down to make a bridge, but the bridge didn't fit right. His mouth was a glittering mixture of mercury and nickel. Dan was advised to have his dental work reconstructed with biocompatible materials, but for him this was not an option. He had already invested $20,000 in his teeth and couldn't bring himself to have them redone. Natural oral chelators and homeopathic remedies for removing heavy metals from his body tissues were therefore recommended instead. He was also advised to go on a liver cleanse diet. (See "Heavy Metal Poisoning" and "Environmental Illness.")

Dan was an excellent patient. Besides homeopathic chelators, he took enormous amounts of greens, including two or three green drinks a day. He said his stools had turned lime green. Remarkably, three months later, his thyroid levels had returned to normal, allowing him to avoid a devastating surgery. More than three years later, he reports that he is still in good health and that his cholesterol, blood pressure, and thyroid levels are all normal.

Chronic Fatigue Syndrome

Chronic fatigue syndrome (CFS) now affects as much as 7 percent of the population and is on the rise.[220] Besides a debilitating, chronic exhaustion not relieved by rest, its symptoms can include sore throats, painful or swollen lymph nodes, muscle and joint pains, headaches, sleep disturbances, and impaired short-term memory and concentration. People with CFS report feeling sick all the time, have chronically swollen glands, and toss and turn all night, rarely getting a good night's sleep. Although they are enormously tired, they can look healthy and energetic, subjecting them to the further burden of not being believed.

CONVENTIONAL DIAGNOSIS AND TREATMENT

Originally, CFS was assumed to have a viral cause and was described as chronic Epstein-Barr-virus syndrome or chronic mononucleosis. Its designation was changed to "chronic fatigue syndrome" (CFS) or "chronic fatigue/immune depression syndrome" (CFIDS), when researchers concluded its cause was unknown.[221] The invading viruses originally thought to cause the disease were merely taking advantage of an immune system weakened from some other cause. No conventional therapy has proven effective in controlled clinical trials with prolonged follow-up in curing CFS.[222]

THE HOMEOPATHIC APPROACH

Although there is no recognized, conventional cure, many cases are on record in which CFS has been cured.

Dr. Bruce Waller was a medical doctor who had a remarkable success rate in treating it with *homeopathy*. He learned directly from Dr. Reinhard Voll, the German medical doctor who developed EAV, the forerunner of electrodermal screening. (See Chapter 2.) Dr. Waller, over eighty and retired, treated hundreds of people in the back room of his trailer, using homeopathy in a way that diverged from its classical approach but was dramatically effective. He maintained that CFS is the end result of a deep suppression of the immune system, preventing the body from fighting its bacterial, viral, or parasitic invaders. As a result, it is liable to have a number of them cohabiting with it at any one time. The result is layer upon layer of disease. Cure requires clearing these layers away one by one.

The typical patient history involves some extreme stress (for example, a car accident) combined with a period of antibiotic use. The result is an abnormal immune system response. A case of this type involved a top athlete under unusual physical and mental stress while in training for the Ironman event, who was then bitten by a dog. He developed CFS after he was given several courses of antibiotics for the bite.

According to homeopathic theory, the suppression of the immune system resulting in chronic fatigue is often a direct result of antibiotic use. Homeopaths say the drugs don't actually kill bacteria but merely push the invaders deeper into the system. A healthy person who comes in contact with a bacteria or virus will get a healing response—runny nose, thick mucus, cough, headache, and so forth. People with CFS are too sick and their immune systems are too suppressed to react.

Dr. Waller's approach was to peel off one layer of disease at a time, treating each for about a month before moving on to the next. Here are some of the layers that could require peeling:

- *Coxsackie* is a virus that stays in the spine, usually causing hip pain or pain along the spinal column. With trauma, it moves to the brain. The trauma is often a car accident, but it can also be a fall or head trauma. The result is foggy thinking and headaches. Patients may want to talk so desperately that they break down and cry; but while they have something to say, they can't pull their thoughts together well enough to say it.

- *Brucella*, a bacteria found in cattle, causes muscle aches and pains, inflammation, aching joints, and swollen lymph glands. The pain of CFS is usually from this bacteria, unless the patient has fibromyalgia. (See "Fibromyalgia.")

- *Peptostrep*, a bacteria found in the sinuses, ears, and throat, is the cause of repeated sinus infections in CFS patients. Each course of antibiotics pushes the bacteria deeper into the sinuses and makes the next infection deeper and heavier.

- *Mononucleosis* is a bacterial infection reported in the histories of perhaps 60 percent of CFS patients. The infection appears to be one of the first assaults to their immune systems.

- *Giardia and other parasites* contribute to the constant gas, bloating, and indigestion problems of CFS patients. Their immune systems are so run down that they easily pick up parasites. Parasites can puncture the digestive tract, allowing macromolecules to slip undigested into the bloodstream, where they strain the immune system.[223]

- *Candida* is treated by many practitioners as a separate disease, but it is more likely to be just one more symptom of an overwhelmed immune system. Candida is one of the last deficiency states to be cleared for good, since until the immune system is working well, the yeast will come right back.

- *Chemical hypersensitivity syndrome* can complicate the condition. Poor oxygen uptake to fatigued muscle tissue results in an abnormal sensitivity to chemicals and environmental toxins—perfume, paint, carpets, and so forth. (See "Environmental Illness.")

- *Allergies* to foods, molds, chemicals, and a long list of other allergens can also be underlying factors.

- *Pneumonia, herpes, Lyme disease, toxic dental work,* and *exposure to environmental toxins* are other conditions the practitioner should look for in the history of a CFS patient.

Each of these layers, said Dr. Waller, needs to be addressed separately. His approach was to use homeopathic remedies, but other practitioners have eliminated specific layers of the disorder with other natural treatments.

CFS Traced to Parasites and Eliminated

David said he had been hopelessly tired and rundown for 14 years. Two doctors had told him he had parasites, but conventional drugs hadn't resolved his problems, even though he had taken them for a number of months instead of the usual three weeks. What did work was a course of homeopathic and herbal parasite remedies. After this simple treatment, he reported a dramatic reversal of his symptoms and a surge of energy he had never before experienced. (See "Parasites.")

CFS Cured by Neutralizing Allergies

Allergy specialist Devi Nambudripad, D.C., L.Ac., R.N., Ph.D., describes the case of a 34-year-old woman on disability, who had been diagnosed with chronic-fatigue syndrome by a famous specialist. The woman had been treated for two years without relief. She had then tried megadoses of vitamin and mineral supplements, but her condition had only gotten worse. Dr. Nambudripad tested her and discovered that she was allergic not only to many health foods (whole wheat, oat bran, bran flakes, and the like) but to particular vitamin/mineral supplements she was taking. Her allergies were neutralized by a method involving reprogramming the brain's negative patternings. She was then able to return to work full time.[224]

HORMONE AND ANTIOXIDANT THERAPY

Dr. Majid Ali, a medical doctor who has worked extensively with chronic-fatigue syndrome, observes that DHEA levels are usually reduced in chronic-fatigue states. DHEA is a primary adrenal hormone that is a precursor to other hormones in the body. Dr. Ali maintains that replacement therapy with DHEA improves the overall energy level and reduces symptoms. Accelerated oxidant injury in chronic fatigue states causes dysfunction of the thyroid and other hormonal systems, and laboratory abnormalities clearly evidence dysfunction in DHEA and the adrenal gland. Accelerated oxidant injury is attributed to the increasing burden of toxins in our water, air, and food.[225]

Dr. Anthony Martin states that the antioxidant *pycnogenol* is also of particular benefit to victims of CFS and fibromyalgia. It wasn't until he stumbled on pycnogenol that he was able to help those patients.[226]

ARE YOUR DENTAL FILLINGS CAUSING CFS?

CFS symptoms have been resolved not only by doctors but by dentists. In their book *Toxic Metal Syndrome*, Drs. Casdorph and Walker assert, "[C]hronic fatigue/immune suppression syndrome (CFIDS) is directly connected to amalgam fillings. . . . Positive response against CFIDS is experienced by the patient and witnessed by the dentist within two weeks of amalgam removal."[227]

Sherry Rogers, M.D., another specialist in the field, explains that heavy metals cause fatigue because they sit in the enzymes on the membrane and inside the mitochondria where energy is synthesized inside cells. Heavy metals displace essential minerals such as zinc, magnesium, manganese, copper, and iron, so the enzymes can no longer function normally.[228]

Faulty dental work can also cause chronic fatigue by impairing the bite. When the bite is "off," so is the temporomandibular joint (TMJ), which has an energetic relationship with areas all over the body.[229] Dissimilar metals in the mouth also create a "battery effect" that interferes with the body's own electromagnetic field, creating fatigue and other symptoms.

Replacing the metals in the teeth, however, requires careful protocols. What the dentist uses for a replacement material is important. Plastic composite materials may also be hazardous, though in a different way. For a thorough discussion of this subject, see Ellen Brown, Richard Hansen, D.M.D., *The Key to Ultimate Health* (La Mirada, California: Advanced Health Research Publishing, 1998).

Chronic Fatigue Reversed

A 50-year-old male hairdresser complained he was so exhausted he could hardly get through his workday. A careful patient history revealed that his health had started to fail after the installation of two gold crowns alloyed with palladium. He said he couldn't afford a complete dental overhaul, but he agreed to get the two gold crowns replaced with a wholly biocompatible material called Degussa porcelain. When this modest modification made him "a new man," he was so impressed that he sold some family assets to finance a complete dental upgrade, not only for himself but for his wife.

Colds

More progress has been made in the drug treatment of disease in this century than in all the rest of medical history. Yet virtually no progress has been made in the battle against the common cold. Most people still get two or three colds a year, and they still last a week or two, regardless of method of treatment.[230]

OVER-THE-COUNTER DRUGS

Americans spend over two billion dollars a year for over-the-counter cough and cold remedies, although these drugs have no effect on the length of the disease. Although drugs often seem to ease the pain, this impression can be the result of an acquired addiction to them. Topical decongestants can instantly open the nasal passages for a breath of fresh air, but "rebound congestion" follows two or three hours later. The nasal passages swell to worse than their original condition, so the sufferer can sleep through the night only with another dose of the drug. Meanwhile, cold and cough remedies can produce side effects, and this problem is compounded in the popular products consisting of a combination of drugs. Most of these remedies include several ingredients in fixed combinations. Typically, you don't need the multiple drugs they contain; but you will experience all of their side effects, which are multiplied in combination.

PRESCRIPTION DRUGS

Well over a million prescriptions a year are written for antibiotics for colds. Yet *colds are caused by viruses, and antibiotics have no effect against these marauders.* The professed justification is prophylactic: to treat any bacterial infection that *might* arise. The problems with this theory are that if an infection does develop, the bacteria will have had an opportunity to become resistant to the antibiotic; and the patient runs the unnecessary risk of developing an allergic reaction to the drug.

NATURAL ALTERNATIVES

That science has found no "cure" for the common cold is considered by homeopaths to be as a good thing. They contend its symptoms are natural cleansing processes that should not be suppressed. The coughing and sneezing that characterize it are the body's attempt to get rid of offending irritants. If these symptoms are suppressed with drugs, toxins can be driven inward, where they do even greater damage. Any attempt to suppress the symptoms of a cold merely prolongs the disease. You're likely to find that when you give up drugs for the treatment of a cold, the condition will become more tolerable of its own accord. If you can refrain from starting on decongestants, the overall course of your congestion will be more manageable. When you let your colds "run their course," they should get progressively milder and farther apart as your body succeeds in its attempted housecleanings. Meanwhile, there are effective natural remedies that can ease cold symptoms without side effects.

Many people believe that early-stage colds can often be knocked out completely with a homeopathic product made by Dolisos called *Cold and Flu*

Solution Plus. (Make sure the label says "Plus." There is also a plain Cold and Flu Solution.) Use one tablet every 15 minutes for the first hour, then one tablet every hour for the next four hours, then one tablet four times daily.

If this product is not available, try a combination of Alpha CF by B&T and *Oscillococcinum* by Boiron. Mix two tablets of Alpha CF and one tube of Oscillococcinum in an eight-ounce glass of water. Drink two ounces every 15 minutes until the water is gone. Make another mixture in water in the same proportions, and drink two ounces every hour until the water is gone.

In the meantime, take other reasonable precautions to boost your immune system. (See "Immunity.") Remember that you probably got sick in the first place because you were run-down.

For other useful homeopathic formulas for colds of various types and stages, see Appendix.

CHINESE HERBAL REMEDIES

Chinese doctors use different herbal remedies for a cold depending on its stage and symptoms. They view the first stage as being on the "outside"—the surface of the body. The symptoms are chills, aches and pains, headache, possibly a slight sore throat, stiff neck, an aversion to cold or wind. The cold that has progressed beyond this stage goes "inside" and turns "hot," producing fever and yellow-green sputum. It can go to the sinuses and cause a sinus infection, or to the chest and cause bronchitis. Appropriate Chinese remedies for various stages and types of colds follow. All Chinese formulas should be taken with warm water for best results—not mixed with water, but drunk down with it.

> *For the cold that is just beginning:* At this stage, there is a sensation of being either hot or cold. There may be sore throat, mild fever, body aches, headache. The appropriate remedy is *Gan Mao Ling*.
>
> *For the second-stage cold:* When your cold has set in a little more—you are feeling a little worse and anticipate feeling quite miserable tomorrow—the appropriate Chinese formula is *Yin Chiao*. Take three to four pills three to four times daily with warm water or add to boiling water as a tea.
>
> *For the cold that has gone to the sinuses:* Stopping the sinuses from running will cause suppression that will lead to sinus infection. *Sangchu* tablets will clear the sinuses without drowsiness and without causing sinus infection later on. (See "Sinusitis.") Take three pills three times daily.

For the cold that has gone to the eyes and the head: In this type of cold, the eyes usually get red or are very sensitive to light, and the sufferer gets headaches. The appropriate remedy is *Ming Mu Shang Ching Pien*. Take four pills two times daily.

For the flulike cold with nausea: When the cold goes to nausea, severe aches and headache, good results may be obtained with *Gan Mao Ling*.

For bronchitis: Where there is deep phlegm in the chest and rattling on coughing tending toward bronchitis, take *Ping Chuan*, ten pills twice daily. For full-fledged bronchitis, with cough and deep rattles in the chest, take *Hsiao Keh Chuan*, two pills three times daily. This formula also comes in the form of a cough syrup.

For a cold with fever: *Zhong Gan Ling* is effective for sore throat and high fever, body aches, and strep throat. Fever is the distinguishing trait for this remedy.

When you are coughing up yellow or green phlegm: The Chinese maintain that this symptom indicates that the cold has gone deep into the body and has gotten very "hot," making the phlegm turn yellow. Constipation is often present as the body fluids are burned off. The remedy is *Ching Fei Yi Huo*. Take three pills two to three times daily.

For strep throat: *Lieu Shen Wan*, when given for a very sore throat with fever, has been known to cure the condition in a single day.

For laryngitis and hoarseness: People who have tried *Laryngitis Pills* keep coming back for more. They say the remedy really works. Also good for laryngitis and hoarseness is homeopathic *Phosphorus*.

WESTERN HERBS

Elderberry extract (Sambucus nigra), a popular herbal remedy for colds, has been shown in clinical studies to stop the spread of the colds virus.

Echinacea is another popular herbal option. It is quite effective if taken at the right stage of a cold—on the first day of symptoms—but taken at the wrong stage, it can actually make symptoms worse. At the first stage of a cold, echinacea stops the pathogens from getting into the body. But once they are in, it will trap them inside. People who complain that they have been sick with a cold for several weeks ("It just won't seem to go away") frequently turn out on questioning to be taking echinacea.

This herb should be taken only when you feel as if you "might be coming down with something." Once you are sick, it's too late. The remedy is a good one to take when you are not sick but people around you are. At that stage, it strengthens the "qi" and protects the body from invasion.

Licorice-root tea is good for opening the bronchioles of the chest. But drinking large amounts can cause water retention and increase blood pressure, so limit your intake to about three cups a day.

NUTRITIONAL REMEDIES

Zinc gluconate has been shown in clinical studies to help at the first stage of a cold. *Vitamin C* and *colostrum* are also highly effective. For other immune system boosters, see Appendix.

Some physicians favor the use of old-fashioned remedies: chicken soup; mixtures of spirits, honey and lemon juice; hot milk and honey; or herbal teas. Studies have shown that hot drinks can actually make you feel better during a cold, by increasing the flow of nasal secretions.[231]

Cold Sores, Canker Sores

Cold sores (fever blisters) and *canker sores (aphthous ulcers)* are two of the most common infections of the mouth. An important difference is that canker sores aren't contagious, while cold sores are. Cold sores may be accompanied by fever, swollen neck glands, and a general achy feeling. Canker sores are rarely accompanied by fever or other signs of illness.

Cold sores are caused by the *herpes simplex* virus, which is thought to be present continually on the skin of most people. Infections result only when resistance is low, as from a cold, sunburn, shock, dental or sinus infections, or menstrual problems. Cold sores may appear anywhere on the skin but occur most frequently on the lips, nose, chin, cheeks, mouth, and eyes. There are two principal strains of *herpes simplex* virus. Type 1 is the usual cause of cold sores; but Type 2, which is generally limited to the genital region, may also produce cold sores on the face. Touching cold sores can result in spreading the virus to new sites on the body or to other people, so it's important to keep hands off and avoid kissing. Once you get oral herpes, the virus remains in a nerve near the cheekbone, and out-breaks can recur. As with genital herpes, oral herpes outbreaks have been linked to emotional stress, as well as to fever, illness, injury, and overexpo-sure to sun.

The cause of canker sores is unknown, but they may be due to aller-gy, nutritional deficiencies or defects in the immune system.

CONVENTIONAL TREATMENT

Products are available for symptomatic relief of cold sores and canker sores. Antiseptic powders and ointments may be used to prevent secondary infec-tions, and various lotions and powders can relieve pain and itching and hasten drying. But there is no pharmaceutical "cure." *Acyclovir (Zovirax)* may be used topically, but the blisters tend to recur.[232]

THE NUTRITIONAL APPROACH: LYSINE

The best-known natural alternative is the amino acid lysine. Dosage is one gram every four hours at the outset, or 500 mg twice or three times a day to prevent recurrences. The remedy works, and it's definitely prefer-able to Zovirax; but it still addresses only the symptoms.

HOMEOPATHIC AND HERBAL REMEDIES FOR COLD SORES

Homeopathic remedies not only can heal cold sores but can prevent them from coming back. *Calendula and Hypericum Ointment* by Boiron clears the blisters up quickly, while *Natirum Muraticum (Nat Mur)* 6x keeps them from recurring. Take the *Nat Mur* at the onset of symptoms, four pills four times daily. Although the cold sores may seem at first to be recurring more often but healing faster, in a few months they should be gone for good. For stubborn cases, a single dose of herpes-simplex home-opathic nosode may also be given. Other effective homeopathic options include *Cold Sores* by NatureBio and *Cliniskin H* by CompliMed (good for herpes).

Other natural topical remedies that aid in healing cold sores include herbal *Goldenseal and Propolis Cream* by Eclectic Institute, *Licgel* by Scientific Botanicals, and *Erpace* by Dolisos.

Recurring Cold Sores Eliminated

An eight-year-old girl was miserable with recurring cold sores. She broke out with them every couple of weeks. Conventional treatment could not break this cycle. What did was the homeopathic remedy *Nat Mur 6x.*

Jeff, 29, also had repeated cold sores until he was tipped off to *Nat Mur.* Six months later, he returned to say he hadn't had a cold sore since. Even when he forgot to take the remedy on a trip to Chicago, where he always gets cold sores, he returned unscathed.

Pleasures of Holiday Eating Restored

A man visiting from out of town complained that an open and bleeding cold sore on his lip was hampering his ability to enjoy the great food in Sun Valley. He went home with *Calendula and Hypericum Ointment.* He came back the next day expressing amazement: His lip was entirely healed, without a trace of the sore.

NATURAL TREATMENT FOR CANKER SORES

Homeopathic Borax 6x helps rapidly heal canker sore blisters. Take three pills three times daily. Another homeopathic remedy that heals canker sores and takes the pain out of them is *Hydrastis MT* (mother tincture), diluted at the rate of one part to ten parts distilled water. Rinse with the liquid, then spit it out.

According to Chinese medical theory, cold sores are caused by too much "heat" in the body, which comes out as sores on the tongue and in the mouth. If you are prone to canker sores, avoid acidic and spicy foods and any foods to which you may be allergic.

Communicable Diseases

Communicable diseases include *diptheria, measles, rubella, mumps, pertussis (whooping cough), polio, tetanus,* and *chicken pox.* Their symptoms in childhood are usually mild, and contracting them once generally affords immunity for life. The exceptions are whooping cough, which can affect adults but is not so serious in adults as in children; and the *herpes zoster* virus, which causes chicken pox, and can become reactivated in adulthood as *shingles*. Unlike whooping cough, shingles is much more serious in adults than chicken pox is in children. (See "Shingles.")

CONVENTIONAL PREVENTION: VACCINES

Between 1911 and 1935, the four leading causes of death among American children aged 1 to 14 were diphtheria, measles, scarlet fever, and whooping cough. The dramatic decline in these epidemics since that time has been attributed to mass vaccine programs, in which antibodies are developed in the body in reaction to inoculation with the inactive virus.

Childhood immunization is now considered so important that parents refusing to have their children vaccinated, even for religious religions, can be held subject to charges of child abuse. But critics observe that injecting an infant, whose immune system is still immature, with viruses that he can't defend himself against can have long-term health consequences. The chief suspect is the MMR (measles-mumps-rubella) vaccine, from which serious complications have been reported. While *Physician's Desk Reference* says complications are "very rare," the critics dispute this contention. They observe that complications may not show up until much later and are hard to trace; and reactions that were rare when the studies were first done may not be today, because infants are second- or third-generation vaccine recipients, with potentially heightened reactions when rechallenged with the vaccine.

There are now a minimum of 250,000 *autistic children* in the United States, a 10- to 15-fold increase since immunization came into vogue. Dr. Bernard Rimland, founding director of the Autism Research Institute, blames childhood vaccine programs for the epidemic. Childhood autism is caused by *encephalitis (brain inflammation)* affecting the limbic system of the brain. The MMR is incubated in chick embryo culture, where researchers suggest the virus becomes programmed to produce antibodies against the protein of the myelin sheath of the chick and then of the child.

Critics also maintain that the benefits of vaccines have been overrated. With the exception of polio, the major contagious childhood killers of the first half of the twentieth century had declined by 95 percent before mass vaccine programs were instituted. This decline is attributed to better housing with less crowded conditions after the Depression, better nutrition, and better public health measures.[233]

WARNING: Children with chicken pox and other viral illnesses should never be treated with aspirin, due to the risk of Reyes syndrome. For that and other downsides of lowering a fever with aspirin, see "Fever."

ALTERNATIVE TREATMENT

To ease the discomfort of chicken pox, *tea-tree oil* can be applied to the pox. Specific homeopathic remedies are also available. A German Staufen remedy for chicken pox, if given right when the pox break out, can make the case a very mild one. You shouldn't give this remedy before the pox break out, however, since you want your child to have a mild case of the disease to develop an immunity to it.

Staufen remedies are also available for each of the other communicable diseases.

AN ALTERNATIVE APPROACH TO PREVENTION

Homeopathy works on the same principle as vaccines: It inoculates the body with a tiny bit of the toxin, stimulating the production of antibodies that fight the disease. Homeopathy has the advantage, however, that so little of the original toxin is left in the remedy that the patient can't accidentally contract the disease from it or be burdened with its latent toxic effects. Homeopathic remedies are essentially water; they work vibrationally rather than chemically. (See Chapter 3.) German homeopathic remedies by Staufen are available for preventing and treating each of the childhood communicable diseases named earlier, including shingles.

Congestive Heart Failure

Congestive heart failure results when the heart is too weak to pump as hard as it should, causing blood to back up into the lungs and veins. The annual death rate for people with the condition is from 15 to 60 percent of sufferers, and it is reaching epidemic proportions. Hospital admissions for congestive heart failure more than doubled from 1979 to 1991, reaching 822,000 by that year.

Julian Whitaker, M.D., suggests that the increased use of beta blockers explains the epidemic. Beta blockers and calcium channel-blockers are the mainstays of conventional drug treatment for high blood pressure, heart disease, angina, and cardiac arrhythmias.[234] Ten to twenty million people are on beta blockers, which act by slowing the heart's pumping. This is exactly what happens in congestive heart failure: the heart pumps too slowly to move the blood sufficiently to nourish the body. Calcium-channel blockers don't seem to be any better: a recent study linked them to a 60 percent *increase* in the risk of death from heart disease. (See "Hypertension.")

DRUG TREATMENT

If drugs are of questionable value in preventing congestive heart failure, they have a proven track record for increasing survival in people who already have the condition. Even with everything medicine has to offer, however, the prognosis of these patients is generally quite poor. Conventional treatment begins with rest, diuretics combined with a low-salt diet to reduce fluid retention, and digitalis drugs to strengthen the heart. If that doesn't work, vasodilators may be added.

Vasodilator drugs work by redistributing blood volume and by lowering pressure and reducing volume in the failing left ventricle of the heart. Options include *oral nitrates (isosorbide), nitrates plus hydralazine, ACE inhibitors (captropril and enalapril), prazosin (Minipress),* and *calcium channel antagonists (Procardia).* Only two of these options have been shown to increase survival in patients with congestive heart failure, however, and then only when combined with digitalis and diuretics. One of these proven options is enalapril. (Captopril, another ACE inhibitor, would probably work as well.)[235] The other proven drug regimen is isosorbide nitrate combined with hydralazine.[236] These vasodilators carry serious risks and patients must be monitored carefully, but in these extremities the risks are no doubt worth hazarding.[237]

Digitalis drugs are obtained from plants and have been around for centuries. Used historically as rat poisons and arrow poisons in large doses, they are fatal to humans. Since there isn't much difference between the dose that speeds up the heart and the dose that stops it altogether, overly aggressive use of digitalis can be hazardous. In one study, long-term use of digitalis after heart attacks was actually found to increase mortality in the four to six months following the attacks. Even if the drugs are expertly administered, your chances of suffering from digitalis toxicity are 5 to 15 percent. Warning signs include nausea, vomiting, stomach pain, sleepiness, headache, depression, and irregular heartbeats.[238] Despite these risks, digoxin (Lanoxin), the most popular of the digitalis drugs, ranks high on the list of best-selling prescription pharmaceuticals.

NONDRUG ALTERNATIVES

A placebo-controlled randomized double-blind study demonstrated that Hawthorn berry (Craetagus), a powerful herb containing antioxidants called OPCs, significantly improves heart rate and endurance and reduces symptoms in patients with cardiac insufficiency, *without reported side effects*. Other researchers finding significant improvement in heart function from this herb suggested it was appropriate for use instead of digitalis for patients who did not yet need that powerful but toxic drug.[239]

Co-enzyme Q10 is another nutrient with documented effectiveness in strengthening the heart in patients with congestive heart failure.

Another safe, proven treatment is Dr. Dean Ornish's diet plan for advanced heart-disease patients. Dr. Ornish, a San Francisco cardiologist, upset conventional wisdom by proving that the fatty plaque deposits blocking the coronary arteries of heart patients with advanced disease could be made to shrink using natural therapies alone. The therapies used in his study were a strict low-cholesterol diet, meditation, and yoga.[240] For details and for a long list of other natural remedies beneficial to the heart, see "Atherosclerosis."

Constipation

Constipation is defined as an irregular retention or delay in bowel movements, but "irregular" is a relative term. The bowel habits of apparently normal people may vary from three stools a day to only one in four or five days.[241]

At least, so says conventional wisdom. Julian Whitaker, M.D., asserts that virtually everyone in the United States is constipated, at least compared to people in the African bush. He observes:

> On a high-meat, processed-food diet with almost no dietary fiber, the stool is always well-formed, tubular (like a sausage), and generally a chore to pass even for the "unconstipated." . . . The healthy human stool is not formed at all. It is wet and bulky. Two English physicians, Henry Trowell and Dennis Burkitt, spent most of their careers in Africa, and took note of the African's voluminous, moist, unformed stool. It spread out in a circle on the ground like cow droppings. They went around and measured the diameter of these stools, even weighed some, and concluded that the size of the human stool was inversely proportional to the size of hospitals![242]

Besides improper diet, the causes of constipation can range from poor childhood training, poor toilet facilities, and pregnancy to serious diseases causing actual blockage of the intestines; for example, certain cancers of the bowel or adhesions.

DRUG TREATMENT

Another major cause of constipation, ironically, is laxative use. Laxatives diminish your natural muscle reflexes, so peristalsis occurs only with stronger and stronger stimulation. The drugs can also irritate and inflame the lining of the bowel, cause anal fissures and hemorrhoids, and deplete your body of important substances including water, calcium, potassium, and magnesium. Water loss causes dehydration, calcium loss weakens the bones, and potassium and magnesium loss weakens the muscles and heart.

Laxatives to avoid are the stimulant, lubricant, and saline varieties. *Ex-Lax*, the stimulant type, forces evacuation by stimulating the nerves controlling the bowel muscles. The FDA has concluded that Ex-Lax is so unhealthy that it recently pulled this popular laxative off the market. Lubricant laxatives coat the stools with mineral oil or olive oil. *Saline laxatives*, including *Epsom Salt* and *Milk of Magnesia*, pull water into the bowels. These laxatives are not only irritating but, if used for long, can upset the body's mineral balance. The best pharmaceutical products are the bulk-forming and stool-softening varieties that encourage normal bowel function. The bulk formers (such as *Metamucil*) generally contain psyllium seed, while the stool softeners (such as *Doxiden*) generally contain docusate.

Nutritional Solutions

Wheat bran can aid constipation by softening stools, preventing straining, increasing the weight of stools, and speeding intestinal transit time.[243] But relying on pure wheat bran can be dangerous, since it irritates the delicate lining of the intestines and can inhibit mineral absorption. Fortunately, the same laxative effect can be achieved by eating whole foods containing *fiber*. Raw vegetables, raw and dried fruits, and most beans and whole grains are high in fiber. They create a heavy intestinal mass that travels quickly through the intestines. The standard prescription for constipation given by Dr. Whitaker is two carrots and two apples per day, totaling about 16 grams of dietary fiber. He observes that peristaltic contractions squeeze bulk along the digestive tract the way you squeeze toothpaste out of a tube. Without bulk there is nothing to squeeze, and bowel function halts.[244]

Beneficial bacteria (*acidophilus* and *bifidus*) in yogurt or capsule form can also aid elimination. In a study of bedridden elderly people, stool frequency improved after they ate bifidus-supplemented yogurt. When the yogurt was withdrawn, stool frequency again became poor, demonstrating that supplementation needs to be long-term and continuous.[245]

Other Natural Remedies

Greens and green-type nutritional supplements can help clean the liver, add fiber, and facilitate bowel movements. Green supplements include *chlorella, spirulina,* and *blue-green algae. Aloe* is also good. Taking spirulina or chlorella twice a day typically results in normal bowel movements in about four days.

Rhubarb is another good laxative. One suggested recipe is three stalks of rhubarb blended with a cup of apple juice, one quarter peeled lemon, and a tablespoon of honey.[246]

For chronic constipation, homeopathics can help. BHI makes a good homeopathic combination called *Constipation.*

Other strong but helpful bowel cleansers include *OxyCleanse, Perfect 7,* and *MagOxide.*

THINGS TO AVOID

Foods to reduce or avoid are those devoid of fiber. That means animal foods, especially cheese, and refined foods, especially sugar. Drugs can also trigger constipation. Common offenders include codeine, antihistamines, diuretics, antispasmodics, narcotics, sleeping pills, antidepressants, tranquilizers, iron supplements, cholesterol-lowering drugs, and antacids containing aluminum or calcium compounds. It's also important, of course, to avoid haste, allowing time for nature to take its course and to respond when it calls.

Coughs

A cough is a protective reflex for eliminating foreign substances that block the airways. The effectiveness of this mechanism was dramatically illustrated in the case of an Indiana man with a bullet in his chest that was too risky to remove. He reportedly coughed the bullet up in church.[247]

There are two types of cough, "wet" and "dry." "Wet" coughs are productive: they're bringing something up. "Dry" coughs are "unproductive" and are liable to be a sign of sinus problems. Coughs go with colds, but the cough accompanying a cold can last for weeks after the cold is gone. Other conditions for which coughs can be a symptom include postnasal drip, allergies, viral infection, sinus infection, asthma, gastroesophageal reflux disease (GERD), lung cancer, and the use of ACE inhibitors to treat high blood pressure and heart problems. *Coughs with high fever, wheezing, pressure in the head, dizziness, or painful teeth should be checked by a medical professional.*

DRUG TREATMENT

The FDA warns that drugs that suppress the protective cough reflex can do more harm than good. *Cough suppressants* are recommended only for dry coughs. They aren't recommended for smokers or for people with asthma, emphysema, and other conditions involving overproduction of secretions, since these coughs, while chronic and annoying, are still "productive." That means most coughs are best left alone.

Assuming, however, that you want to suppress yours, there are ingredients the FDA says are effective for the purpose. They include *codeine, dextromethorphan,* and *diphenhydramine hydrochloride (Benylin),* derivatives of the narcotic morphine that work by drugging the brain. The main drawbacks of codeine are that it can be addictive and very constipating. Dextromethorphan isn't addictive, but overdoses can produce bizarre behavior. And diphenhydramine hydrochloride can make the user very drowsy, making driving a car or operating machinery hazardous. The FDA has labeled other cough-suppressant ingredients safe in recommended doses, but not of proven effectiveness in suppressing coughs. Some of these ingredients can also be toxic when children overdose on them.

Unlike suppressants, which deaden the cough reflex, *expectorants* encourage it. Some do this by stimulating the vomiting reflex; others irritate the stomach; others act on the bronchial-tube nerve endings. If your cough is already "productive," however, you probably don't need expectorants; and even if you do need them, few ingredients are approved by the FDA as both safe and effective for the purpose. The FDA recommends that cough remedies, if used at all, be taken as single ingredients rather than in fixed-combination products, which generally increase the risk of side effects without increasing effectiveness. You're unlikely to need all the ingredients, and even if you do, they're unlikely to be in the proportions appropriate for your particular condition.[248] Sometimes the drugs in combination cough and cold products actually cancel each other out. An example are the cough remedies that combine an expectorant, which stimulates the cough reflex, with a suppressant, which deadens it. You get the side effects of two drugs and the effectiveness of neither. The most popular single-ingredient expectorants are *Robitussin, Terpin Hydrate,* and *Potassium Iodide Solution.* (Robitussin PE and Robitussin CF are combination products.) *Benalyn* is another single-ingredient cough remedy, but the ingredient is an antihistamine (benadryl), which works mainly by making you drowsy.

NATURAL REMEDIES

Fortunately, good natural cough remedies are available. *Chestal* by Boiron and *Cough* by Natura Bio are two popular and effective options.

Aromatherapy—the essential oils of plants—can also be effective in alleviating symptoms. Try rubbing your chest with *essential oil of eucalyptus* or *myrrh*.

Another way to loosen nasal secretions is by breathing the steam from a vaporizer or hot shower.

For other effective natural remedies, see "Colds."

Cytomegalovirus

Cytomegalovirus (CMV) is a common sexually transmitted virus in the herpes family. It generally causes no symptoms, but it can cause severe infections and even death in infants of infected mothers, who may not even know they have the disease. It has also been linked to Epstein-Barr-virus-associated infectious mononucleosis, characterized by fever, malaise, myalgias, arthralgias, and abnormal liver tests. CMV infections have been found in the gastrointestinal tract, liver, lungs and nervous system. The main concern for patients with CMV is that the disease can turn into chronic-fatigue syndrome.

DRUG TREATMENT

Conventional medicine has no effective cure for CMV. A strong antiviral drug is used, but only in severe cases involving AIDS patients.

ALTERNATIVE TREATMENT

Staufen makes an effective homeopathic remedy specifically for CMV called *Cytomegalie*. It's best to seek the help of a qualified practitioner, however, to make sure there are no underlying problems that also need to be corrected. CMV is complex and is usually the result of multiple assaults on the immune system. Stress, trauma, poor diet, and toxins all contribute to breaking down the body's resistance, allowing the virus to flourish.

Depression

An estimated 15 million Americans are clinically depressed. One in five women and one in ten men will experience at least one major episode of depression in their lives; and in a third of them, the condition will be chronic. Depression is attributed to genetics, developmental problems, or psychosocial factors; but for many cases, there is no clinically understood cause. Besides lowered mood, symptoms may include feelings of guilt, worthlessness, or hopelessness; loss of energy, appetite, or sex drive; headache; and disturbed or excessive sleep. Related disorders include *panic attacks, bipolar disorder* (alternating manic and depressed phases), and *seasonal affective disorder* (caused by too little sunlight in winter months).

Where no other cause can be found, hormones are likely suspects, at least in women. Premenstrual and premenopausal women are notorious for being moody and depressed. The stress hormone (cortisol) and the sex hormones (estrogen and progesterone) come from the same hormone chain. Thyroid hormone can also play a role.

DRUG TREATMENT

Amphetamines have been used for 50 years to give the depressed a "lift." But controlled trials have failed to establish that the drugs relieve depression significantly better than placebos do.[249] Amphetamines were later replaced with other drugs, including the *monoamine oxidase (MAO) inhibitors* and the tricyclic and other *antidepressants*. But in some cases the newer antidepressants actually posed a greater risk to health than the amphetamines, especially for the elderly and the medically ill.[250] People on MAO inhibitors need to watch their diets and avoid foods rich in tyrosine, including alcohol, cheese, red meat, and yeast extract.

Prozac (fluoxetine) ushered in a new line of antidepressants called selective serotonin reuptake inhibitors (SSRIs), which also includes *Zoloft* and *Paxil.* Serotonin is a mood-elevating neurotransmitter, a natural "upper" that mediates depression. The drugs don't actually produce serotonin but are serotonin "enhancers." They act by inhibiting a natural process, the reuptake of serotonin by the neurons.

Prozac is not an amphetamine, but in some ways it acts like one. Unlike the older antidepressants, it's more likely to wake you up than to put you to sleep, and it's more likely to cause weight loss than weight gain. Prozac is being used to treat not only depression and anxiety but addiction, bulimia, overweight, and a host of other ills. It isn't sedating, and it has significantly fewer side effects than the older antidepressants; but it can still have significant side effects. The most common are sleeplessness, nervousness, nausea, and anxiety. Prozac decreases both sexual interest and the ability to perform, and some 3.5 percent of patients who weren't suicidal before treatment get that way on the drug. Others get jittery and restless or experience tremors, symptoms reminiscent of amphetamines. Too much serotonin can trigger something called "serotonin syndrome," which involves lethargy, confusion, flushing, sweating, and muscle jerks. In severe cases, it can be fatal. Withdrawal can also be difficult, producing disturbing symptoms described as "a bad case of the flu."[251] Prozac works only 60 percent of the time (compared to a potential 80 percent with appropriately prescribed tricyclics). And it's a relatively new drug with a track record that is still developing. Enthusiasm for it rivals the sixties craze for Valium, which now heads the list of dangerously addictive drugs.[252] Prozac has already been implicated in more than a hundred civil suits and 30 criminal suits involving allegations that it caused violent behavior including murder and suicide. Despite these hazard warnings, the FDA has declined to withdraw this very lucrative drug from the market.[253]

Nutritional Alternatives

Prozac's side effects result from the way it works: It inhibits a natural process, throwing the system out of balance. The natural, balanced way to get serotonin is with its precursors, the amino acids *L-tryptophan* and *L-tyrosine*. Tryptophan is the most effective serotonin producer currently known, and for nearly half a century it was used as a safe and natural alternative to pharmaceutical tranquilizers. It was inexpensive and readily available. Then in 1989, after decades of incident-free use, it was removed from the market by the FDA. The ban was precipitated by reports of serious side effects and deaths, tragedies traced to contamination in a manufacturing process involving genetic engineering used by a particular Japanese manufacturer during late 1988 to early 1989. A study reported in the *Journal of Clinical Investigation* in November of 1990 showed that animals given this Japanese batch of tryptophan developed symptoms like those resulting in the human deaths, while pure grade L-tryptophan produced no such symptoms.[254] The FDA nevertheless kept even pure-grade L-tryptophan off the market until recently. But L-tyrosine remains noncontroversial and readily available. For safe sources of L-trytophan, try pumpkin seeds or turkey.

Inositol, a cousin of glucose, has also been shown to be an effective treatment for depression, as well as for panic disorder and mental illness. Researchers in the seventies discovered that the level of inositol in the spinal fluid of depressed people tends to be much lower than it is in other people.[255]

Magnesium levels also tend to be low in people who are depressed. Low magnesium levels heighten the nerve impulses that lead to nervous conditions. Supplementing with magnesium can help in cases of depression accompanied by panic or anxiety.

Phosphatidylserine and *5-HTP* are other nutritional supplements shown to help alleviate depression.[256]

B vitamins can also help lift the spirits and are particularly important for women under stress. For adrenal stress, try *Bragg Liquid Aminos*, a tasty supplement used as a condiment on food.

HERBAL ALTERNATIVES

The market favorite among natural remedies for depression is an herb called *St. John's wort* (*Hypericum perforatum*). In Germany, physicians write around three million prescriptions a year for this herb—25 times as many as for Prozac. A review of 23 controlled studies published in the *British Medical Journal* in August of 1997 concluded that St. John's wort works nearly three times better than a placebo and as well as prescription drugs in countering depression, without the unwanted side effects accompanying drugs. Mild, reversible side effects did occur in some patients, but they were far less frequent or serious than pharmaceutical antidepressants.[257] Millions of Germans have used St. John's wort with no reported deaths from its use.

For people with depression and anxiety, a combination herbal product called *Nutrizac*, containing St. John's wort and other herbs, is quite popular and effective.

Other effective herbal remedies for depression include *Skullcap and Oats* by Eclectic Institute, *Rescue Remedy* and other Bach flower remedies, and the herbs *kava kava* and *valerian*.

THE ORIENTAL APPROACH

In Chinese medicine, a major cause of depression is considered to be liver stagnation. The liver energy gets sluggish and makes the body sluggish, not wanting to move. The emotions become dull, depressed, and irritated.

The Chinese herbal formula for liver stagnation is called *Hsiao Yao Wan*. It stimulates the liver energy to work more actively, relieving the stagnant feeling. Depression typically lifts within a few days. American-made versions have the brand names *Relaxed Wanderer* and *Bupleurum & Peony*.

Chinese doctors also move the liver energy with greens. *Chlorophyll* and *milk thistle* are good for this purpose. An excellent product called *Ultimate Green* by Nature's Secret includes chlorella, blue-green algae, barley grass, wheat grass, spinach, alfalfa, kale, and turnip greens.

If depression is also linked to anxiety, palpitations, nightmares, or panic attacks, the heart meridian is usually involved. For a heart meridian that is out of balance, appropriate Chinese herbal formulas are *Anmien Pien*, *Pai Tzu Yang Hsin Wan*, and *Hu Po Yang Xin Dan*.

OTHER NATURAL REMEDIES

Exercise has been shown to increase brain concentrations of serotonin and norepinephrine. Running is well known for the "runner's high." However, jogging carries certain risks as you get older, including blood clotting, which can increase the risk of strokes and heart attacks; flat feet; varicose veins; and uterine prolapse. Walking, swimming, and low-impact aerobics are safer alternatives.[258]

Another way to raise brain levels of serotonin is to change your diet. Researchers at MIT found that women who binged on high-carbohydrate foods before menstruation experienced relief of depression, anger, tension, tiredness, and moodiness. These effects were attributed to an elevation in serotonin levels.[259] You should avoid sugary foods, however, since they can wreak havoc on your blood sugar level. Erratic drops in blood sugar can cause both depression and binging. The best carbohydrates are whole grains—oatmeal and other whole-grain cereals, whole-grain breads, rice, and potatoes.

Supplemental *estrogen, progesterone,* and *thyroid hormone* can also elevate the mood. Natural forms are better than synthetics. See "Menopause," "Hypothyroidism."

In the homeopathic line, *Aurum metallicum* is a specific homeopathic for suicidal depression.

For mood swings, good herbal remedies are available. For these and other natural remedies for depression, see Appendix.

For SAD, full-spectrum lights or blue light, customized colored glasses, and homeopathic *melatonin 12x* help give relief.

For bipolar disorder, patients who didn't respond to drug treatment with lithium were found in a recent study to respond to treatment with *choline*.[260]

Homeopathic lithium (something quite different from the drug) is also good for depression.

WARNING: Suicidal depression is a severe condition that should be treated only by an experienced health professional.

Diabetes

The seventh leading cause of death in the United States, diabetes is a chronic condition in which too much sugar is in the blood. Sixteen million Americans, or about 15 percent of the population, are diabetic; and another 21 million have impaired glucose tolerance, a prediabetic condition. Diabetes results from insufficient production of or an inability to make use of insulin, the hormone that helps sugar get into the tissues. Prolonged hyperglycemia (elevated blood sugar) is a risk factor for the development of such chronic complications as visual loss, kidney failure, high blood pressure, cardiovascular disease, and neurological disorders. Among U.S. adults aged 20 to 74, diabetes is the leading cause of noncongenital blindness and kidney failure; and poorly managed diabetes increases the risk of a heart attack or stroke by 600 percent. Early warning signs include excessive thirst, urination, and hunger; sudden weight loss; fatigue; nausea and vomiting; blurred vision; and numbness in the extremities.

Diabetes that begins in childhood, called Type I or *insulin-dependent diabetes mellitus (IDDM)*, is nearly always due to severe insulin deficiency. Its victims produce little or no insulin, so they must obtain the hormone by artificial means. IDDM is an autoimmune disease, which results when confused antibodies mistake the beta cells in the pancreas for foreign invaders and destroy them.[261] Researchers writing in *The Archives of Diseases in Childhood* in November of 1997 pointed to childhood immunizations as a possible cause. Childhood infections were found to reduce the probability of acquiring IDDM. The suggested explanation is that the immune system has to keep busy. If it doesn't have infections to react to, it reacts to the body of the host.[262] (See "Communicable Diseases.")

Fortunately, childhood-onset diabetes constitutes only 5 to 10 percent of all diabetes cases. The other 90 to 95 percent are Type II or *noninsulin dependent diabetes mellitus (NIDDM)*, which doesn't show up until adulthood. People with NIDDM may actually have normal or even elevated levels of insulin; the hormone just isn't working properly. Why isn't certain, but the chief predisposing risk factor is obesity. Research now suggests that Type II diabetes is a lifestyle disease that is both preventable and reversible. In traditional societies such as the Australian Aboriginal and Pacific Island populations, urbanization has resulted in a dramatic increase in NIDDM during this century. Between 10 percent and 35 percent develop the disease when they move to the city (compared to only 3 percent of Caucasians of European descent). The condition in diabetic Aborigines has shown dramatic improvement when they returned for as few as seven weeks to their traditional diet of legumes and other whole, natural foods.[263]

Hypoglycemia is the flipside of diabetes: low blood sugar. Eating sugary foods causes the body to secrete large amounts of insulin. In the hypoglycemic person, the sugar is used up before the insulin is, causing the blood sugar to drop too low.

DRUG TREATMENT

Serious cases of diabetes at the beginning of this century inevitably led to severe dehydration, coma, and death. Then it was discovered that the disease could be treated with extracts of the pancreas, the organ that releases insulin. Advances since then have progressively improved the treatment. Type I diabetics still must test their blood-sugar levels and inject themselves with insulin several times a day (usually before meals and before bed) and keep their blood-sugar levels stable by eating at regular times and avoiding sugar or sugary foods; but new single-step devices allow hourly monitoring of blood-sugar levels and more accurate insulin dosing, and newer forms of insulin afford better control. Too much insulin can cause blood sugar to drop dangerously, inducing a frightening, dreamlike state called an insulin reaction. A long-acting insulin called NPH helps avoid this reaction by reducing blood sugar gradually, imitating the body's own natural drop. For some patients, new battery-powered insulin pumps imitate the body's insulin release by pumping a steady stream of the hormone through a tube implanted under the skin. The main problem with the pump is the price— about $4,000, with insulin adding another $60 a month.[264]

DRUGS THAT CAN CAUSE DIABETES

Some drugs can actually induce diabetes in otherwise-normal people. Known offenders include steroids, birth-control pills, and diuretics. Diabetes or impaired glucose tolerance often develops during antihypertensive therapy with diuretics; and often, the condition does not go away when treatment is discontinued.[265] Other drugs can either increase blood-glucose levels or decrease them, thus increasing the risk of hypoglycemia in combination with sugar-lowering drugs. Leading offenders that diabetics should avoid are listed in the figure below.[266]

Drugs That Can Affect Blood Sugar Levels

BLOOD GLUCOSE LEVELS ARE DECREASED BY:

Aspirin and other salicylates
Phenylbutazone (a nonsteroidal anti-inflammatory agent)
Coumarin anticoagulants
Ethanol (in alcoholic beverages)
Sulfonamide antibiotics
Trimethoprim (for urinary tract infections)

BLOOD GLUCOSE LEVELS ARE INCREASED BY:

Caffeine (in large quantities)
Corticosteroids
Diazoxide
Ephedrine
Estrogen
Furosemide and thiazide diuretics
Lithium
Nicotinic acid (in large doses)
Phenobarbital
Phenytoin
Rifampin (for the treatment of tuberculosis)
Sugar-containing medications
Thyroid preparations

Nondrug Alternatives

Although insulin injections have improved, correcting the underlying problem is obviously preferable where possible. Besides the inconvenience of the treatments, whether lowering blood sugar with drugs reduces the risk of diabetic complications remains to be proved. There is some evidence, in fact, that oral sugar-lowering drugs actually *increase* the diabetic's risk of death from coronary heart disease, the main cause of premature death in diabetics. Recent research shows that high circulating levels of insulin can be destructive to the arteries.[267] For diabetics without symptoms or with only mild disease, nondrug solutions involving diet, nutritional supplements, and exercise are safer and more satisfactory alternatives.

Dietary Solutions

For many adult-onset diabetics, simply shedding 10 to 20 percent of body weight has dropped elevated blood sugar to near-normal levels.[268] Even for diabetics who need insulin, dietary change can reduce and sometimes even eliminate insulin requirements.

This was shown in a landmark study in which the carbohydrate intake of diabetics was nearly doubled by substituting high-fiber complex carbohydrates for animal foods. Diabetics on low doses of insulin managed to give up the drug altogether, and those on high doses substantially reduced their prescriptions.[269] The high-carbohydrate, high-fiber diet recommended in this study represented a radical reversal in diabetic theory. Since carbohydrate is what sugar is made of, eating it was formerly assumed to raise the blood sugar. Early recommendations therefore involved *reducing* carbohydrate and increasing fat and protein. But that diet tended to cause weight gain rather than weight loss, and its excess fat contributed to the risk of heart disease. Complex carbohydrates (whole grains and beans) are digested more slowly than simple carbohydrates and actually help regulate blood-sugar levels. Fiber also helps regulate glucose metabolism by delaying glucose absorption from the intestines. A high-fiber diet takes longer to be digested, and sugar from the food is absorbed over a longer period. Soluble fibers are particularly effective at regulating blood sugar. They improve glycemic control, reduce fasting plasma-glucose levels, reduce insulin requirements, and lower cholesterol and triglyceride levels. Fiber also helps keep your weight down. It fills you up with fewer calories and gives you more opportunity to chew.[270]

Beans and other legumes that are slowly digested and absorbed are particularly good foods for diabetics. Studies show that diets based on legumes improve diabetic glucose and insulin profiles and that slow-release carbohydrate can help relieve the symptoms of the disease. Legumes remain the traditional staples in parts of the world such as Africa and India where diabetes is uncommon.

The ideal diabetic diet is also low in fat. Fat not only adds pounds but can impair insulin activity. Two thirds of the fat in the American diet is derived from animal foods, while all of its fiber comes from plant foods. Diabetes is most prevalent in beef-eating countries. In one study, for men who ate meat daily, the risk of developing diabetes was four times as great as for those who ate it once a week or less. Interestingly, no such association was found with the consumption of eggs, milk, or cheese, although those foods are also high in saturated fat.[271]

REGULATING BLOOD SUGAR NATURALLY

Diabetics are known to have low levels of chromium, an essential mineral involved in blood-sugar regulation. Supplementing with *chromium picolinate* helps even out the blood-sugar level, preventing dramatic highs and lows not only in diabetics but in people with hypoglycemia (low blood sugar).

Anecdotal reports of improvement after chromium supplementation were discounted by the medical mainstream, until a 1996 Department of Agriculture study produced results that were called "spectacular." The difference between it and earlier studies was that chromium picolinate was given in 1,000 microgram (mcg) doses—five times the standard dose. The test subjects were 180 Type 2 diabetics in China (where nutritional supplements are rarely taken, so effects would be easy to document). High doses restored normal glucose and insulin levels and eliminated the classic signs of diabetes in nearly all of the subjects.

The researcher heading the study observed, however, that most diabetics need only 400 to 600 mcg of chromium daily. He warned that diabetics with longstanding disease or complications won't benefit from chromium and that diabetics who want to try it should first consult with their doctors, since insulin intake may have to be reduced. Chromium is recommended not only for diabetics but for hypoglycemics and for people with impaired glucose tolerance, in whom it might help prevent the development of full-blown diabetes. By lowering insulin resistance, blood cholesterol, and blood pressure, it also seems to lower heart-disease risk.[272] Chromium is not recommended, however, for men with enlarged prostates.

Insulin Needs Reduced

Pat, a hospital receptionist, was diagnosed with diabetes at 48. After she began taking chromium picolinate, she was amazed not only at how much better she felt but at how she could maintain her blood sugar with only half the medication she was taking previously.

OTHER NUTRITIONAL AIDS

Recent research indicates that *alpha lipoic acid*, a powerful antioxidant found naturally in spinach and other foods, can lower glucose levels by 20 to 30 percent.[273] Recommended daily dosage is 20 to 50 mg for nondiabetics and 300 to 600 for diabetics.

Besides insulin, the pancreas makes other enzymes, including amylase to break down starches, lipase to break down fat, cellulase to break down vegetable fiber, and protease to break down protein. Diabetics are liable to be low in these enzymes, impairing proper digestion. Supplementing with *digestive enzymes* can help (two or three with each meal). Homeopathic remedies can also stimulate the pancreas to make its own enzymes; for example, Pancreas M-17 by Futurplex (ten drops three times daily).

Supplementing with *magnesium* (found to be low in diabetics) and the trace mineral *vanadium* is also recommended.

An excellent combination nutritional and herbal product is *Diabetrol* by Cardiovascular Research.

HERBAL AND HOMEOPATHIC REMEDIES

The herb *milk thistle*, containing the antioxidant *silymarin*, was shown by Italian researchers to significantly drop and stabilize glucose levels without hypoglycemic episodes. The herb also helps with the utilization of insulin, reducing the amount needed.[274]

In Chinese medicine, the herb *Chrysanthemum* is used to treat diabetes. *Stevia Rebaudiana*, a sweetener, is an herb of the Chrysanthemum family. Stevia in its natural form is 10 to 15 times sweeter than common table sugar, and in extract form it's 100 to 300 times sweeter. Yet it doesn't affect blood-sugar metabolism. Studies have verified that Stevia aids in reducing plasma-glucose levels in normal adults.[275]

Another herb that is growing in popularity with diabetics is one used for centuries in India to support the pancreas and help regulate blood-sugar, *Gymnema Sylvestre*. It should be taken with water 15 minutes before each meal: one capsule with a small or low-sugar meal, two with a larger or high-sugar meal.

A homeopathic remedy called *Syzgium Jambolanum* can also help.

Insulin Injections Avoided

A 36-year-old dietitian sought help after being diagnosed with diabetes a month earlier. The woman had a family history of diabetes, and insulin had been prescribed, but she felt the doctor had been too cavalier about the whole matter. He had not given her an adequate explanation concerning how she had gotten it or how she could help herself. She started taking chromium, 200 mcg with breakfast and lunch. She also took homeopathic *Syzgium Jambolanum 3x* (five drops in water three times daily), and the trace mineral *vanadyl sulphate* (five drops three times daily). Within two weeks, she was off insulin and controlling her diabetes with her diet. She continues to be very careful about her diet and her doctor visits but is grateful that she no longer has to give herself injections.

NATURAL REMEDIES FOR HYPOGLYCEMIA

Hypoglycemia (low blood sugar) is corrected by the same natural blood-sugar balancers as is diabetes (high blood sugar). Chromium picolinate taken with lunch and dinner can help balance out the blood sugar. Protein should be eaten with every meal. Almonds are particularly good. Sugar should be avoided.

OTHER NATURAL BLOOD SUGAR REGULATORS

Exercise can aid in the control of diabetes. It not only helps burn up excess calories but improves glucose utilization and cardiovascular performance. WARNING: Major changes in activity levels may require a change in drug dosage. Otherwise, increased exercise can trigger hypoglycemic episodes.

Sunlight is another natural insulin. When diabetics have been exposed to sunlight treatments, their blood sugar has dropped and the sugar in their urine has decreased or disappeared. Acetone bodies also decreased or vanished. Natural sunlight seems to produce the best results. *As with exercise, diabetics need to enter a sunbathing program gradually and to keep in close touch with their doctors, since the insulin-like effect of sunlight is so dramatic that it can precipitate a hypoglycemic episode when compounded with insulin injections.*[276]

Diarrhea

Diarrhea is characterized by frequent, loose, watery stools, sometimes with cramping and vomiting. But these symptoms aren't something that should normally be suppressed, since the body is trying to get rid of things it's better off without. In infants and small children, diarrhea can cause dangerous dehydration. But even in those cases, suppression isn't recommended, since the drugs can mask the signs of very serious illness.[277]

Travelers' diarrhea (locally designated "Montezuma's revenge," "the Aztec two-step" or "Delhi belly") is always caused by something you ate that your body rejects. If you suppress the eliminatory process, the bacteria will remain inside and can be responsible for serious infectious diseases such as typhoid and cholera. Even if you're not traveling, if your diarrhea is merely the occasional bout, it's likely to be from food poisoning and shouldn't be suppressed. And if it's more than the occasional bout, it may signal a more serious condition that also should not be masked with drugs.

PRESCRIPTION DRUG TREATMENT

Even if you wanted to suppress your diarrhea with a drug, it would be hard to find one that is really safe and effective for controlling the condition. Prescription drugs are effective—in fact, they can bring bowel function to a grinding halt, by drugging the nerves that trigger it—but the result can be hazardous. Bacteria and other toxins remain in the body to wreak their own havoc, and the drugs contain narcotics that can lead to dependency. Prescription remedies should never be used for mild cases of diarrhea or for more than two or three days. They should also not be used by young children, since the drugs can be very toxic.

Lomotil and *Motofen* are popular prescription remedies that are quite effective but are narcotics that can be addicting and even fatal if taken in large amounts. They contain agents that are chemically related to the narcotic meperidine (Demerol). To discourage potential addicts, a bit of atropine is added to give the drugs unpleasant side effects. But the result is some unpleasant side effects, most commonly dizziness and sedation. Others include headache, restlessness, depression, nausea, and vomiting.[278]

Paregoric, another narcotic drug, is an opium tincture that works so well it's liable to make you constipated. It can also cause nausea, and if used for long periods, it can be addicting and can cause diverticular disease by permanently stretching the intestinal wall.

OVER-THE-COUNTER DRUGS

Imodium (loperamide) is an over-the-counter diarrhea drug that until recently was sold only by prescription. Like the prescription remedies, it can cause constipation by bringing peristaltic activity to a halt; and it can have other side effects, including drowsiness, fatigue, dizziness, dry mouth, and abdominal discomfort.

Most other over-the-counter antidiarrheal drugs, while safer than prescription drugs, lack evidence of effectiveness according to the FDA.[279] In animal studies, the active ingredients in *Kaopectate*—kaolin and pectin—haven't significantly reduced the number of bowel movements, the amount of cramping, or the amount of fluid lost. And *Donnagel*, which also contains these ingredients, adds several others that haven't been proven effective and have unwanted side effects. Kaolin and pectin products do seem to ease discomfort, however, perhaps by firming the stools; and they're considered safe. Another over-the-counter option, which the FDA considers more effective, is *polycarbophil (Mitrolan)*. It's actually a bulk-forming laxative, which eases the discomfort of diarrhea by firming the stools. It has the amazing ability to absorb 60 times its weight in water.[280]

DIARRHEA DRUGS FOR TRAVELERS

For travelers' diarrhea, a 1994 British study found that treatment with one 500-mg dose of the broad-spectrum antibiotic *ciprofioxacin (Cipro)* significantly reduced the severity and duration of symptoms.[281] For the downsides of antibiotics, see discussion under "Infection, Immunity."

Pepto-Bismol, another useful drug for travelers' diarrhea, is available over the counter and is generally considered safe. It contains bismuth, which kills bacteria; and travelers report that it works not only as a treatment but as a preventative. Downsides are that the amounts required to be effective are large, potentially resulting in salicylate poisoning, with side effects similar to those from an overdose of aspirin; and if you're taking the drug preventatively, it could be constipating.

NATURAL ALTERNATIVES FOR CHILDREN WITH DIARRHEA

For small children with serious diarrhea, the American Academy of Pediatrics recommends oral electrolyte solutions (*Ricelyte, Pedialyte, Rehydralyte*). Popular choices such as fruit juice, water, Gatorade and jello, on the other hand, are not recommended, because their water, salt and sugar contents aren't in the proper proportions.[282]

For children old enough to eat solid foods, bananas, rice, applesauce, toast, and tea are easy to digest and may help stop fluid loss. Home-made applesauce is preferred over the store-bought variety. Better yet, grate a raw, peeled, and cored apple to the consistency of applesauce. Apples contain *pectin*, an ingredient that helps stop diarrhea. Pectin is contained in over-the-counter antidiarrheal medicines such as Kaopectate and Parapectalin, but it's destroyed by cooking.[283]

Oriental doctors recommend drinking *rice water* to firm up the stools.

Although oral rehydration (replenishing fluids) prevents deaths from dehydration in children, it doesn't decrease the duration or amount of diarrhea. A study published in 1994 in *Pediatrics* (the journal of the American Academy of Pediatrics) investigated whether homeopathic treatment would do so. The researchers observed that acute diarrhea is the leading cause of pediatric deaths and complications worldwide, and that inappropriate use of antibiotics for this illness is widespread in developing countries. Homeopathy, a nontoxic and accessible alternative, is also in widespread use in developing countries. The researchers found that the remedies worked. A statistically significant decrease in the duration of diarrhea was seen in a study group given homeopathic treatment.[284]

RESTORING AND MAINTAINING FRIENDLY INTESTINAL FLORA

In Japan, diarrhea is successfully treated in children by feeding them fermented dairy products to which large amounts of *bifido bacteria* have been added. Research has shown that beneficial bifido bacteria help control diarrhea and other intestinal problems by establishing a healthy microfloral balance. Some U.S. dairies have also begun adding bifidus, along with *acidophilus*, to yogurts.

In one study, children with chronic diarrhea were given traditional drug therapy, antibiotics, and special diets; yet their diarrhea persisted for as long as ten weeks. When the children were given bifido bacteria preparations, their conditions improved in three to seven days. In another study, adults with diarrhea were given bifidus-supplemented yogurt three times daily along with antibiotic treatment. After three days, the patients had less abdominal discomfort and fewer bowel movements than without bifidus supplementation.[285]

Acidophilus Relieves Drug-induced Diarrhea

The American Journal of Psychiatry reported the cases of two women in whom persistent diarrhea had begun after taking the antidepressant sertraline (Zoloft). Symptoms were relieved with acidophilus, a bacterium found in yogurt and other fermented milk products and sold in capsules and tablets. When one of the women stopped supplementing with acidophilus, her diarrhea recurred. She found that one daily dose was sufficient to relieve her symptoms, as long as she ate yogurt along with it.[286]

ELIMINATING PARASITES

Parasites may also be an unsuspected cause of diarrhea. Treating them can resolve the condition. (See "Parasites.")

Chronic Diarrhea Cured

A 29-year-old sculptor complained that he had had chronic diarrhea and stomach problems for more than four years. He had taken conventional drugs for these problems, but the relief was temporary at best. After a four-week bout of diarrhea, he couldn't take it anymore and sought alternative treatment. His diarrhea and upset stomach were cured completely with the parasite remedy Para A and the German homeopathic remedy for giardhia.

HOMEOPATHIC ALTERNATIVES

For food poisoning, a single dose of homeopathic *Salmonella 200x* will often relieve even severe cramping and nausea. Another useful homeopathic remedy for cramps, nausea, vomiting and pain resulting from food poisoning is *Arsenicum Alba 6x*. Take 2 pills every 15 minutes, up to 6 doses.

Travelers' diarrhea can be relieved with the homeopathic remedy *Vermicillin* by CompliMed or *Ver* by Deseret.

Busy Travel Agent Cured with Simple Homeopathic Remedy

A 52-year-old travel agent returned from Europe with painful stomachaches and a constant feeling of fullness. Just the thought of eating, she said, made her nauseous; but she couldn't do the full four-week program, as she was off on another adventure. Homeopathic *Ver* alleviated her pains so that she could travel; and after six weeks on it, she reported having no recurrence of symptoms. Five months later, she still had had no recurrences.

WHAT TO AVOID

If you're prone to diarrhea after eating foods that leave your friends unaffected, you may have a food allergy or intolerance. This problem can also underly irritable-bowel syndrome, a condition characterized by constipation, diarrhea, or both alternately. Try switching to a bland diet, then adding foods of which you're suspicious back in one by one until you pinpoint the offenders. To replace lost fluids, drink plenty of water or juice diluted with water (but not heavily sugared drinks).

Even if you're not allergic to milk in your normal state, milk products can aggravate an active case of diarrhea and should be avoided. Dairy products contain lactose that is hard to digest. Caffeinated beverages should also be avoided.

You should also avoid drugs that you don't have to take. Drugs that can cause or aggravate diarrhea include antibiotics, antacids containing magnesium (such as Maalox and Mylanta), laxatives, and medications for high blood pressure and irregular heart beat.

Overdosing on vitamin C can also cause loose stools, although this isn't necessarily bad. The Vitamin-C Flush popular with alternative practitioners involves using heavy doses of the vitamin for the express purpose of flushing out toxins.

*E*ar Infections ("Otitis Media"), Hearing Problems

Despite aggressive treatment, otitis media, or middle-ear infection, has reached epidemic proportions in American children. Called the bread and butter of the pediatrician, its treatment grosses at least $1 billion annually.[287]

Chronic middle-ear effusion (fluid in the ears) underlies the most frequently performed operations of childhood—myringotomy (surgical incision of the eardrum, with or without the insertion of tubes), tonsillectomy, and adenoidectomy. Myringotomy is sometimes elected because the parents are afraid that reduced hearing from chronic fluid in the ears will impair learning. But recent studies show that the effectiveness of these operations is very limited and that they should be reserved only for children who are severely affected. They can mean further trauma to the eardrum, prolonging the time required for the ear to heal, and they don't shorten the duration of pain. In most cases, the condition eventually clears by itself without surgery, presumably because the skull and eustachian tubes have grown.[288]

Drug Treatment

Standard drug treatment for ear infections is with antibiotics, but the ailment often fails to respond even to repeated courses of these drugs.[289] The majority of ear infections are caused by viruses, for which antibiotics don't work; and the widespread use of antibiotics has led to the widespread development of antibiotic-resistant strains of bacteria.[290]

A landmark Swedish study involving 2,145 patients showed that for the majority of ear infections, antibiotics may do more harm than good. Not only did ear infections not go away any faster when treated with the drugs, but children treated with them were 30 percent more likely to have a recurrence of the infection. For those treated with antibiotics from the first day of the disease, recurrences were 40 percent more likely. The chance of a repeat infection within a month of the previous one was more than twice as great in children treated with antibiotics as in those not treated. And in those treated with antibiotics from the first day of the disease, it was nearly three times as great.[291]

The researchers noted that ear infection recurrences are on the increase and concluded that routine early administration of antibiotics may be responsible. The drugs depress the immunological response to bacteria, preventing the development of natural antibodies and interfering with the development of natural immunity. That explains why the earlier they're given, the more frequent are relapses of the disease. Antibiotics also permit overgrowths by resistant Candida microbes, which then produce toxins that can weaken the immune system and further reduce the child's resistance.[292] (See "Candidiasis.")

Results of this Swedish study were confirmed in a study reported in the *New England Journal of Medicine* in 1987. Over 500 children with middle-ear infection were given either (1) an antibiotic alone (the popular amoxicillin), (2) that antibiotic along with a decongestant-antihistamine, or (3) a placebo. After four weeks, no significant differences were found in the children's conditions.[293] Neither drug provided any advantage over no drugs at all, confirming earlier research.[294] Other studies of children with otitis media with fluid in the ears have found that the majority of cases resolved by the following month without treatment.[295]

HOMEOPATHIC ALTERNATIVES

Then doesn't mean you have to ignore your suffering child who is screaming and pulling at her ears. Effective natural remedies are available to ease pain while the ears heal.

One is *Mullein Oil Ear Drops*. Mullein has narcotic properties. While it's a strong painkiller, it doesn't produce the lightheadedness or psychological aberrations of narcotic drugs. Applied directly in the ear, it quiets irritated nerves, relieves pain, and soothes inflammation. Other helpful herbs are *echinacea* and *elderberry*.

Home remedies when you can't make it to an herb shop include a few drops of plain fresh *onion juice*, squeezed in a garlic press right into the ear. Cotton can be applied afterwards to hold the juice in. Fresh-squeezed *garlic oil*, warmed on a spoon over the stove, is also good.

An excellent homeopathic combination popular in France for ear infections is a product called *ABC*. The letters stand for *aconite, belladonna* and *chamomile*, the three main homeopathic remedies for soothing ear pain and promoting healing. Given as often as every 10 or 15 minutes at the onset of pain (or in young children when they start pulling on their ears), it can eliminate ear pain with as few as two doses. ABC is available in the

United States from MPI, or its ingredients can be purchased separately and taken together. Other good products are *Earache Pain Relief* by Natra-Bio and *Chamilla* by BHI. Take one pill every hour for severe pain, or one pill three times daily.

Children's homeopathic expert Kathy Arnos recommends *acidophilus* and daily *flaxseed oil* for children with ear infections. If the child is moody or irritable, she always looks at the teeth. She feels the majority of childhood ear problems are related to teething. Homeopathics are available that can speed the eruption of the teeth: *Cal Carb 200x* (give three pills three times in one day, then stop) or *Cal Phos 6x* (three pills two times daily for one week).

Another solution to ear pain that is controversial but growing in popularity is ear candling. Mothers report that when ear candles have been used on children with ear problems, the pain disappears immediately. For a fuller discussion, see "Tinnitus, Hearing Impairment."

Endometriosis

Endometriosis is a condition involving the abnormal growth of uterine tissue outside the uterus, causing chronic pelvic pain, disabling periods, internal scarring, and infertility. Affecting five million American girls and women from ages 11 to 50, it is the second most common gynecological disorder requiring hospital treatment and is a leading cause of hysterectomy. The condition is generally considered incurable.[296]

The endometrium, or lining of the womb, bleeds every time menstruation occurs. In women with endometriosis, endometrial-like tissue migrates to other parts of the body (usually the ovaries, tubes, and peritoneum), where it behaves like the endometrium: it bleeds. But the blood can't escape, so it tends to form adhesions, which become inflamed and scarred and make the organs stick together.

Endometriosis may be asymptomatic and may regress without treatment. For this reason, when it's discovered accidentally and produces no symptoms, it shouldn't automatically be treated. More commonly, however, the condition is not only symptomatic but so painful that victims sometimes report harboring thoughts of suicide.

Drug Treatment

Analgesics, hormonal drugs, and surgery are the usual conventional treatments, but none is a cure.

Analgesics relieve discomfort but don't affect the cause. The condition usually returns when pharmaceutical hormones are discontinued, and the drugs have unwanted side effects. *Birth-control pills* relieve the symptoms of endometriosis but may also be responsible for inducing it, through a sort of rebound effect when the drugs are discontinued. A drug called *Lupron (leuprolide acetate)* is sometimes given to induce menopause, since endometriosis tends to improve after that passage. But while the drug may successfully eliminate the pain of endometriosis, its cost is premature menopause; and the drug tends to be given to women who are still young. It induces hot flashes and can cause bone pain, weakness, and numbness in the lower limbs during the first few weeks of treatment.[297] Women who take it also seem to age overnight.

The radical surgical alternative—removal of the ovaries—also brings on premature menopause. The transition can be so sudden as to bring on severe symptoms, causing the patient to resort to hormone replacement therapy, which can then reactivate the endometriosis. Surgery also leads to adhesions, which further impair function of the female organs.

Most doctors recommend getting pregnant, which generally eliminates symptoms, perhaps because progesterone levels are particularly high during pregnancy. But symptoms can recur several years after delivery. And endometriosis victims tend to have trouble getting pregnant. Whether endometriosis actually causes infertility isn't clear, but the two conditions tend to go together.

Tracking the Cause

In Chinese medicine, endometriosis is attributed to the body's Qi energy flowing the wrong way; for example, from the use of tampons or from having sex during menstruation. The tampon theory has recently gained scientific credence, but for another reason: Most tampons contain dioxin. The Endometriosis Protection Agency reports a close association between levels of dioxin in the body and the incidence and severity of the disease. Dioxins are chlorinated hydrocarbons that are airborne byproducts of manufacturing processes involving chlorine, including those for making plastics, PVCs, solvents such as drycleaning fluid, pesticides, and drugs.

Apart from the air, the major source of dioxins for humans is animal fat (meat and dairy), where the chemicals become concentrated after grazing animals ingest them. Dioxins are also byproducts of the chlorine-bleaching process used to whiten paper, rayon, cotton, and other materials, including the fibers used in most feminine hygiene products. Dioxin can remain in the pulp once it is bleached and, like DDT, collect in human fatty tissue.

A bill to fund research on the possible health hazards of dioxin in feminine products was recently introduced into Congress. The bill followed reports in the media of a possible link between the amounts of dioxin found in tampons and sanitary pads and various ailments, including not only endometriosis but cancers of the cervix, ovaries, and breast.[298]

Endometriosis is one of a number of diseases linked to environmental endocrine disruptors—synthetic chemicals that mimic natural hormones. Hormones act like keys in a lock. When they are replaced by hormone mimics, the locks don't turn and normal body functions are blocked. Besides dioxins, other hormone mimics are found in spermicides. (See "Bladder Infection.")

TREATMENT WITH NATURAL HORMONES

Despite official pronouncements of incurability, cases of endometriosis have been cured. One key to cure is *natural progesterone*. Endometriosis can be stimulated by estrogen and is characterized by high blood levels of estrogen, indicating a hormone imbalance. Progesterone balances estrogen levels and is a precursor to other hormones, normalizing their activity in the body. *NOTE: For menstruating women, natural progesterone should be used only from ovulation to the period.* See "PMS."

Endometriosis Cured with Natural Progesterone

Sandy was only 19 when her gynecologist recommended a hysterectomy. He said her endometriosis was so severe she would never have children anyway. But Sandy's father, Bruce, was one of the developers of a natural progesterone cream called *ProGest*. He decided to try to correct her hormone imbalance with that newly developed product. The experiment saved her uterus and gave Bruce a grandchild. Sandy had had only four periods since she was 16, but she had a normal period the next month; and at 29, she delivered a normal, healthy baby.

Herbal Treatment

In Chinese medical theory, liver stagnation contributes to endometriosis by causing hormone imbalance. This imbalance can be corrected with a Chinese patent formula called *Hsiao Yao Wan* in combination with a Liver Cleanse Diet. (See "Liver Disease.") *NOTE: Hsia Yao Wan also increases bleeding, so its use should be stopped from three days before the period is due until after the period has ended.*

The Chinese herb *keishi-bukuryo-gan* has been shown to suppress adenomyosis (ingrowth of the endometrium) in mice.[299]

Herbs can also be used to regulate hormones. Hormone levels should be checked by a practitioner experienced with herbal remedies to determine which levels are out of balance and which herbs are appropriate for balancing them.

Homeopathic Treatment

Homeopathy is another alternative for stimulating the body to rebalance the disturbed hormone levels linked to endometriosis. The appropriate remedy depends on the case, but a good beginning in most cases is a combination remedy by Boiron called *Cyclease*. *Mag Phos 6x* can also help stop the pain of cramps. The underlying endometriosis should then be treated with constitutional homeopathic remedies specific to the patient.

Homeopathic Relief from Endometriosis

Shelley, a 24-year-old hairdresser, had such painful endometriosis that she had considered taking her own life. Every month she dreaded her period. She had to plan for it and take time off work, since she got such severe cramps that she couldn't stand on her feet. The cramps started about two days before her period and continued until it was in its second day.

She had the odd habit of lying naked on the cold bathroom floor to get relief, a symptom that was important in selecting a constitutional remedy. With Shelley's type of endometriosis, "cold" feels better than "hot" (for example, a heating pad or hot-water bottle). Hospital emergency room personnel are familiar with the woman who has gone into shock and has been found naked and unconscious on the bathroom floor.

Shelley had to work for many years with natural remedies before her cramps were entirely under control, but it took only a few months before she was able to live with them. Her endometriosis has now been under control for many years. The remedies that worked in her case were a German homeopathic called *Endometritis Tuberculosa*, and a Chinese herbal formula by Seven Forests. Shelley, too, had been told by a number of doctors that her case was so progressed that she could not have children, but after a program of homeopathic and herbal remedies specific for her condition and personality type, she recently delivered a nine-pound baby boy.

OTHER NATURAL ALTERNATIVES

Acupuncture can help balance hormones and relieve symptoms.

Sitz baths may give symptomatic relief. Alternate between sitting in a hot bath for three minutes and a cold bath for thirty seconds.[300]

Recommended dietary modifications include avoiding foods to which you are allergic, alcohol, sugar, and processed and heavily chemicalized foods, all of which can inhibit immune function.

Recommended nutritional supplements include *vitamins A, C, E, and B6 with B-complex;* the minerals *calcium, magnesium, zinc,* and *selenium; evening primrose oil* and *chlorophyll.*

CAUTION: Evening primrose oil increases bleeding, something menstruating women with endometriosis already do too much of. Evening primrose oil should not be taken immediately before or during the period.

Environmental Illness, Liver Stagnation

The typical victim found to be "environmentally ill" complains of being enormously tired and run down, barely able to function; yet medical testing finds nothing. Only after careful questioning is the problem revealed: The liver has become so overburdened with accumulated toxins that it can't "keep up." Unsuspected immune system assailants may include pesticides sprayed in the house, on the lawn, or on a nearby golf course; formaldehyde and other chemical fumes from the upholstery in a new car, new carpeting, paint, fire retardants in a new mattress, or dry-cleaning fluid; petrochemicals in perfumes, dyes, plastics, or synthetic rubber; the chlorine in swimming pools; the metals and plastics in dental materials. These accumulated toxins overwhelm the body and the immune system. The diagnosis is established when detoxification measures reverse the problem.

Chemical and metal toxicities have also been linked to more serious diseases with unknown causes. Cases of Parkinson's disease, multiple sclerosis, lupus, and Alzheimer's disease have been traced to pesticide exposure, pharmaceuticals use, and heavy metals accumulated in brain tissues. For techniques for eliminating heavy metals from the body, see "Heavy-Metal Poisoning."

An increasing but unrecognized problem is sensitivity to molds and fungi, which can linger after the rainy season and blow through heating and air conditioning systems from musty basements into the rest of the house. A recent study traced brain damage in infants to this source. (See "Asthma.") Natural remedies are available that are designed specifically for this problem.

DETOXIFYING THE LIVER

All of the toxins that come into the body have to be broken down by the liver before they are excreted. The liver also has the task of breaking down hormones. In women, hormone levels are highest from ovulation to the menses, so the liver is most stressed at that time. The liver has its work cut out for it just detoxifying the normal products of metabolism. When extraordinary environmental toxins and drugs are added to that load, it breaks down. Chinese doctors say that when the liver gets so overwhelmed it can't do its job, the internal movements of the body stagnate. The Chinese patent remedy for moving liver stagnation is *Hsiao Yao Wan*.

Foods that stimulate drainage of the liver help detoxify the system; foods high in sulfur and selenium act as antioxidants; foods high in inositol and choline help the liver eliminate excess fat. Good choices include watercress, mustard greens, red and black radishes, wheat grass juice, dandelions, parsley, apples, artichokes, beet and beet greens, carrots, Brussels sprouts, horseradish, garlic, cabbage, cranberries, Swiss chard, kale, and celery.

Dr. Bernard Jensen, a naturopathic pioneer, also recommended skin brushing: brush you skin with a dry brush to remove dead skin to help the body release toxins and dead skin before bathing.

THE LIVER-CLEANSE DIET

This detox program is specifically designed for cleaning the liver:

1. Begin each morning with the juice of half a lemon squeezed into warm water.
2. Eat only whole, fresh foods—no preservatives, coloring, or fillers (all found in processed foods). Emphasize green vegetables, the foods that stimulate the liver to release and process toxins. Limit protein to 30 grams a day.
3. Drink at least 64 ounces (8 glasses) of distilled water while on the detox diet. (Distilled water isn't recommended, however, for more than seven days.)
4. Drink the juice of fresh mixed greens (parsley, celery, carrot) at least twice a day. If you can't find these drinks or make them yourself, drink chlorophyll in water or juice, two to four ounces daily.
5. Throughout the day, drink unfiltered apple juice and detox tea.
6. Exercise or walk briskly at least 20 minutes a day. (If you aren't used to regular exercise, don't overdo it.)

Acetaldehyde Sensitivity Reversed

Virginia, in her late twenties, was under tremendous stress from starting two new businesses; but she was doing well financially. She used some of her new earnings to buy a new car, paint her bedroom, and buy a new bed. Suddenly she got quite ill and couldn't sleep, but no medical cause could be found. After questioning, her problems were determined to be stress and sensitivity to the chemicals in the new car upholstery, paints, and new mattress. The recommended treatment was the Chinese herbal formula *Hsiao Yao Wan*, a homeopathic remedy called *Acetaldehyde*, and the Liver-Cleanse diet. After two weeks on this program, she was happy to report that her energy level and sleep habits had returned to normal.

DETOXIFYING CHEMICAL TOXINS

Homeopathic remedies are also available for neutralizing chemical toxins. A new line of products is specifically designed for detoxifying particular chemicals in the body.

House plants can also help clean toxins from the air. Some plants thrive on the same chemicals that are poisonous to humans. See Chart.[301]

Chlorine Sensitivity Reversed

A mother complained of bad acne in her nine-year-old daughter, who seemed too young for the problem. Questioning revealed that her acne was aggravated whenever she went swimming. The recommended treatment was a New Vista homeopathic remedy called *Chlorine*, which is specifically formulated for eliminating chlorine from the system. The remedy worked and the girl's acne cleared up, except on the days that she swam. The mother then started giving her daughter the remedy before and after swimming. She reports the girl has had no further acne problems since.

DETOXIFYING MOLDS AND FUNGI

Homeopathic remedies can also neutralize the toxic effects of molds and fungi.

Baffling Family Ailment Reversed

A mother complained that her whole family seemed continually to be sick. Despite the usual preventive measures, Sam, her nine-month-old baby, got repeated colds. On questioning, the mother said they were living in condos converted from an old hotel in Sun Valley. In its dilapidated former state, the roof had leaked water into the walls. The walls had been painted, but black mold was still evident. Worse, the family was using a humidifier every day. The windows would get wet with water from it. The baby's room was a breeding ground for toxic molds and fungi. A remedy called *Mold and Fungus* by Molecular Biologicals was recommended for the whole family, and they all reported feeling better after taking it. They were advised, however, that as long as they lived with the "maintaining cause," they were never going to have strong immune systems. They finally broke their lease and moved, and say they have never felt healthier.

Charlie, the attorney who helped this family get out of their lease, had a similar problem. He felt exhausted, was losing his memory, couldn't think clearly, and was so disoriented he was having trouble doing his work. He'd been to all the best doctors and clinics, including Johns Hopkins and the Mayo Clinic. But after trying everything they could think of, the doctors told him there was nothing more they could do. Then an environmental specialist discovered molds and fungi growing in the air conditioning over Charlie's desk. They were a particularly bad variety, which emits fumes that are toxic to the brain. Charlie moved to a new office in another building and was much improved, except when he handled files brought from his old office. The toxic fumes were evidently on the files. His solution was to xerox all his files and use the copies. Again he was improved, but still not cured. After a week on *FNG* by Deseret and *Mold and Fungus* by Molecular Biologicals, he reported that he was back to feeling like his old self. He continues to be well, except when directly exposed to molds or fungi.

Eye Problems

"Pink eye," or bacterial conjunctivitis, is an eye infection that causes only mild discomfort but can produce copious discharge and redness. It typically begins in one eye but can move to the other if precautions aren't taken. Viral conjunctivitis usually includes fever, malaise, redness, and copious discharge from the eye. Contaminated swimming pools are a common source of infection.

Other common minor eye ailments include styes, dry eyes, torn corneas, night blindness or poor night vision, and redness or tiredness from overwork. The more serious chronic degenerative eye diseases—cataracts, macular degeneration and glaucoma—are discussed under those headings.

NOTE: If you are having chronic eye problems, you should see an ophthalmologist (medical doctor specializing in eye diseases).

OVER-THE-COUNTER DRUG TREATMENT

Over-the-counter eye medications are widely advertised as removing redness, but these drugs can have unwanted side effects. Cases of blindness have actually been reported from their misuse.[302] Drugs dropped into the eyes reach the general circulation; and since the contact time with the eye is often only a fraction of a minute, eye medications are highly concentrated. They drain rapidly back into the mucus membranes of the nose, where they can enter the bloodstream and reach the heart, lungs and other organs without being detoxified. Daily use can also make your eye problems worse, since like many other drugs, they can produce a rebound reaction that makes your eyes redder and more irritated than before you started using them. The popular *Visine* and similar products contain an agent called tetrahydrozoline HCl, which makes the tiny blood vessels in the eyes constrict. This temporarily clears minor redness due to irritants; but if you use the medicine repeatedly, your eyes react by dilating. This can lead to a vicious cycle of worsening eye redness and dependency on the drops. A better option is the *Murine* formulation that omits this vessel-constricting medication. (Note: there are two Murine formulations, one with the medication—called Murine Plus—and one without.) Better yet, omit the drops, rest your eyes and avoid irritants. If your problem persists, it may indicate something more serious that requires a doctor's attention.[303]

PRESCRIPTION DRUG TREATMENT

Prescriptions are often given for minor eye redness or inflammation, but these drugs can have even more dangerous side effects. Options include steroids (*prednisolone* or *dexamethasone corticosteroid* eye drops or ointments), antibiotic eye drops or ointments *(bacitracin, gentamicin, ofloxacin, ciprofloxacin, norfloxacin)*, and *sulfacetaminde* drops or ointments (*Bleph-10, Sulf-10, Sodium Sulamyd, Cetamide*).

Sulfa drugs carry the warning that a significant percentage of Staphylococcus bacteria—the usual suspects for eye infection—are resistant to them. A significant number of people are also allergic to them, and "severe sensitivity reactions have been identified in individuals with no prior history of sulfonamide sensitivity." Adverse reactions can include headache, local irritation, burning, stinging, and bacterial and fungal corneal ulcerations. Worse yet are corticosteroids and corticosteroid/antibiotic combinations. Corticosteroids suppress inflammation; and when inflammation is reduced, resistance is lowered and secondary infections can occur. The drugs can also cause glaucoma and cataracts. (See "Glaucoma.")

Drugs used by ophthalmologists to dilate the pupils have also been associated with glaucoma, as well as with certain rare but serious systemic side effects. *Cyclopentolate hydrochloride*, one of these drugs, has produced central nervous system effects when applied in the eyes, including visual hallucinations and schizophrenic and psychotic reactions. The reactions were usually in children and involved formulations containing strong concentrations of the drug. A similar drug, *phenylephrine hydrochloride*, has been associated with uncommon but severe cardiovascular and other side effects. It should be used with caution or not at all in patients with heart conditions or diabetes and in lightweight children.[304]

HOMEOPATHIC REMEDIES

Safe, effective homeopathic remedies are available that can clear pink eye in just a couple of days. *Eye* by BHI is particularly good. It contains several homeopathic medicines, including *Euphrasia*, which clears redness from the eye. Also good is *Optique* by Boiron, which contains not only *Euphrasia* but *Calendula*, a remedy for healing the eye. These individually-packaged eye drops remain sterile and contain no preservatives.

Torn Cornea Healed in a Single Day

Gary, a local bookstore owner, managed to tear his cornea while removing his contact lenses when his eyes had become dry, causing the top layer of his eye to pull out with the contact lens. A torn cornea is very painful and can take more than a week to resolve on its own; but Gary reported being healed in a single day, taking *Calendula 6x* (four pills four times daily) and using *Optique* eyedrops topically twice daily.

HERBAL AND NUTRITIONAL REMEDIES

All *antioxidants* are beneficial for the eyes. They include alpha-lipoic acid, coenzyme Q10, cysteine, glutathione, melatonin, selenium, superoxide dismutase, vitamin A and beta-carotene, vitamin C, vitamin E, zinc, and oligomeric proanthocyanids (OPCs). OPCs are powerful antioxidants found in grape seeds and pine bark (pycnogenol). Both are sources recommended for the person using the computer all day.

Most of these antioxidants are contained in a combination nutritional product good for vision problems called *Ocudyne II*. It also contains *lutein*, a carotenoid found to prevent cataracts and macular degeneration. (See "Cataracts.")

HERBAL REMEDIES

Herbs high in antioxidants include *bilberry, ginkgo biloba*, and *green tea*.

Bilberry, an herb shown in studies to increase night vision, was reportedly used by the Air Force to sharpen the vision of night pilots charged with dropping bombs.

The herb *eyebright* (*euphrasia*) is also good for any eye problem: pink eye, tired eyes, puffy eyes, and so forth. It comes as capsules, bulk herbs, tinctures, and more. It can be drunk as a tea, and the tea bags can be placed on the eyes.

LIGHT THERAPY

Full-spectrum lighting is important for the eyes. Glass windows and lenses filter out beneficial components of the sun's rays. Dr. Jacob Lieberman recommends spending at least an hour each day outdoors, regardless of the weather. You need not be in the sun—being in the shade or on a screened porch is fine—but for this therapy to work, you should not wear sunglasses, prescription glasses, contact lenses, or suntan lotion. If you are in the sun, it's best to avoid the rays between 10 A.M. and 2 P.M. and not overdo them at other hours. If you must be out in the bright midday sun for more than 30 minutes, Dr. Lieberman recommends sunscreens, but not those containing PABA. A recent FDA report concluded that 14 out of 17 suntan lotions containing PABA could be carcinogenic.[305]

*F*ever

Hippocrates considered fever a therapeutic process designed to "cook out" invaders. His attitude prevailed until the 1900s, when aspirin was introduced. By the turn of the twentieth century, drug companies were promoting aspirin for its ability to reduce fever as well as pain, which seemed to go together. Ultimately, mass advertising turned public sentiment against this natural cleansing process.

Today, fever is one of the most common symptoms prompting parents to bring their young children to the doctor. The popular fear is that fever will cause brain damage. Several investigators who carefully reviewed the literature, however, failed to confirm this adverse effect. The only possible exceptions were in cases of meningitis or encephalitis; but the relationship was uncertain, since those conditions can cause brain damage independent of the effects of fever. In any case, fever won't cause brain damage below 108 degrees; and temperatures that high are extremely rare.[306]

New research supports Hippocrates. A little fever does a body good. Studies show that it cripples many temperature-sensitive viruses. In laboratory experiments, artificially induced fevers have decreased the death rate among infected animals. Conversely, *lowering* their temperatures has *increased* the death rate. Fever evidently fights disease by means of a substance called interleukin-1 (IL-1), which is released from white blood cells when a foreign agent invades the blood. Fever raises the thermostat in the hypothalamus, probably by activating prostaglandins, the substances aspirin suppresses. (See "Pain.") IL-1 speeds the production of the immune system's T cells, which augment natural killer cell activity. When the temperature rises from 98.6 to 102 degrees Fahrenheit, T-cell production increases by as much as 20 times. When aspirin is given to rabbits in doses sufficient to prevent fever, the killing activity of their neutrophils (a type of white blood cell) is inhibited. High body temperatures also strengthen the effect of interferon, a natural protein that combats viruses.[307]

Fevers can be harmful in certain circumstances. They can pose an unnecessary stress on patients with heart or lung disease; they can cause confusion and delirium, especially in the elderly; they can reactivate fever blisters; and they may be harmful to the fetus during the first three months of pregnancy. They can also provoke seizures in children prone to them. However, drugs aren't usually effective in preventing this type of seizure, since by the time the fever is recognized, the seizure is already in full swing. Fortunately, these seizures are harmless.[308]

NOTE: The medical recommendation is to get a doctor's advice for any fever over 103 degrees or for one above 100 degrees that lasts more than three days, especially if accompanied by a very sore throat.

THE CONVENTIONAL APPROACH

Aspirin was the usual treatment for fevers for decades, until it was discovered that the aspirin treatment of viral infections can cause Reye's syndrome. One of the top ten child killers, Reye's syndrome usually develops several days after a viral infection—flu, chicken pox, or a cold. Half its victims die, and some who live through it wind up permanently brain damaged. The brain damage erroneously linked to the natural fever process seems in these cases to have been caused by the drugs given to treat it. Symptoms to watch for are persistent vomiting, listlessness, drowsiness, personality changes, disorientation, delirium, convulsions, or loss of consciousness.

Because of the risk of Reye's syndrome, *acetaminophen* (*Tylenol* and others) is now generally recommended instead of aspirin for reducing fever in children. Aspirin, acetaminophen, and ibuprofen are all about equally effective in reducing fever, but acetaminophen is considered the safest. Mothers of children prone to seizures with fever are generally told to give them acetaminophen prophylactically whenever a fever develops. But caution is necessary here too, since acetaminophen can lead to hepatic necrosis and other liver problems if taken chronically or in large doses. Even for short-term use in normal children with viral infections (the most common cause of fevers), there is now evidence that acetaminophen may do more harm than good. In one study, 68 children with chicken pox were given either acetaminophen or a placebo four times a day for four days. On the second day of treatment, children in the acetaminophen-treated group were more active than those in the placebo group; but on the fourth day, the treated children itched more, and their chicken pox took a day longer to scab over. The data suggested that the effects of fever were actually beneficial in fighting off the virus, and that fever should be allowed to run its course.[309]

Some pediatricians routinely treat fevers with antibiotics, even before they have laboratory evidence of bacterial infection. But most fevers will go away by themselves without treatment; and even if they wouldn't, antibiotics wouldn't work on them, since only 3 to 15 percent of fevers are caused by bacteria. The rest are caused by viruses, on which antibiotics aren't effective.

A study in the *New England Journal of Medicine* concluded that routine treatment of high fever with standard oral doses of antibiotics (in this case amoxicillin) in small children was unwarranted, except when actual laboratory evidence of a bacterial infection justified it. The study involved 955 children aged 3 to 36 months with temperatures over 102.2 degrees Fahrenheit but without apparent local infection. Blood cultures established that only 2.8 percent of the children had bacterial infections caused by disease-producing organisms. There was no evidence that early antibiotic treatment prevented new, serious bacterial infections (meningitis, pneumonia, and so on), which weren't statistically different in the treated and control groups. And the antibiotics themselves produced side effects, including diarrhea and rash.[310]

THE ALTERNATIVE APPROACH: FEVER AS THERAPY

Before antibiotics, patients with syphilis were deliberately inoculated with typhoid bacteria to induce fever. This treatment was thought to speed recovery by inhibiting the syphilis bacteria from reproducing. In European hydrotherapies, fever is still intentionally induced for its cleansing effects. Heat treatment, or hyperthermia, has also been used successfully as a form of cancer therapy. A famous German cancer specialist reported that in a swampy area in Italy where malaria was rife, cancer was unknown. When the area was dried out, the malaria disappeared, but cancer became a problem. The doctor postulated that the high fevers common in malaria had stimulated the natural defenses of the residents so cancer couldn't develop.[311]

HOMEOPATHIC REMEDIES

Fevers serve beneficial functions, but treatment of high childhood fevers is still recommended, as they can be uncomfortable and can lead to seizures. Homeopathic remedies are the ideal first choices, since they don't interfere with the natural efforts of the body but work vibrationally on the cause. Homeopaths treat the whole symptom picture, not just the fever. Here are some common symptom complexes and their appropriate homeopathic remedies:

- *Belladonna 6x to 30c:* For the child who is restless, with a very hot face, who feels better with cold applications. Give the remedy every 15 minutes for 2 hours, or until the fever has come down.

- *Ferrum Phos 6x to 30c:* For the child with a temperature but no localized symptoms. Give 2 to 3 pills, at intervals of 15 to 60 minutes as needed, up to 5 doses.

- *Aconite 6x to 30c:* For the fever that comes on suddenly, often after exposure to wind or cold. The person is usually thirsty. Give 2 pills every 15 minutes as needed, up to 5 doses.

An effective homeopathic combination product by Boericke & Tafel is *Fever Reducer.*

HERBAL REMEDIES

Effective Chinese herbal formulas are also available for treating fever. They include:

- *Zhong Gan Ling* by Zand: For a cold with fever. The adult dose is 2 dropperful in water 3 times daily. K'an also makes a formula by the same name.

- *Liu Shen Wan*: For fever with strep throat. This formula has been known to eliminate severe strep throat symptoms in a few hours.
- *Antiphlogistic Tablets*: An effective Chinese patent remedy for sore throat or tonsillitis accompanied by fever.

Fibromyalgia

Fibromyalgia is a baffling disease characterized by chronic generalized muscle pain, stiffness, and weakness, which tends to be worse in the morning. It afflicts women ten times more frequently than men. Patients with the condition, which is very hard to diagnose, were once simply dismissed as neurotic. Fibromyalgia is now recognized as a medical syndrome, but the cause and cure still remain mysteries. For unknown reasons, the muscles start making too much fibrin, the stuff the body uses to protect itself. The fibrin is what makes the muscles painful to the touch. Often physical pressure that doesn't hurt at the time is quite painful a couple of hours later. The condition usually begins when a person who is already under stress undergoes some further trauma—the woman already run down with chronic fatigue or stress who gets in a car accident or has a bad fall—prompting the body to overreact in producing its protective fibrin.

CONVENTIONAL TREATMENT

Until the last couple of years, conventional treatment was symptomatic, with analgesics, antidepressants, anesthetics, or corticosteroids, drugs that merely mask or suppress the problem without addressing the underlying cause. Recently, drug treatment has been developed involving *glycerol glycolate*, the main ingredient in *Robitussin* cough syrup. Taken in very high doses over a long period of time, the drug dries up the fluids in the body and stops fibrin production. One problem is its side effects, which can be more daunting than the disease. Another problem is that for a large percentage of patients it doesn't work. It's also an expensive and lengthy therapy that has to be used daily. If you skip a day or two, you're back to where you started. Still, it does work for some people.

NUTRITIONAL AND HERBAL TREATMENT

The leading alternative treatment is a combination of *malic acid* (magnesium maleate) and *boswellin* (an Ayurvedic herb). Malic acid alone can help fibromyalgia pain, but the combination is more effective. One downside is that the treatment has to continually be repeated (every six hours). If the remedy is stopped, the pain returns, indicating it is still only masking pain. But it does avoid the side effects of the conventional drugs and is more effective than ordinary analgesics and antidepressants.

Another nutrient found to benefit fibromyalgia patients is the antioxidant *pycnogenol*.[312]

A surprisingly effective protocol that has been known to work when all else fails is one produced by a multilevel marketing company called Life Plus, which uses products called *Lyprinex* (consisting of special oils) and *Proanthonols* (strong antioxidants). Both are taken at very high doses for the first month. The first month's treatment is thus quite expensive (around $300); but in subsequent months, the dosage and cost are reduced.

Dancer Returns to Work

Before she got sick, Anna was a dancer. She was used to working out several hours a day. Then she developed chronic-fatigue syndrome. She got fibromyalgia after getting in a car accident in her early forties. She became so stiff and sore, she couldn't work at all. She tried the Robitussin glycerol glycolate treatment, but found the side effects to be worse than the disease. Malic acid gave her significant relief. However, she still couldn't exercise at the level she was used to, and she had to take the remedy continually without skipping a dose. When she was told about the Lyprinex and Proanthonols protocol, she decided to try it despite its high cost. She checks in every couple of months. She is back at work full time and says she is amazed at how much better she feels.

HOMEOPATHIC TREATMENT

British studies have shown that the homeopathic remedy *Rhus tox* is also effective in reducing the pain of fibromyalgia.[313]

First Aid:
Trauma, Bruises, Wounds, Cuts, Sunburn, Burns

Household injuries and minor traumas are everyday occurrences. Simple natural remedies are available that can heal injuries and reduce trauma to the body. Many people seek natural treatment for sports-related injuries, not only because the cost of going to the emergency room is so high and making a doctor appointment is difficult, but because they have had such good luck with the remedies.

Western herbal remedies useful to have on hand for emergency first aid are discussed in Chapter 4. Less well known, but remarkably effective, are some Chinese herbal and homeopathic remedies:

FOR OPEN OR BROKEN SKIN. Homeopathic *Calendula*, made from the marigold flower, rapidly promotes healing of the skin. Dramatic responses are often reported with this amazing ointment.

Open Sore Healed Overnight

A woman who had had a leg amputated and was wearing a prosthetic device was worried because it was rubbing on her skin and causing an open sore. Her doctor had proposed giving her antibiotics and cutting the sore open. What worried her was that this was the very procedure that had caused her to lose the leg originally, after she'd had a skin infection that kept getting worse and that had finally gone to the bone. An ointment of homeopathic *Calendula* and *Hypericum* was recommended as a natural alternative. She returned the following day very happy to report that the remedy had caused the open sore to heal overnight, without cutting or drugs.

TO STOP BLEEDING. A remarkable Chinese formula that stops bleeding when nothing else seems to work is *Yunnan Pai Yao*. It was used by Vietnamese soldiers, who put the powder on their wounds to avoid leaving a bloody trail when they got shot. It can be taken orally (two capsules every hour until bleeding stops) or applied topically to the wound. Even severe cuts will heal in just a few days—but faith is required. At first, the wound gets inflamed and looks infected, but this purging is followed by rapid healing.

Sliced Finger Healed in Four Days

A cook at a Mexican restaurant accidentally sliced off a chunk of his index finger. But he said he didn't have time to go to the hospital emergency room. Instead, the wound was cleaned and *Yunnan Pai Yao* was poured on it. When he returned four days later, he came with lunch, to show his appreciation for how well his finger had healed in such a short time.

FOR TRAUMA. *Arnica montana* is a highly effective homeopathic remedy for trauma and injury to the body.

When you need more than a single remedy, *Trauma* by CompliMed contains not only *arnica* but *bellis* for blunt trauma, *symphytum* for broken bones, *rhus tox* and *ruta grav* for muscle aches and pains, *calendula* to promote healing, and *hypericum* for nerve pain. It comes as a liquid and can either be taken orally or applied topically to the injury.

Other good topical homeopathic remedies for injuries include *Trauma One* and *Traumeel* (available either as a topical cream or as oral tablets and drops). *Trauma One* contains *arnica* to stop the body from overreacting to trauma, *bellis* for blunt trauma, *chamomilla* for stress, to relax and calm, *echinacea* to build the immune system, *hypericum* for nerve pain, *calendula* to promote healing, *rhus tox* for muscle pain and stiffness, *ruta grav* for sore muscles and tenderness, and *symphytum* to promote bone healing (for broken bones).

Arnica also comes as an oil, gel, cream or ointment, great for a massage to relax sore muscles after an injury or workout. *CAUTION: Never apply to broken skin.*

FOR SPRAINED ANKLES. Sprained ankles have been known to heal with remarkable speed using this combination approach:

1. Take *Trauma* orally, 10 drops every 15 minutes for one hour, then 10 drops every hour for 4 hours, then 4 times daily.

2. Apply the Chinese patent formula *Te Tah Wan* to the sprained ankle or injury. The remedy comes as a waxed ball containing an herbal paste wrapped in cellophane. Open the ball, remove the paste, add a few drops of water, and heat to a smooth consistency. Paint the ankle or injury with the paste, cover it, and keep it covered for 24 hours.

3. To further promote healing, try applying magnets to the acupuncture points above and below the injury.

FOR BURNS AND SUNBURN. Homeopathic *Cantharis* and *Causticum* are effective remedies for burns.

"Untreatable" Road Burn Healed

A man in excruciating pain said he had skidded along the road in a motorcycle accident and had "roadburn" over the top half of his body. He "couldn't get away from the pain," but his doctor said there was nothing to be done. The man was given three pills of *Causticum 30x*. Within minutes, he said the pain had eased. In a day there was remarkable visible improvement, and in a week the burn was almost totally gone. The man was enormously grateful for the speed with which it had healed.

Flu

The "flu" is a very contagious upper respiratory infection caused by the Influenza virus. Symptoms include generalized achiness with a runny nose, sneezing, cough, headache, sore throat, weakness, chills, fever, and possibly vomiting and diarrhea. Flu epidemics hit most frequently in the winter or early spring and are responsible for 30,000 deaths a year in the United States.

CONVENTIONAL PREVENTION AND TREATMENT

Because the flu is caused by a virus, antibiotics won't work on it. The usual treatment is simply rest with plenty of fluids and a painkiller such as *Tylenol*.

WARNING: Children with flu should not take aspirin, due to the risk of Reye's syndrome. See "Fever."

For prevention, *flu shots* are heavily promoted; but the flu shot is specific for certain strains and won't work on "surprise" epidemics of unanticipated strains. Julian Whitaker, M.D., warns strongly against this prophylactic measure in any case. Unlike for childhood diseases, in which a single course of vaccination is considered good for a lifetime, flu shots must be repeated every year; and tampering with the immune system is risky business. Fifty percent of people who get the shots, according to some studies, have complications; and for a small percentage, they can be life-threatening. In anticipation of a swine-flu epidemic in 1976, a vaccine aimed at that scourge caused thousands of cases of Guillain-Barre syndrome, a very serious neurological disease that can be fatal; yet the swine-flu epidemic never hit. There are safer and more effective ways to prevent flu.[314]

NUTRITIONAL ALTERNATIVES

Dr. Whitaker observes that in a Canadian study, taking vitamins and minerals cut the incidence of sick days by nearly 50 percent—more than with the flu shot, without side effects or risks. An excellent preventative is the *Jarrow Pak Plus*, a comprehensive vitamin/mineral/herbal supplement that covers the gamut of these requirements.

A specific nutrient shown to cut flu incidence nearly in half in elderly and chronically ill people is *N-acetylcysteine (NAC)*. In a study reported in 1997 involving more than 200 people, the percentage getting flu symptoms dropped from 51 percent to 29 percent in those taking NAC; and in people who did get symptoms, severity and duration were significantly reduced.[315]

Flu Cycle Broken with Vitamins and Minerals

Jerry, a 32-year-old contractor who works outdoors in the cold, complained that he was prone to getting severe flus and colds lasting six to eight weeks every winter. He started taking the Jarrow Pak and, each time he returned for more, was excited to report that he hadn't yet gotten sick. He was able to negotiate the entire winter season without catching either the flu or colds.

HOMEOPATHIC REMEDIES

Homeopathic *Oscillococcinum*, the largest selling flu remedy in France, was shown in a clinical study to be significantly better than placebo in treating the flu.[316] The remedy comes in a package containing six little tubes of tiny granules. The best way to use it is to take one tube at the onset of symptoms, then put another tube in a glass of water and sip it slowly over the next six hours. Boiron, the manufacturer, recommends taking one tube every week during flu season as a preventative instead of flu shots.

A cheaper alternative that is good to take when you first feel you are getting sick is Dolisos *Cold and Flu Solution Plus*. Take one tablet every 15 minutes for the first hour, then one every hour for four hours, then one pill four times a day.

The German homeopathic company Staufen also makes a number of effective influenza remedies specific for each year. Other options are *Influenza* by Complimed and *Virus* by Deseret.

Heart Symptoms Reversed with Flu Remedy

A dramatic case involved a man who had never been well since he had the flu in 1983. He had heart symptoms and palpitations and was short of breath. Staufen's homeopathic *Flu 1983* caused all his symptoms to disappear.

HERBAL AND OTHER NATURAL ALTERNATIVES

Herbs are also good for preventing and treating flus and colds, including *echinacea, garlic, goldenseal, ginger,* and *peppermint.* An extract of the herb elderberry was shown in an Israeli study to cut recovery times from the flu in half.[317]

Sleep, fluids, and stress control are also important. For other remedies to boost the immune system, see "Colds and Infection, Immunity."

Food Poisoning, Salmonella

Food poisoning is on the increase. Symptoms usually appear within hours of eating infected foods and include nausea, vomiting, and diarrhea. Many strains of bacteria can be responsible. The highly publicized deaths of children who ate meat at a popular fast-food chain in Seattle were traced to *E. coli.* The other leading offender is *Salmonella.* Sometimes the infectious agent is never known.

Antibiotic overuse is blamed for the increasingly serious nature of this problem. Antibiotics are routinely fed to animals to increase their growth, giving antibiotic-resistant strains an opportunity to develop. If you ingest one of these strains when you happen to be taking an antibiotic, the drug will wipe out all but the resistant bacteria. These bacteria will then take over in the gut, resulting in a "superinfection" that can be life-threatening.

CONVENTIONAL TREATMENT

The conventional approach is to treat food poisoning with more antibiotics. But antibiotic-resistant strains of the responsible bacteria are also on the increase, and antibiotic-resistant bacterial infections aren't easily treated. This is particularly true if the bacteria have developed a resistance to the "broad-spectrum" antibiotics, leaving your doctor with the difficult task of determining which of a range of elusive infectious agents he or she is dealing with.

HOMEOPATHIC TREATMENT

Homeopathic remedies are quite effective for treating food poisoning. Particularly good is a German homeopathic remedy in ampule form called *Salmonella* by Staufen. A good combination product is *Salmonella* by Hanna Kroeger. An effective single remedy for salmonella and other food poisonings with cramping, diarrhea, and nausea is *Arsenicum Alba* 6c to 30c. Take two pills every hour for four hours. (See also "Diarrhea," "Nausea, Vomiting.")

Food Poisoning Relieved Homeopathically

A 34-year-old woman had just spent four days in the hospital with severe diarrhea, nausea, and vomiting and had been released feeling no better than when she was admitted. The hospital personnel were certain she had some form of food poisoning, but they weren't sure how to treat it because they weren't sure of its cause. Within four hours of taking the German remedy *Salmonella* by Staufen, she felt much better. By the next day, all of her gastrointestinal symptoms were gone. Her son, though not nearly as sick as she was, had also had diarrhea for two weeks and was given a dose of the same remedy. His diarrhea also cleared.

Two sisters who had gotten sick in a restaurant and had suffered with gastrointestinal complaints for two days before seeking a remedy were given Hanna Kroeger's homeopathic *Salmonella* and also reported feeling better within hours.

Fungal Infections, Athlete's Foot, Jock Itch

Athlete's foot and *jock itch* are fungal infections that get their names from the fact that they tend to get picked up in gyms. Athlete's foot manifests as a rash or patch of cracked, scaly, very itchy skin. Jock itch is the same fungus spread to the groin.

Fungal infections can also affect other parts of the body. *Onychomycosis*, a painful fungal disease of the toenails and fingernails, particularly affects the elderly and has increased by a factor of four in the last 20 years. In one survey, it struck nearly half of patients over 70.

Difficult-to-treat fungus cases are generally a sign of systemic infection with *Candida albicans*. They indicate that the immune system is impaired. (See "Candidiasis.")

DRUG TREATMENT

Antifungal creams such as *Tinactin* or *Lotrimin* are the conventional remedies for athlete's foot and jock itch. For best results, soak the feet for ten minutes in warm salt water before applying the cream. Over-the-counter antihistamines may also give symptomatic relief.

For onychomycosis, the drugs used until recently were griseofulvin and *ketoconazole*; but side effects ranging from annoying to serious, along with a high relapse rate, made doctors reluctant to prescribe them. A new line of broad-spectrum oral antifungal agents are promoted as working quickly and safely on fungal conditions. The drugs include *itraconazole (Sporanox), terbinafine (Lamasil),* and *fluconazole (Diflucan).*[318] New research indicates, however, that these drugs, too, can be hazardous; and they're very expensive and need to be taken for months. The popular Diflucan has been linked to a remote but serious risk of liver damage. (See "Candidiasis.")

NATURAL ALTERNATIVES

A currently popular natural anti-infective that is less toxic than drugs is *colloidal silver* (silver suspended in a liquid medium). It can be used topically as a spray or taken orally if the spray is insufficient to eliminate symptoms. It works in difficult cases, but like antifungal drugs, it doesn't necessarily cure the problem for good; and while it doesn't have serious reported side effects like the drugs, silver is still a heavy metal, with unknown long-term effects.

Other natural topical agents that effectively kill fungi and parasites without side effects are *tea tree oil* and a combination Chinese product called *Wo oil*. Wo oil may also be used for cleaning under the nails with a scrub brush to help eliminate parasites.

Homeopathic fungus remedies can boost your immune system sufficiently to allow it to eliminate fungal infections permanently. Effective options include FNG by Deseret and *Fungisode* and *Molds, Yeast and Dust* by Molecular Biologicals.

Elusive Fungus Cured Homeopathically

Lynette had a distressing fungus under her arms, contracted after using a particular deodorant. The colloidal silver spray eliminated her symptoms, but the infection kept coming back. The problem went away permanently after she took homeopathic *FNG*.

PREVENTION

Recommended measures for preventing athlete's foot and jock itch include drying your groin and feet thoroughly with a towel or with a low-set blow dryer (dry the feet last if using a towel to avoid spreading the fungus), putting antifungal powder in shoes and on the feet, showering in sandals, changing shoes and socks frequently, and wearing loose-fitting cotton boxers rather than tight-fitting briefs.[319]

For prevention and treatment of Candida, see "Candidiasis."

Gallbladder Disease, Gallstones

The gallbladder is a small organ located on the upper-right-side of the abdomen under the liver. It stores bile, which is excreted by the liver to break down fats in the digestive tract. Ninety percent of all gallbladder problems are due to gallstones, which afflict 20 million Americans. Gallstones result when cholesterol precipitates out from the bile and forms crystals. Minerals, bile pigments, and calcium are then deposited around the crystals. Symptoms of acute inflammation of the gallbladder include severe steady pain and tenderness in the gallbladder area, nausea and vomiting, jaundice, and fever. An acute attack is often precipitated by a large fatty meal and is typically described as a sudden, severe pain in the gallbladder area that radiates to the back between the shoulder blades.

Epidemiological studies suggest that gallstones are largely a disease of civilization. Americans, with a high incidence of stones, have bile that is nearly saturated or supersaturated with cholesterol. The bile of rural Africans and Japanese, by contrast, is almost always highly unsaturated. The late Denis Burkitt, M.D., a renowned medical missionary-researcher-clinician, stated that during his twenty years of surgery in Africa, he removed only two gallbladders from Africans, at a time when Americans were losing those organs at the rate of 1,000 per week.

CONVENTIONAL TREATMENT

Gallstones are so common that at one time, the gallbladders of symptom-free patients were removed by some doctors just as a preventive measure. But enthusiasm for the surgery was tempered when a landmark 1982 study found that most people with gallstones never develop symptoms. A review published in the February 1993 *New England Journal of Medicine* found that even for people with recurrent gallstone pain, the problem may resolve spontaneously without surgery after several months. Intolerance to fatty foods, bloating, and flatulence are often attributed to gallstones, but the only symptoms for which surgery is now considered medically necessary are a specific type of abdominal pain called biliary colic (a steady pain in the upper right side of the abdomen) and jaundice.[320]

In the 1980s, alternatives to surgery were developed that destroy gallstones with strong drugs or shock waves. But gallbladder surgery may still be considered preferable, because unless the gallbladder itself is removed, the gallstones will often return. Stones cause pain when they get stuck in the bile duct. This can't happen when the gallbladder has been removed, because the bile is then secreted directly into the intestines.

THE SURGICAL ALTERNATIVE

Gallbladder surgeries jumped by 20 percent after 1988, rising to the third most popular major operation in the country after Caesarean section and hysterectomy. Not that gallbladder disease had suddenly increased; the operation just became more marketable. 1988 was the year laparscopic cholestcystectomy was introduced. This "band-aid" surgery involves only a tiny cut instead of the six-inch abdominal incision required for standard gallbladder surgery, substantially reducing pain and recovery time. Enthusiasm for it, too, was tempered, however, when the complication rate suddenly skyrocketed. Surgeons were learning to perform the surgery at weekend seminars and returning to do it on their patients. Laparoscopic surgery, it seems, is much more sophisticated than the old operation, since the internal organs are no longer exposed to plain view. Because the surgeon has to "see" through a laparoscope, errors can go undetected. The patient may be sewn back up while potentially fatal bleeding continues inside.[321]

THE APPROACH OF ORIENTAL MEDICINE

Risks of the procedure aside, Oriental doctors maintain that gallbladder surgery merely compounds the patient's problems and worsens his or her symptoms, by throwing the gallbladder meridian further out of balance. Western medicine diagnoses gallbladder disease only when the condition is so acute that surgery is already necessitated. In Chinese medical practice, diagnosis is made long before the gallbladder is in such serious condition that it needs to be removed. Early warning signs include belching, burping, nausea, and problems digesting fat or fried foods.

LiDan by K'an is a classic Chinese formula that dissolves stones without surgery. The remedy is appropriate for people who have problems digesting fat and who feel worse after a fatty meal. It should be used for approximately three weeks, and may be followed by the Gallbladder Flush (see page 181).

Another herbal formula, called *LiDan Pian*, has been used by the Chinese for thousands of years to dissolve gallstones. The formula, which is composed of pig bile, is anecdotally reported to be as effective as the prescription drug derived from ox bile, at much less cost (about $4 per week).

Gallbladder Surgery Avoided with Chinese Remedy

A distraught woman sought a remedy after getting a sonogram indicating that she had gallstones. Gallbladder surgery had been scheduled for a few days later, but she said she would do anything to avoid it. She postponed her surgery and took the *LiDan* herbal liquid faithfully for four weeks. Then she had another sonogram. The result so surprised her doctor that the woman asked for a copy of the report: It indicated that her stones had completely disappeared.

THE HOMEOPATHIC APPROACH

Homeopathic remedies can also reverse gallbladder disease before it becomes so acute as to require surgery. An excellent combination product is CompliMed's *Liver and Gallbladder Homeopathic Formula.* It can help even people who have had their gallbladders removed, since the problem is not with that organ alone but results when the gallbladder is deprived of energy from some other source, causing the organ to no longer work properly. The homeopathic formula rebalances the body, clearing the energy field around the gallbladder area. The recommended dose is ten drops three times per day.

Stomach Ailments Relieved with Simple Remedies

Maria had been suffering for weeks from burping, bloating, stomach pains, low energy, heartburn, and nausea. She was awakening between 2 A.M. and 4 A.M. feeling anxious and unable to sleep. She said her first attack had begun after a lunch consisting of a large helping of French fries—the only thing she had eaten that day. On questioning, however, she recalled having had "stomach problems" off and on for years. She had never been able to eat a fatty meal without being uncomfortable for days afterwards.

Maria had seen a medical doctor, who had run tests; but he had found that her gallbladder, while inflamed, had no stones. He had therefore ruled it out as the source of her stomach problems. Instead, he had put her on a stomach acid-blocking drug called *Prilosec*. (See "Ulcers.") The drug had eased her symptoms somewhat, but it masked rather than addressed her underlying condition. In the ordinary course, her inflamed gallbladder would have continued to deteriorate until it needed to be removed.

To Chinese doctors, Maria's symptoms were the classic signs of first-stage gallbladder disease. The liver and gallbladder are considered to share energy. When the liver is in a state of excess (for example, in women with PMS), the gallbladder is in a state of deficiency. The "time of the liver" is from 2 A.M. to 4 A.M., a factor reflected in Maria's inability to sleep at that time.

She was given the Chinese herbal formula *LiDan* and CompliMed's *Liver and Gallbladder Homeopathic Formula*. Several days later, she reported that she was finally sleeping through the night and that her stomach symptoms and belching were gone.

THE GALLBLADDER FLUSH

The gallbladder flush is controversial. *The Encyclopedia of Natural Medicine* states that "stones" passed in this way are actually a complex of minerals, olive oil, and lemon formed within the gastrointestinal tract, and that large amounts of olive oil will contract the gallbladder and increase the likelihood of a stone blocking the bile duct.[322] Yet good resulted have been had with the gallbladder flush, particularly when preceded with a three-week course of *LiDan* to break up the stones.

Paul Pitchford's version of the gallbladder flush consists of sipping a mixture of two-thirds cup warm olive oil and one-third cup fresh lemon juice at bedtime, then sleeping on the right side. In the morning, the stones usually pass in the stool.

Dr. David Williams' protocol is a bit more complicated but seems to be more effective. It includes taking *Di Sodium Phosphate* (available to doctors from Standard Process. Follow these steps exactly:

1. Monday through Saturday noon, drink apple juice or apple cider to capacity (without sugar or additives and not from concentrate). Take vitamin and mineral supplements with meals. At noon on Saturday, eat a normal lunch.

2. Three hours later, take two teaspoons of Di Sodium Phosphate dissolved in an ounce of hot water. Follow with orange juice, if desired, for taste.

3. Two hours later, repeat Step 3.

4. Drink citrus fruit juices for dinner.

5. At bedtime, drink either 2 cups unrefined olive oil followed by grape-fruit juice or 2 cups warm unrefined olive oil blended with 2 cups lemon juice.

6. Go immediately to bed, lying for 2 hours on your right side with your knee pulled up close to your chest.

7. An hour before breakfast the next morning, take two teaspoons of Di Sodium Phosphate dissolved in two ounces of hot water. Eat normally thereafter.

Full Recovery from Pain

Dan, 47, was a restaurant owner who had sold his business so he could ski all winter. But he had been forced to abandon that plan after he began experiencing serious pain in his neck and shoulders. His medical doctor had given him pain pills and muscle relaxants, but they didn't seem to help. Massage and chiropractic treatment had also given only temporary relief.

Dan's neck and shoulder pain was the key to his care. Digestive ills aren't the only signs of gallbladder ailments. Upper-back pain, shoulder pain, or abdominal pain are often-overlooked symptoms that can also signal the condition. CompliMed's *Liver and Gallbladder Homeopathic Formula* and a Gallbladder Flush resolved his pains and allowed him to return to the slopes.

DIETARY SOLUTIONS

Denis Burkitt, M.D., attributed the low incidence of gallbladder disease among rural Africans to fiber. They eat enormous amounts of it, while Americans on refined-foods diets eat unnaturally little. Fiber binds bile acids in the intestines so that they can be eliminated in the stools rather than resorbed and returned to the liver. Since bile acids are made from cholesterol, more cholesterol must be used to replace its loss in the bile, leaving less cholesterol available for forming stones.

A drug called chenodeoxycholic acid, derived from ox bile, is often given to dissolve gallstones, but it has side effects and is expensive. Cereal fiber in the diet increases the production of chenodeoxycholic acid naturally, helping to keep bile in solution.

Fortunately, to increase your fiber intake, you don't have to dump indigestible wheat bran on your foods. Cellulose, another class of beneficial fiber, is found in such tasty foods as cantaloupe, bananas, apples, and other fruits and vegetables.[323] Dr. Burkitt's dietary suggestions for avoiding gallstones (as well as diverticulosis, kidney stones, and many other "Western" diseases) included substituting complex carbohydrates for fiber-depleted carbohydrates (white sugar and white flour). Complex carbohydrates include whole-grain breads (wheat, rye, oats, corn, and millet), whole-grain cereals (wheat bran, oat bran, and corn bran), and high-fiber vegetables (potatoes, carrots, beans, Brussels sprouts, and onions).

Certain specific foods are also beneficial for preventing and treating gallstones. There is evidence that soybean products not only guard against stones but dissolve those that have already formed.[324]

Paul Pitchford, in *Healing with Whole Foods*, recommends apples (particularly green apples) to help soften stones; radishes to help remove stones and deposits from the gallbladder; and pears, parsnips, seaweed, lemon, limes and turmeric to hasten gallstone removal. He also suggests a two-month course of three to five cups of chamomile tea daily, along with five teaspoons of fresh flax oil added to food.[325]

Gastritis, Heartburn, Esophageal Reflux, Hiatal Hernia

Gastritis, or inflammation of the stomach lining, can produce indigestion, diarrhea, and stomach pain. *Esophageal reflux* is a digestive complaint resulting when acid escapes from the stomach into the esophagus. A hiatal hernia results when the esophagus becomes herniated, or pushed out, usually from eating something large and hard to swallow. A common offender is the popular antibiotic *Vibramycin (doxycycline)*, a large pill that can injure the esophagus. *Heartburn* is a burning feeling in the chest near the heart, sometimes mistaken for a heart attack. Heartburn actually has nothing to do with the heart but results when stomach acid enters the esophagus.

WARNING: A heart attack can also be mistaken for heartburn. You should call your doctor if you experience heartburn symptoms along with shortness of breath, problems swallowing, sweating, dizziness, vomiting, diarrhea, fever, bloody stools, or severe abdominal pain.

CONVENTIONAL TREATMENT

Faced with evidence that ulcers are caused by the bacterium *H. pylori* and are curable with antibiotics, manufacturers of the H_2-blockers (*Tagamet, Zantac, Pepcid,* and the like), are now promoting their blockbuster drugs for symptomatic relief of gastritis and other less serious stomach complaints. The H_2-blockers work by blocking the flow of stomach acid. The problem with using these drugs for gastric distress is that this symptom is often caused by *insufficient* stomach acid. (See "Indigestion.") In those cases, the H_2-blockers are merely augmenting the condition. In any case, the drugs, which need to be taken repeatedly, aren't addressing the underlying problem. New research indicates that *H. pylori* can be responsible not only for ulcers but for gastritis that doesn't reach the ulcer stage.[326] H_2-blockers are also expensive and can have insidious long-term side effects. (See "Ulcers.")

NATURAL ALTERNATIVES

For gastritis and indigestion, many herbal remedies are available. Particularly good are the Chinese herbal formula Pill *Curing, peppermint oil* (add a couple of drops to warm water), *peppermint tea, ginger tea,* or a slice of *ginger* boiled in water. For other remedies, see "Indigestion" and the Appendix.

For heartburn, Boiron and Hylands both make homeopathic products called Heartburn that are effective. For many people, heartburn is aggravated by carbohydrates and soft drinks. Some people have reported that their heartburn resolved on an Atkins-type diet, high in protein and low in carbohydrates. Another useful suggestion is to wear looser jeans. Tight pants are thought to contribute to heartburn by forcing acid into the esophagus.

For hiatal hernia, several patients have reported that a nutritional remedy called *Probioplex* by Metagenics healed their hernias in a week or two. Take one to two tablespoons three times a day for one to two weeks.

STUBBORN HIATAL HERNIA HEALED
WITH NATURAL PRODUCT

A 52-year-old man complained of chronic heartburn and a stubborn hiatal hernia that had afflicted him for over a year. He began taking *Probioplex* by Metagenics. A week later he returned to report the amazing results: for the first time in a year, he hadn't had any pain or sensation in that area. He felt his hiatal hernia was completely healed.

Genital Herpes

The *Herpes simplex* virus belongs to the group of large DNA viruses that includes *varicella-zoster virus*, *Epstein-Barr virus*, and *cytomegalovirus*. Herpes lesions are painful, recurring blisters that break and form crusty sores, shedding millions of viruses that are extremely contagious. The disease can promote cervical cancer in women and can kill infants who contract it from their mothers at birth. Half the victims of neonatal herpes die, and half the survivors develop serious brain damage or blindness. Genital herpes is usually caused by the Herpes simplex virus-2 (HSV-2). However, it is increasingly caused by the virus that causes cold sores, HSV-1. HSV-2, in turn, can be responsible for blisters on the mouth. (See "Cold Sores.")

To prevent spreading the disease, infected people need to be able to recognize a recurrence when it hits and to studiously avoid sexual contact while the lesions are present. The viruses may emerge before the blisters do, but there is often a feeling of tingling, itching, or general ill health that warns of an impending outbreak.

DRUG TREATMENT

There is no effective conventional cure for genital herpes. Symptoms can be reduced by an expensive drug called *acyclovir (Zovirax)*, at least on the first attack. For patients with frequent recurrences, acyclovir is sometimes given orally three to five times a day and topically up to every three hours. This regimen can reduce the frequency of recurrences by as much as 75 percent; but it doesn't prevent them, and its long-term safety and effectiveness are unknown. *WARNING: Acyclovir should not be used by women who are pregnant or who might become pregnant.*

Anesthetics aren't recommended for herpes, even though the lesions can be very painful. The lesions need to be kept clean and dry, and anesthetics can counteract the desired drying effect.[327]

NATURAL ALTERNATIVES

The most popular natural treatment for herpes is the amino acid *L-lysine*.

Lysine works, and it's definitely preferable to Zovirax; but it still addresses only the symptoms. A German homeopathic remedy by Staufen called *Herpes Simplex* actually clears the disease in patients with frequent, recurring herpes outbreaks.

If the Staufen remedy doesn't work, the problem is likely to be due to a staph/strep infection inside the herpes lesions. The bacteria are taking over after a breakout. For these cases, a remedy called *Staph-Strep* by Staufen needs to be taken in combination with the *Herpes Simplex* homeopathic.

Treatment with these remedies is generally followed by a particularly bad outbreak, but this is a good sign: The virus, which sits on the nerve endings, is being cleared from the body. This healing crisis is liable to occur any time from a week after treatment is started to a week or two after it is completed. The longer the disease has been suppressed with drugs, the worse the outbreak is likely to be; but after that, outbreaks generally cease or are limited to a few manageable incidents when under unusual stress.

People with occasional minor outbreaks report that *Cliniskin H* by CompliMed is also effective, taken at a dosage of ten drops every fifteen minutes at the onset for one or two hours. If the remedy is taken before the lesions actually manifest, they often won't break out at all. If taken after the outbreak, the remedy should be continued four times daily until the lesions are gone.

Herpes Cleared with Homeopathic Remedy

Two women seeking help for herpes complained they were having severe outbreaks every two weeks. They had tried everything, including L-lysine and ample doses of Zovirax, but nothing seemed to help. They were given the Staufen homeopathic remedy. Within two weeks both had unusually bad outbreaks (the homeopathic clearing). One woman never got another outbreak. The second woman did get one, when under unusual stress from a wedding; but she reported that this incident, which formerly would have been incapacitating, was minor and manageable.

RELAXATION TECHNIQUES

Meditation and positive thinking may also help keep outbreaks under control. Studies have confirmed anecdotal evidence linking outbreaks to psychological stress. In one study, the stress of taking a medical-school exam was found to activate latent herpes. Another study found that men who were anxious, depressed, or lonely had higher levels of herpes antibodies in their blood than did men who were in better spirits. Since antibody levels go up during periods of reactivation, higher levels are thought to reflect a depressed immune system that is unable to keep the virus under control.[328]

Genital Warts

A million cases of genital warts are reported each year. They can occur, among other places, on the anus, penis, urethra, vulva, vagina, or cervix. Genital warts are caused by infection with the human papilloma virus (HPV), which is linked to genital cancer; and they can significantly increase the risk of cervical cancer. Genital warts are sexually transmitted, but the source is sometimes hard to trace, since the warts may not show up for 2 to 18 months after exposure. In one study of women aged 15 to 50, HPV was found in 10 percent of those with normal Pap results and in 35 to 40 percent of those with abnormal smears.

CONVENTIONAL TREATMENT

Genital warts are easily removed with topical drugs, laser surgery, or freezing. The problem is the high rate of recurrence. Removing the warts doesn't eliminate the virus, which can remain latent in the skin. Repeated treatments may be necessary.[329]

Recommended preventive measures include abstention, regular checkups and condoms; but there is some evidence that HPV is so small that it can penetrate a condom and may be transmitted through it.

HOMEOPATHIC TREATMENT

A German homeopathic remedy called *Condylomata* by Staufen clears not only the warts themselves but the underlying infection. The remedy should be taken at the rate of one ampule every three days for a month. Any warts that have been burned off are liable to reappear, but don't panic; that's how the remedy clears the virus from the body. Sex should be avoided during this process, since infections that have reached the surface of the skin can be contagious.

Although no clinical studies are available to prove it, homeopaths feel that clearing the system of HPV in this way also substantially reduces the risk of contracting cervical cancer.

Shocking Infestation of Genital Warts Cleared

A woman confided that her vagina had been covered with hundreds of warts, described by her appalled gynecologist as the most rampant case he'd ever seen. The woman had also suffered from chronic fatigue syndrome for years. Her system was so run down that she had no immune reserves left to fight off the virus. She had previously undergone a series of extremely painful laser treatments to burn the warts off, but they had now returned. When the Staufen homeopathic remedy further aggravated them, she wasn't too happy, but she was assured that it was merely a cleansing and that the warts would go away. To her relief, in about two months they did, and they have not returned.

Gingivitis, Periodontal (Gum) Disease

Periodontal or *gum disease* results when the "periodontium" (the gum tissue and bone supporting the teeth) becomes inflamed, attracts bacteria, and becomes infected. Other names for periodontal disease or closely related conditions include *pyorrhea, gingivitis, trench mouth,* and *periodontitis.* If allowed to progress untreated, the gum fibers that hold the teeth in place may disintegrate. In the worst-case scenario, the teeth can actually fall out.

CONVENTIONAL TREATMENT

Periodontists treat the condition by scraping tartar or calculus (hard stone-like deposits) from the teeth and their roots and curetting the gum tissue. Surgery is done in advanced cases to eliminate pockets of infection and irritants. Gingivectomy involves actually cutting away gum tissue. Open-flap surgery is done to eliminate deep infection. Where the bone has been eaten away, bone grafting is performed. Downsides of these procedures are that they are lengthy, uncomfortable, and require a high degree of technical skill. Scraping the gums can take from four to eight hours. Common complications of periodontal surgery include sensitivity of the teeth to heat, cold, and sweets caused by the additional exposure of the roots; and an unesthetic appearance of the teeth, which tend to retain food around them after meals.

THE HERBAL ALTERNATIVE

A simple home alternative that can obviate the need for these drastic invasive procedures is *tea tree oil.* Applied topically, it has produced quite remarkable results in all kinds of gum or periodontal problems. If the gums are receding, it can be applied directly to the gums. Tea tree oil toothpaste can also help.

"Irreversible" Gum Disease Reversed

Tea tree oil was recommended to a patient who sought help for *lichen plantus,* a common fungal gum disease that her dentist had pronounced incurable. She couldn't believe the result and neither could her dentist: The tea-tree oil made the condition completely disappear.

OTHER NATURAL OPTIONS

Bleeding gums usually indicate vitamin C deficiency. Supplementing with this vitamin should be pursued before resorting to anything more invasive, since it usually cures the condition. Recommended dosage is 2,000 to 4,000 mg a day. The gums should improve in about two weeks.

A good combination homeopathic product for all types of gum problems is *Gum Therapy* by Quantum.

For relief from toothache and dental trauma, see "Toothache."

Glaucoma

Glaucoma is estimated to affect at least two million Americans and to be responsible for $1.9 billion in medical costs annually. The condition is characterized by an increase in pressure within the eyeball sufficient to damage the optic nerve, which carries images from the eye to the brain. Visual loss caused by glaucoma can lead progressively to blindness; but the rate of visual loss among people with ocular hypertension is so low that it's hard to estimate how many would actually experience blindness in their lifetimes, with or without treatment.[330]

Causes of glaucoma include injury, cataracts, and inflammation in the eye. Glaucoma can also be caused by drugs, including steroids and certain drugs that dilate the pupils. An Italian study found that the use of corticosteroid eye drops increased the risk of developing ocular hypertension or glaucoma by *700 percent. Corticosteroids increase fluid pressure in the eye, making them the primary iatrogenic (drug-induced) cause of glaucoma.* Not only steroids dropped in the eyes but those taken by mouth or applied to the skin, including steroids in asthma inhalers and low-dose topical steroids to treat eczema, have been implicated. Mild corticosteroids can produce glaucoma within months, while more potent steroids can produce it within weeks; and up to a third of these drug-induced cases are irreversible.[331] Other drugs known to be toxic to the optic nerve include ibuprofen, aspirin, tranquilizers, antidepressants, antidiabetic drugs, and certain antibiotics.

New research indicates that the primary cause of most cases of glaucoma is actually vascular disease. It's systemic rather than a local condition. That means the ideal treatment is not to the eyes but by measures that balance and support the whole body.[332]

DRUG TREATMENT

To avoid blindness, a lifelong daily drug regimen is conventionally prescribed. But the drugs have disturbing side effects, and the most common type of glaucoma—chronic or open-angle glaucoma—is asymptomatic, causing no pain or immediate disability. As a result, glaucoma patients can lose interest in taking their medications, a temptation as many as half of them fall into.

To foster patient compliance, ophthalmologists felt it was particularly important to find a drug that was easily administered and had few side effects. *Timolol (Timoptic)*, a beta-blocker approved for opthalmologic use in 1978, seemed to be the answer. Its most popular predecessor, *pilocarpine*, generally had to be administered four times a day and caused side effects including burning and stinging on application, brow aches, and visual disturbances. Timolol and its companion beta-blockers, *betaxolol* and *levobunolol*, had few eye-related side effects, and they had to be administered only once or twice a day.[333]

Timolol soon became the most commonly used anti-glaucoma medicine in the world. But while its local side effects were minimal, it proved to have serious systemic side effects. By 1987, 2,000 cases of systemic toxicity from timolol had been reported to the National Registry of Drug-Induced Ocular Side Effects. These side effects were the same as those seen with beta-blockers taken orally, including severe heart and breathing problems, low blood pressure and slowed heartbeat, acute suicidal depression, and major personality disorders requiring hospitalization, even death from heart failure or acute asthmatic attack.

Drugs dropped into the eyes reach the general circulation. And since the contact time with the eye is often only a fraction of a minute, eye medications are highly concentrated. They drain rapidly back into the mucus membranes of the nose, where they can enter the bloodstream and reach the heart, lungs and other organs without being detoxified.[334] Unfortunately, the eyedrop drugs considered most indispensable—those for the treatment of glaucoma—are also those that can do the most damage.

Ironically, there is now evidence that anti-glaucoma eyedrops actually contribute to glaucoma. All of these drugs (as well as many other eyedrops and contact-lens-cleaning solutions) use the preservative benzalkonium chloride, which enhances absorption of the medicine by making the cornea more permeable. As long as the cornea is permeable (leaky), it can't heal itself. The preservative accumulates, producing toxic effects that further damage the eye.

Compounding the problem is the fact that diagnosis of glaucoma is difficult. Tests comparing the diagnoses even of trained ophthalmologists have found widely differing results. Visual-fields tests, requiring the patient to respond to a flashing light, are confusing to the elderly. Patients who fail the test run the risk of being put on a drug regimen that, if they didn't have glaucoma to start with, may precipitate its development. A Center for Health Care Policy Research report concluded there is no solid evidence that medical therapy for open-angle glaucoma or ocular hypertension reduces the risk or progression of field defects and that medical therapy subjects patients to unnecessary risks and is a waste of money.[335]

Meanwhile, timolol remains the conventional drug of choice for glaucoma. It is not recommended, however, for patients with asthma or a history of asthma, chronic obstructive pulmonary disease, cardiovascular disease, or those taking oral beta-blocking drugs.[336]

THE NATURAL WHOLE-BODY APPROACH

New research indicates that ocular hypertension has the same causes as ordinary hypertension, and that it should be treated in the same way—by measures designed to ease fluid pressure throughout the body. Timolol, a beta-blocker, is a blood-pressure-lowering drug, but better than using drugs is dietary change and nutritional supplementation to support the body's own efforts at normalizing fluid pressure. (See "Hypertension.")

Recommended dietary measures include a largely vegetarian diet that adds cold-water fish and eggs. A 1949 Duke University study found that greater reductions in eye-fluid pressure could be brought about by a low-fat rice-based diet than by drugs.[337]

An herbal supplement that reduces ocular pressure is *coleus*. A variety of mint used by ancient Hindu practitioners for disorders including asthma, heart disease, and high blood pressure, it can be purchased in oral capsule form under the ayurvedic Indian name *forskohlii*. Recommended dosage is 200 to 400 mg daily.

Another natural pressure-lowering supplement is magnesium, called "nature's calcium channel blocker." The recommended dose is 400 mg daily.

Bill Sardi, who wrote an excellent series of articles on glaucoma, also recommends the following daily supplements: vitamin B12 (1,500 to 2,500 mg), vitamin C (500 to 1,000 mg), vitamin E (400 IU), coenzyme Q10 (30 mg), beta carotene (25,000 to 40,000 IU), zinc (15 to 25 mg),

N-acetyl cysteine (200 to 600 mg), ginkgo biloba (100 to 240 mg), omega 3/omega 6 oils (1,000 to 3,000 mg), vitamin B6 (50 mg), vitamin B1 (25 to 50 mg), folic acid (400 mcg), quercetin (500 mg), choline (100 mg), and ginger (100 mg). Other recommended measures include to limit alcohol and saturated fat (meat and milk products), eat five servings of fresh fruits and vegetables daily, exercise, lose weight, wear UV-blocking sunglasses, and avoid optic nerve toxins—steroids, aspartame, tobacco, and certain drugs.[338]

Gonorrhea

Around one million cases of gonorrhea are reported each year, but the actual annual incidence is estimated to be at least twice that figure. Homosexual men are at highest risk. Thirty percent of those who visit VD clinics are found to have the infection. In women, untreated gonorrhea can lead to infertility or pelvic inflammatory disease.

Another potential complication is *gonococcal arthritis,* the most common form of arthritis caused by an infectious agent. The first symptoms are fever, chills, and body aches. If left untreated, the condition develops into full-blown arthritis, with rapid destruction of cartilage and bone.

Gonorrhea may produce no symptoms; but if they appear, they develop one to three weeks after exposure. They include difficult or painful urination and, in men, penile discharge; or in women, a yellowish vaginal discharge, bleeding between periods or after intercourse, and pain in the pelvic area during intercourse. Gonorrhea isn't detectable by Pap smear but requires other specialized tests.

DRUG TREATMENT

Gonorrhea was once easily treated with penicillin, but antibiotic-resistant strains have increasingly frustrated standard treatment. The availability of other antibiotics still makes it 95 percent curable, but in many areas, only one or two effective drugs are now available, and these may soon be obsolete.[339] (See "Infection.")

Homeopathic Treatment

Homeopaths warn that even when treated with antibiotics, gonorrhea can result in "miasms"—deep, lingering, chronic conditions that are transmitted to offspring and affect the overall health of both parent and child for the rest of their lives. Children of a parent with gonorrhea often have psychotic tendencies. Homeopathic remedies clear the miasms along with the disease.

Gonorrhea victims are required by law to see a doctor, who must report each case to the health department. As a result, patients diagnosed with gonorrhea generally wind up on antibiotics. But even if antibiotics are used, homeopaths maintain that homeopathic treatment should be sought from a qualified practitioner, to resolve not just the infection but any inherited miasms contributing to it. The practitioner will choose the appropriate constitutional remedies based on a detailed patient history.

Prevention

Condoms, diaphragms, and spermicides containing nonoxynol-9 may help reduce the spread of the disease, but nonoxynol-9 is a synthetic estrogen mimic that can have other side effects. (See "Uterine Prolapse," "Bladder Infection.") The safest course remains abstinence or careful selection of sexual partners.

Gout

Gout, or gouty arthritis, is an arthritic condition producing an acute pain in the joints. It is caused by a faulty processing of uric acid, resulting in an accumulation of uric-acid crystals in body tissues. Repeated attacks can lead to destruction of bone. The typical attack involves a sudden severe pain in a joint—the big toe, ankle or knee—usually in the early morning. The joint swells and the skin over it turns purple. The pain tends to go away during the day and to come back at night, lasting for about a week. Gout affects one percent of Americans, 95 percent of them men. Genetics is a factor, and so is diet. Uric acid and its salts are the end products of the breakdown of nucleoproteins, which come primarily from ingested animal products.[340]

People often have gout without realizing it. It is often misdiagnosed as simple knee or foot pain. If your feet hurt with your first steps in the morning, you may have gout.

DRUG TREATMENT

Aspirin, the conventional first treatment for arthritis, merely exacerbates gout, since it causes the *retention* of uric acid. Other nonsteroidal *anti-inflammatory drugs,* however, don't have this effect and may be used. For acute attacks of gout that don't respond to milder drugs, *corticosteroids* may be used.

For long-term treatment, the drug most often prescribed is *allopurinol,* which stops the formation of stones and slows kidney damage by reducing the uric acid in the blood. Its drawbacks are that it can trigger acute attacks of gout when first used, and it can produce rash, hives, sleepiness, upset stomach, diarrhea, and headache. Alternative drugs include *phenylbutazone, indomethacin,* and *colchicine.* Colchicine, a derivative of the meadow saffron plant, is the least toxic and has been used for centuries by gout sufferers.

THE CHERRY CURE

Cherry juice is a dramatically effective gout treatment. It stops uric-acid crystals from forming. For prevention, eat 10 to 15 cherries each day or drink cherry juice.

Remarkable Cherry Cures

A 45-year-old contractor would not let his wife, a professional reflexologist, give him a foot massage because it was so uncomfortable. His knees had hurt for ten or twelve years, but he hadn't thought of gout. When it was suggested as a possibility and cherries were suggested as a remedy, he tried them. Within three days, his knees had stopped hurting; and about a week later, he enjoyed his first foot massage. When he stopped eating the cherries a couple of weeks later, his knee pain came back. He reports that his knees give him no trouble as long as he keeps eating cherries.

Another man had been so crippled with chronic gout that he had been relegated for years to a wheelchair. A week after he was advised to start eating cherries, he was up and about. "My God," he said in disbelief, "I can walk after all these years."

HOMEOPATHIC OPTIONS

Cherries work for prevention, but for an acute attack of gout, something more will be needed. An excellent homeopathic regimen includes the remedies *Belladonna 6c, Colchicum 6c,* and *Nux Vomica 6c.* Take them as follows: three tablets of Belladonna 6c, followed 30 to 60 minutes later with three tablets of *Colchicum 6c,* followed 30 minutes later with three tablets of *Nux Vomica 6c.* Acute attacks are generally relieved in about two hours. Repeat this routine two to three times daily for three days.

Arthritis by BHI is a combination homeopathic that can also help alleviate pain and swelling.

Gout Symptoms Disappear in Two Hours

A woman limped in complaining of a pain in her toe that she'd had for three weeks. She hadn't known what it was until someone suggested gout. She was given the three homeopathic remedies for gout and reported that all of her symptoms and pain were gone in two hours.

OTHER HERBAL AND NUTRITIONAL REMEDIES

Andrew Weil, M.D., recommends *burdock tea* to retard the formation of crystals and clean the blood. Burdock-root capsules can also be taken (two capsules three times a daily).

Celery seed capsules or tea are an effective herbal gout remedy.

Dietary change is recommended to reduce uric-acid production. Many studies have shown the value of a diet free of meat, the major dietary source of uric acid, in relieving both gout and kidney stones.[341] Liver, kidney, brains, and sardines are particularly high in nucleoproteins. Alcohol should also be avoided. Although these foods don't cause gout, they're notorious for provoking acute attacks, particularly when they are overindulged.

Grief

Chinese and homeopathic doctors distinguish grief from clinical depression and treat each differently. Clinical depression is a low emotional state without apparent cause. Grief has a definite cause: a death in the family or other serious loss.

DRUG TREATMENT

Sedatives are typically given to the grief-stricken, and on a temporary basis they can help. But the drugs mask rather than support the grieving process, a cycle that needs to be worked through. Sedatives can drug grief and depression away, but the underlying problem will remain unless the sufferer talks it out and resolves it emotionally.

NATURAL ALTERNATIVES

The Chinese believe that unexpressed grief damages the lungs. While admittedly this sounds like nonsense, anecdotal observations of widows suggest that they do have more lung and breathing problems than other people do, and that these problems generally begin within about a year of their husband's funerals. The wife has had to be strong, make the funeral arrangements, take care of financial matters. She has had no time to grieve; she has work to do. Problems with her health tend to begin about a year later.

Homeopathic *Ignatia* is a natural remedy that can help support and encourage the grieving process. Women who have taken it during a divorce, breakup with a boyfriend, or death in the family report that it has helped them deal with their grief in a constructive way, without sedating the emotions or causing drowsiness.

Skullcap and Oats is an herbal combination product that induces relaxation and calms anxiety. It can be taken as needed, two droppersful at a time.

Rescue Remedy is a Bach flower remedy that is good for any emotional upset. Add four drops to a bottle of water and sip throughout the day.

Grief Dispelled with the Aid of Simple Remedies

A 25-year-old woman was distraught over the illness of her father and the breakup of her three-year relationship with her boyfriend, which had both hit the same week. She could not stop crying even long enough to tell her story. She took *Ignatia 200c* (three pills five times daily), along with *Rescue Remedy* and *Skullcap and Oats*. Two days later, she was another person. She said she felt as if the weight of the world had been lifted from her shoulders. The situation had not changed, but she was handling it better.

*H*air Loss, Dandruff

Hair loss afflicts 35 million American men and 20 million women. For nearly half of all males, it begins in the teens, twenties, or thirties; men collectively spend about $2 billion a year trying to reverse it. Male pattern baldness is linked with genetics and the male sex hormone testosterone. Testosterone combines with a certain enzyme to produce dihydrotestosterone, which inhibits hair follicle function. Female pattern baldness is related to declining levels of female hormones and a relative increase in testosterone. Hair loss can also be caused by drugs (particularly chemotherapeutic agents), scarring from radiation, poor thyroid function, skin disease, stress, poor nutrition, parasites, and high doses of vitamin A. In women, certain hair styles and hair products are also among the usual suspects, including tight ponytails or buns, curling irons and blow dryers, and harsh chemicals in dyes and sprays.

Chronic *dandruff* can also result in hair loss. Dandruff is a condition of the scalp involving the shedding of white flakes of dead skin, commonly caused by a disorder of the sebaceous glands. Other causes are trauma, hormone imbalance, poor diet, and excess sugar.[342]

DRUG TREATMENT FOR HAIR LOSS

The most popular pharmaceutical answer to hair loss is a drug called *minoxidol (Rogaine)* used topically to restore hair growth. Originally prescribed to lower blood pressure, the drug's hair-growing potential was discovered by accident by patients taking it in tablet form. Rogaine was approved for over-the-counter sale for hair loss in March of 1996, but despite substantial hype, it has not proved to be a miracle cure for reversing time's ravages. In controlled trials, it produced "dense" hair growth in only 8 percent of users after a year's application, and only 16 percent found regrowth sufficient to continue the treatment. Some men experienced severe itching, and the long-term effects of the drug are unknown. Up to eight months may be required before effects are noticeable enough to know if the drug will work, and it has to be applied daily for life to keep up its effects, an investment of $45 to $55 per month.[343]

CHINESE HERBS

A natural alternative that is not only cheaper but is claimed by users to be more effective is the Chinese patent formula *Sheng Fa*. The formula will do little for the scalp so bald as to be shiny, but it has quite remarkable effects at early stages of hair loss. The recommended course of treatment is four pills twice daily over a four-month period.

Full Head of Hair Regained

Thomas, 62, sought a hair potion three months after he had taken antibiotics for pneumonia. The drugs had caused a substantial portion of his hair to fall out, and the hair that was left was thin and dull. Two months after completing a four-month treatment with *Sheng Fa*, he returned to show off his beautiful, thick head of hair. He maintained it was fuller and had more body and curl than it had in thirty years.

A man who was nearly bald at the tender age of 25 also reported being delighted with *Sheng Fa*, which had given him back a full head of shiny black hair.

OTHER NATURAL ALTERNATIVES

Natural hormones can stimulate hair growth. Women losing their hair report that applying one-quarter teaspoon of *natural progesterone cream (Pro-Gest)* to their scalps each night has resulted in hair that is thick and lustrous.

An herbal hair product sold in beauty salons that has produced dramatic results is one called *Nixion*. It comes in the form of a shampoo, conditioner, and scalp treatment.

For dandruff, *tea-tree oil shampoos* are available that are very effective. *Evening primrose oil pills* are also recommended as a nutritional supplement at bedtime.

Vitamin products are available that are specially formulated for the hair. Nature's Plus makes *Ultra Hair* capsules. For people who don't like taking pills, it also comes in the form of a tasty morning drink.

The amino acid *cysteine* can promote not only hair growth but hair curl.

Chemotherapy-induced Hair Loss Reversed

At 58, Sheila had lost all of her hair to chemotherapy. She said cysteine caused it to grow back with more body and curl than it had even in her teenage years. At 64, she has beautiful hair that is still her most striking feature.

Headaches, Migraine Headaches, Cluster Headaches

Headaches are rarely life-threatening; but severe, recurrent headaches can prompt thoughts of suicide. Every year, more than 45 million Americans get headaches, and more than $4 billion are spent on analgesics to mask their symptoms.

More than 90 percent of these manifestations are simple *tension headaches.* Tension constricts blood vessels in the head. Tension headaches can be a symptom of anxiety, stress, or physical tension, lack of sleep, overconsumption of caffeine, food allergy, eye strain, fever, hypoglycemia, drug side effects, PMS, dehydration, or trauma. Tension headaches are typically dull and persistent, affecting both sides of the head.

Migraine headaches, on the other hand, are usually on one side of the head. They are severe, recurrent headaches typically accompanied by nausea, vomiting, "auras" (visual disturbances), lightheadedness, intolerance to light, and numbness or tingling in the head or arms. Attacks last 4 to 72 hours and hit an average of one to four times a month. About 17 percent of American women and 6 percent of men get them. Heredity is a factor; one or both parents of most migraine sufferers suffered with them as well.

While migraines mainly affect women, *cluster headaches* mainly affect men. They tend not to last as long as migraines, but the pain can be as severe. They are usually localized on one side of the head and occur in clusters over a period of weeks or months, as in the spring or fall.[344]

NOTE: Sudden severe headaches can indicate something more serious, for example, hemorrhage or bleeding inside the brain. A severe headache with stiff neck and fever could indicate meningitis or meningoencephalitis. Other danger signals are headaches that begin after exertion, straining, coughing, or sexual activity; or those that are accompanied by changes in mental state, drowsiness, confusion, or memory loss.

CONVENTIONAL TREATMENT

Most tension headaches are treated with over-the-counter analgesics (*aspirin, acetaminophen, ibuprofen*). For habitual users, however, the drugs can become progressively less effective and can precipitate a syndrome of "rebound headaches." The sufferer pops more analgesics, but the headache never really goes away. The result is a constant dull headache perpetuated by the drugs intended to relieve it. Over-the-counter analgesics have other unwanted side effects as well. (See "Pain.")

To treat migraines and cluster headaches, prescription drugs are often used. Drugs for cluster headaches include *methysergide (Sansert), corticosteroids* and *ergotamine.* For migraines, *Sumatriptan (Imitrex), ergotamine tartrate,* or *dihydroergotamine (DHE)* may be prescribed.

Imitrex, which is particularly popular, changes serotonin levels in the brain. By 1995, Imitrex was being used by more than two million people worldwide. However, the FDA had received 3,526 voluntary reports by then of suspected side effects, including 83 deaths and at least 273 life-threatening complications. Lawsuits followed. Safety concerns eventually prompted the manufacturer to change its labeling to emphasize that Imitrex should be used only when a doctor has clearly established that a patient is suffering from migraine, and that it should "not be given to patients in whom unrecognized coronary artery disease is likely without a prior evaluation for underlying cardiovascular disease." The question is, how do you recognize patients likely to have "unrecognized" coronary artery disease? Deaths of people who were apparently healthy and had no heart disease detectable even at autopsy have been blamed on the drug. Research also suggests that Imitrex can gradually damage heart vessels in otherwise healthy people.[345]

In July of 1996, a group of Los Angeles physicians reported what appeared to be a safe, inexpensive alternative: a few drops of a solution containing *lidocaine*, a local anesthetic commonly used to treat hemorrhoids and sunburn, placed in the nose. This remedy was found to relieve migraines in 5 to 15 minutes in 55 percent of 81 patients tested. The lidocaine mixture costs only a few cents, compared to $35 for an injection of Imitrex, and the mixture reportedly has no major side effects. One problem with this small study was that the drug wasn't used repeatedly on the same patients. Lidocaine has produced even more impressive initial results with cluster headaches, only to get progressively less effective with each use, apparently because the patient develops a tolerance to it.[346]

Other drugs may be prescribed to prevent migraines, including beta-blockers, calcium-channel blockers, and certain antidepressants and anticonvulsant drugs; but none is very effective for this purpose.

NATURAL ALTERNATIVES

For migraines, the herb *feverfew* has been touted as a miracle cure that can eliminate the need for drugs. British researchers have found that the herb not only cuts the number and severity of headaches but reduces the nausea that goes with them. Feverfew suppresses the release of prostaglandins and histamines, which produce inflammation. In one study, migraine victims who took feverfew capsules for six months were relatively free of migraines, while victims taking a placebo had three times the normal incidence of them. In another study, the herb reduced the incidence of migraines by 25 percent and their severity dramatically.[347]

For simple headaches, simple relaxation can also be effective. Muscle-contraction headaches, including common migraines, may respond to easy neck stretches. Move your head to one side and then the other, resisting against the palm of your hand. If that doesn't work, try rubbing your forehead with *peppermint oil*. This natural antispasmodic and diuretic has been shown in German research to be as effective as Extra-Strength Tylenol in easing tension headaches.[348]

The old-fashioned ice pack to the forehead also works—in about the same amount of time it takes an analgesic to kick in. The ice constricts the swollen blood vessels that cause the head to ache.[349] If the ice pack isn't enough, some sufferers find relief by putting their arms in ice water up to the elbows.

For sinus headaches, hot compresses can relieve pain.

The herbal form of aspirin is *willow bark*. Used by Chinese physicians 2,500 years ago, it contains salicin, nearly the same pain reliever as in aspirin. Another herbal aspirin is *meadowsweet tea*. These herbal options can be just as effective as aspirin at much lower risk. *Magnesium* supplements have also been found to reduce nerve excitability and migraine susceptibility. Low levels of magnesium result in increased nerve cell excitability and pain.[350]

Acupuncture and EMG biofeedback have both been used successfully in the treatment of tension and migraine headaches. Physical therapy, self-hypnosis, and relaxation can also offer relief.[351]

TREATING THE CAUSE

The ideal solution to intractable headaches is to find and eliminate the cause. Migraines may follow particular triggers. They can often be tracked by keeping a log of your headaches and correlating them with your habits. In some women, migraine attacks are linked to the menstrual cycle, suggesting a hormonal cause. Migraines can also be triggered by stress, changes in eating or sleep habits, certain drugs, or environmental irritants. Chocolate, alcohol, caffeine, monosodium glutamate, aged cheese, red wine, artificial sweeteners, nitrites (found in cured meats such as hot dogs, bacon, ham and salami), nicotine, and certain drugs have all precipitated headaches. Migraines have also been blamed on "reactive hypoglycemia"—the plunge in serum insulin levels that follows a precipitous rise after you overdose on sugar.

Other cases of migraine have been traced to detoxing from the materials used in dental restorations. Mercury amalgam is the usual suspect; but Dr. Robert Marshall, a holistic health practitioner in Torrance, California, reports that he has also seen cases in which chronic migraine headaches began with the placing of plastic-composite dental fillings. The condition resolved only when the composites were replaced with a biocompatible material called Degussa high-fusing ceramic, which is almost identical in composition to the human tooth.[352]

Headaches can also be caused by a misaligned bite. Temporomandibular joint dysfunction (TMJ) is a dental condition that results from irritation of the disk connecting the jaw to the skull. If this is your problem, before you succumb to expensive mouth reconstruction, try making a studied effort to relax your jaw. Tension can throw your bite off, resulting in headaches. Your dentist can also fit you with a mouthpiece to wear at night to relieve jaw tension. (See "Temporomandibular Joint Dysfunction.")

Homeopathic remedies are another effective way to reach the cause of recurring headaches.

Remedies that Get to the Root of the Problem

For 24 years, Mary had suffered with severe migraines every week, involving nausea and vomiting for two or three days at a time. She had taken every conceivable drug for them, including Prozac and Imitrex, but nothing worked. The Imitrex was effective at first, but she had to keep increasing the dose, until she was up to 10 or 12 injections per headache. At $40 per injection, this was a prohibitively expensive proposition.

Mary's problem appeared to be emotional. She wasn't getting along well with her husband. She had been married for 24 years—only a few months longer than she had suffered from migraines. Homeopathic remedies were recommended based on her particular symptoms: *Ignatia*, then *Chelidonium*, then *Staphysagria*, then *Lac Caninum*.

At first, the remedies aggravated Mary's emotional symptoms. She cried more. She saw what a disaster her marriage was, a fact she hadn't really faced before. She realized that her husband was treating her unfairly. She started to fight back. The homeopathic remedies re-balanced her life and her outlook. She was no longer attracted to a man who was out of balance in his.

Mary's marriage not only improved after she learned to express herself, but her migraines have decreased dramatically, to about one manageable headache a month. She is still working out her problems. Homeopathic remedies are helping her move past an emotional trap in which she had become "stuck."

CHOOSING THE RIGHT HOMEOPATHIC REMEDY

The remedies that worked for Mary wouldn't work for everyone. They were specific for her constitution. Finding the right remedies usually requires consulting a homeopathic physician, who will take a detailed patient history. You may, however, be able to recognize your symptoms from the following list. Take 3 pills of one of the options listed every 15 minutes for 8 doses. If no relief is felt, a different remedy is needed.

HOMEOPATHIC OPTIONS FOR TREATING MIGRAINES

- *Iris versicolar*—for classic migraine, usually right-sided; pain typically centered in the temple, above or below the eye; vomiting that gives no pain relief; blurred vision preceding headaches; a tight feeling in the scalp.

- *Lac caninum*—for headache on alternating sides, either during one attack or from one headache to the next; occipital headache radiating to the forehead.

- *Lac defloratum*—for migraine preceded by an aura or dim vision; worse with noise, light, menses; nausea and vomiting present with headache; frontal headache with nausea, vomiting and chills; headache better with cold applications, lying down, or in the dark.

- *Natrum muriaticum*—for the throbbing, blinding headache or migraine that can be felt in any location; often right-sided; "feels like a hammer beating the head"; headache from grief; numbness in face or lips; worse with light, in the sun, when reading, before or after menses, with noise, with head injury, between 10 A.M. and 3 P.M.; better lying in a dark, quiet room; better with perspiration and cold applications.

- *Sanguinaria*—for the migraine headache that is better after vomiting, with sleep, or after passing gas; migraine on the right side, typically beginning in the neck on the right side and extending to the forehead and eye.

HOMEOPATHIC OPTIONS FOR CLUSTER HEADACHES

- *Gloninum*—for the pulsating, bursting headache; headache with flushed face and pounding pulses/carotids (arteries in the neck); headache worse from the sun, or that comes and goes with the sun, even without direct exposure; worse from alcoholic drinks, motion, heat, jarring, tight collars; better with external pressure or when lying in the dark.

- *Belladonna*—for migraine that begins in occiput and radiates to the right temple or forehead, settling around the right eye; headache worse after a hair cut; head sensitive to cold, drafts, washing hair.

- *Lachesis*—for pulsating, bursting headache; left-sided headache that can be migraine; headache that begins on the left and moves to the right; headache that comes before the menstrual period and is better after the flow begins; headache with flushed feeling.

HOMEOPATHIC OPTIONS FOR TENSION HEADACHES

- *Aconite*—for the headache that comes on suddenly; headache after shock or fear, exposure to wind or cold; severe headache during fever.
- *Apis*—for head pain behind the left ear, extending to the left eye or temple; the brain feels tired or the head feels swollen; feeling of heat; throbbing pains; better with pressure; worse with motion.
- *Bryonia*—left-sided headache; headache over the left eye extending to the occiput, then to the whole head; worse from coughing, in the morning, when constipated, when ironing; better with pressure or with eyes closed.
- *Gelsenium*—for the headache beginning at the occiput or neck and radiating to the forehead; worse at 10 A.M.; better with urination; head feels very heavy.
- *Ignatia*—for the headache that is worse after sweets; headache pain like a nail driven into the head; headache after grief, characterized by sighing.
- *Coffea*—for headache resulting from coffee withdrawal, strong stimulation or strong emotions; headache worse with music, noise, footsteps; headache or migraine pain like a nail driven into the head.
- *Chamomilla*—for headache from tooth pain, teething, or earache.
- *Lycopodium*—for headache that's worse on the right side, worse from 4 P.M. to 8 P.M. or when trying to concentrate; pain as if temples are being screwed together.
- *Pulsatilla*—for headache or migraine that occurs at the end of the menstrual flow; headache that's worse with menopause, heat, sun; worse on exertion or after emotional stress; better with open air, cold applications, pressure; head pulsates or feels as if it's pressing outward.
- *Silicea*—for headache or migraine that begins in occiput and radiates to the forehead or right side of the head; worse from cold, drafts, mental exertion, menstruation, uncovering the head; better when lying with eyes closed or in the dark, or from warming or wrapping the body.

- *Arnica*—for headache from trauma or concussion; the head that feels bruised or has an aching, sharp pain; worse when stooping.
- *Hypericum*—for the bursting, aching headache; worse in damp and fog; headache from contusions or dental work.
- *Nux vomica*—for the headache of a hangover; worse with noise, light, mental activity, before menses; head highly sensitive to stimulation; allergy headache.

A Combination homeopathic remedy by CompliMed called *Migramed* helps relieve pain if taken at the onset of a migraine headache.

Head Lice

Six million Americans a year contract head lice. These very small but visible parasites live in the hair, cause the head to itch, and are highly contagious.

CONVENTIONAL TREATMENT

The usual treatment is with shampoos or lotions containing *lindane*, a chemical poison (formerly sold under the brand name *Kwell*). The problem is that this chemical is highly toxic not only to lice but to children, and because it's absorbed through the skin without being neutralized in the stomach, it can go right into the bloodstream. (See "Skin Problems.") Lindane is a suspected cause of seizures, brain damage, and worse.[353] Lindane shampoos are intended for use only once or twice. But many mothers become so frantic over the thought that their children have lice that they go overboard and start washing the whole body with it or using it repeatedly.

NATURAL ALTERNATIVES

A safe and effective herbal alternative is *tea tree oil*. Treatment involves putting it directly on the scalp (or on the body for body lice), leaving it for about 10 minutes, then washing off. About 20 drops can then be added to half a bottle of shampoo and used in the child's regular hair washings for a week or two after that.

Tea-Tree Oil Works Where Chemical Pesticide Fails

Two children who were relatives of one of the authors had head lice. Their mother had used Kwell on their heads, but the lice persisted. She wanted to use the drug again but was advised against it due to its toxicity. Instead, she tried applying tea-tree oil, using most of a ten-milliliter bottle for her two children. The rest was added to their shampoo. The lice completely disappeared.

Heart Attack

Heart attacks strike more than 1.5 million Americans a year and kill 500,000 of them. A heart attack is typically caused by the rapid formation of a blood clot, or "thrombus," which blocks the flow of blood in one of the coronary arteries. Clotting can be the result of atherosclerosis, heart-valve disease, inflammation, poor circulation, or extended bed rest.

In an informative January 1998 journal article, Wayne Martin observes that before 1925, heart attacks were practically unknown. Seventy years ago they were blamed on blood clots in the arteries and were called "coronary thrombosis." But *warfarin*, an anticoagulant that breaks up clots, didn't do much to prevent a second heart attack in people who had already had one. Attention therefore switched to cholesterol, and the disease was renamed "myocardial infarction." (See "Atherosclerosis.") When eating polyunsaturated liquid vegetable fats such as corn oil was found to reduce blood cholesterol somewhat, butter was abandoned *en masse* for margarine. Yet heart disease and heart attacks steadily increased.

Ironically, critics are now blaming the epidemic of heart attacks on the widespread use of polyunsaturated vegetable fats once thought to prevent them. Heart attack deaths have increased by a factor of 80 in the same time that polyunsaturated fat use has tripled. The problem with this fat is that the protective antioxidants have been removed during processing. Antioxidants are lost in the modern diet not only in commercial fats but in bleached flour and other processed foods. Homogenization and pasteurization of milk have also been linked to an increased risk of heart disease.

In 1980, cardiologists returned to their first theory and decided that sticky platelets and blood clots were the problem. Everyone over 40 was advised to take aspirin, an anticoagulant, to avoid a heart attack. But doctors began to reconsider this advice, too, when several trials with aspirin merely produced a run of ulcers without preventing heart attacks. Then a large American trial showed that regular aspirin use reduced heart attack incidence by 40 percent in male doctors. A daily aspirin again became the rage. But critics pointed to a subtle discrepancy in this study: Unlike those in which aspirin was ineffective, it used Bufferin, which contains magnesium. Magnesium is a natural vasodilator that reduces platelet adhesion independently of the effects of aspirin.[354]

DRUG TREATMENT

While drug treatment for heart attack prevention remains controversial, drugs for people in the throes of a heart attack have clearly saved lives. Not long ago, doctors couldn't do much to stop a heart attack once it was occurring. Now there are drugs that actually dissolve the clots that bring on a heart attack. Studies suggest that if these clot-dissolving drugs are used within hours of the first symptoms of an attack, deaths can be reduced by as much as 50 percent.[355]

What is controversial is what drug to use. The first contender was a bacterial protein called *streptokinase*. But streptokinase promotes bleeding throughout the body, putting patients at risk of bleeding to death from ordinary tissue damage.

High-tech genetic engineering then produced another clot-dissolving substance from human cells called *tissue plasminogen activator*, or TPA. TPA costs around $2,200 for a single course of therapy, compared to $200 for streptokinase; but TPA dissolves clots at a higher rate. It was therefore assumed to have the advantage that its clot-dissolving action would be more containable in the heart.[356] Studies reported in 1989 and 1990, however, found that the higher rate at which TPA dissolves clots doesn't correspond to a better outcome for heart attack patients.[357]

DRUGS FOR PREVENTION

For people not yet in the throes of a heart attack but at risk because of a tendency to form blood clots, *anticoagulants* are sometimes prescribed. But clinical trials with the anticoagulants *warfarin (Coumadin)* and *heparin* have failed to show an increase in patient survival. Apparently the drugs, while preventing new clots from forming, don't affect clots that are already there.

Meanwhile, the anticoagulants themselves are hazardous. *Warfarin and heparin must be taken exactly as prescribed, and they shouldn't be mixed with other drugs of any sort—prescription or nonprescription—without your doctor's knowledge and approval. Aspirin and warfarin are a particularly bad mix, since both thin the blood and increase bleeding. Acetaminophen used to be considered a safe alternative, but dire results have now been reported even with this combination.*[358]

In the face of these dangers, aspirin as an anticoagulant seemed a truly safe alternative. However, aspirin isn't the ideal solution either. Regular aspirin use can lead to ulcers and other adverse effects. And while a reduction in *heart attack* incidence has been shown in normal middle-aged men regularly using it, an increase in *overall survival* from this habit in this population has not been shown. One reason seems to be that while the drug reduces heart attacks, it also increases a certain type of stroke. When blood clotting is prevented, bleeding times are extended, sometimes to dangerous lengths. The risk of stroke from cerebral hemorrhage, or bleeding, then goes up.[359]

NATURAL ALTERNATIVES

Many natural substances are available that reduce platelet adhesion better than aspirin. Possibilities include *vitamin E* (at 400 IU per day), *vitamin B6* (at over 40 mg a day), *purple grape juice* (at 10 ounces a day), *fish oil*, the gamma linolenic acid in *evening primrose oil*, the oils of *onion* and *garlic*, and *ground ginger* (which, like aspirin, also reduces pain and is highly anti-inflammatory). *Quercitin*—a flavonoid antioxidant found in black tea, onions, and French wine—has also been shown to reduce heart attack deaths. Other nutritional supplements successfully used to treat heart disease include *coenzyme Q10* and *melatonin*. Newer strong antioxidants that are now available as pills include *N acetyl cysteine, alpha lipoic acid,* and *OPCs* or *pycnogenol.*

The British Medical Journal reported in 1997 that men who were deficient in *vitamin C* were 3.5 times more likely to suffer a heart attack than men whose vitamin C intakes were sufficient.[360]

The mineral *magnesium* also reduces heart attack risk. In a study published in the British medical journal *Lancet,* magnesium sulfate given intravenously to patients with suspected myocardial infarction reduced cardiovascular mortality by a remarkable 25 percent.[361]

Antioxidants can be obtained from foods: You just need to eat the whole food, not the processed version. Eat whole-grain bread, whole oatmeal, whole buckwheat, and so forth. Cut down on beef, avoid iron pills, and look for a certified raw-milk source.[362]

In the herbal line, *hawthorn berry* is a heart remedy that has been clinically proven to be effective. For that and other remedial options, see "Atherosclerosis."

HEART ATTACKS AND STRESS

Besides blood coagulation, there is an emotional element to a heart attack. The stereotypical victim grips his chest as he suffers some great shock or fright. Natural remedies can help alleviate this emotional factor. Bach flowers are vibrational remedies that are particularly good for treating emotional conditions. Compare the following two cases:

Heart Attack Precipitated by Surgical Stress

Before he was wheeled into the operating room, a 41-year-old man scheduled for heart surgery got into a violent argument with his brother over the need for the operation. Worse, the surgery was conducted an hour and a half earlier than scheduled, so the man's girlfriend, whom he was expecting, had not had a chance to arrive. The man was so upset when he entered the operating room that he had a heart attack on the table.

Rescue Remedy Called a Lifesaver

A European woman familiar with Bach flowers states that when her husband was in the throes of a heart attack, she gave him *Rescue Remedy*. The remedy calmed the panic induced by not being able to breathe. The man attributed his recovery from this crisis to his wife's ministrations with Bach flowers.

Heavy Metal Poisoning

Heavy metals that have accumulated in the brain have been linked to serious neurological disorders, including Alzheimer's disease, Parkinson's disease, and multiple sclerosis. The link has been established when victims recovered or improved after having the metals removed from their teeth and the residues removed from their tissues.[363]

Why some but not all people exposed to environmental toxins are afflicted with serious diseases may be explained in part by the "compounding effect." The effect was demonstrated in a recent study prompted by the mysterious Gulf War syndrome. When chickens were exposed to toxic chemicals, those exposed to only one chemical showed no outward signs of illness or debilitation. But chickens exposed to any two chemicals exhibited varying degrees of weight loss, diarrhea, shortness of breath, decreased activity, stumbling, leg weakness, and tremors. Chickens exposed to three chemicals showed the most severe symptoms, including total paralysis and death in some cases. *This was true although the total amount of chemicals to which the chickens were exposed was the same in each group.* It was the combination that evidently tipped the scales.[364]

Dr. H. Richard Casdorph and Dr. Morton Walker, in their book *Toxic Metal Syndrome*, state there is a threshold level beyond which toxic metals accumulate in the body. They cite a study involving aluminum-containing antacids. Patients ingesting less than five milligrams per day of aluminum remained in negative aluminum balance. But when the patients' diets were supplemented with antacids, the scales tipped the other way and aluminum was retained in their bodies. Other studies show that the neurotoxicity of aluminum is increased by exposure to mercury and other toxic metals.[365]

Interestingly, breast cancer has been reported to be eight times more likely to develop near where deodorant is applied than anywhere else on the breast. Aluminum is contained in most deodorants, and antiperspirants suppress sweating, trapping toxins inside. Fatty breast tissue is particularly efficient at storing toxins.

The first step in detoxification is to track down and eliminate the source. Usually this means a dental overhaul. But not all patients with MS and other heavy-metal related diseases who have had their silver/mercury amalgam fillings removed have gotten better. One explanation is that the replacement materials (usually plastic composites) can be as disturbing to the body's energy fields as the metals being replaced. Electro-dermal screening (discussed in Chapter 3) indicates that the only universally biocompatible filling material may be a little-known one called Degussa low-fusing ceramic. For a fuller discussion of this issue, see Ellen Brown, Richard Hansen, D.M.D., *The Key to Ultimate Health* (La Mirada, California: Advanced Health Research Publishing, 1998).

Eliminating toxic stressors from the teeth and environment is only half the battle. Toxic residues also need to be eliminated from the blood and tissues. Various natural remedies and detoxification programs are available that can aid this process. For general detoxification of the body, fasting is excellent (see "Aging, Longevity"); but fasting evidently won't eliminate heavy metals from the tissues. Something more is required.

THE NIACIN FLUSH

The niacin flush is a detox treatment that combines exercise and sauna or sweat therapy with the B vitamin niacin. A primary means of eliminating heavy metals from the body is through the skin by sweating. Niacin aids this process by dilating the capillaries. The face turns red and the skin turns hot as the niacin flushes out toxins. In a California study, participants undergoing this treatment experienced significant drops in blood pressure, improvements in vision, increases in IQ points, and lessening of the symptoms of a number of physical ailments, including asthma, allergy, migraine, and hypoglycemia. Participants also reported reexperiencing the smells and physical effects of drugs taken in the past.[366] The program was followed daily for a period of three weeks. It involved 20 to 30 minutes of vigorous exercise (jogging, stationary bicycling, rowing), followed by 30 minutes in the sauna, a 5-minute cooling-off period, then 30 more minutes in the sauna. Sauna times could be gradually increased to two hours. Niacin dosage began at 400 milligrams (mg) spread throughout the day. The dose was then increased gradually to as high as 6,000 mg, depending on tolerance.[367]

NOTE: The niacin "flush" can be quite intense. Test your tolerance gradually. At high doses, niacin should be taken only with medical supervision. Even 400 mg is a large dose; starting at 100 mg would seem more prudent. It's also important to balance niacin intake with a B-complex containing the other B vitamins.

CHELATION

Heavy metals can also be eliminated from the tissues and arteries through chelation—intravenous, oral, or homeopathic. A natural process in the body, chelation is the method by which metals necessary for body functions are transported through the body and in and out of cells. Iron in hemoglobin is a chelated metal; the chlorophyll in plants is a chelate of magnesium. Chelators are substances with extra electrons, or negative charges, that combine with the positive charges of a metal and hold it fast in a clawlike grip. ("Chele" means "claw" in Greek.) Temperature, acidity, and other environmental changes affect this grip, causing the release and exchange of metals, allowing them to be picked up, transported, and released as needed.

IV CHELATION WITH EDTA

EDTA (disodium ethylene diamine tetra-acetic acid) is a chelating substance that has long been used conventionally as a treatment for lead poisoning. Its effectiveness as a treatment for blocked arteries was discovered accidentally in the fifties, when a medical doctor named N. E. Clarke used EDTA to treat tenants in a World War II tenement house in Detroit who had come down with lead poisoning from the paint used on the building.[368] The patients were all elderly, and many had cardiovascular problems. To Dr. Clarke's surprise, when the lead was chelated out of their arteries, their cardiovascular troubles went away.

Ray Evers, M.D., an early pioneer of intravenous chelation therapy, analyzed the heavy metal levels in his patients through hair analysis and 24-hour urine tests. He found that the vast majority of them had some abnormality in heavy metal content, with lead and mercury usually being the highest. Elevated levels of lead were present in nearly all his arthritis patients. Remarkably, chelation successfully relieved their symptoms.

Dr. Evers also found that diseases of the cardiovascular system—the number-one cause of death in industrialized countries—were significantly alleviated with the therapy. These diseases are all caused by the same basic abnormality, a narrowing or closing off of the blood vessels. He postulated that the closing was caused by heavy metals that had built up in the vessels. Conditions that were helped by chelation included arteriosclerosis (hardening of the arteries of the heart), angina (chest pain), strokes and senility (hardening of the arteries of the brain), pain in the limbs (hardening of the arteries of the limbs), multiple sclerosis, cataracts, heart-valve calcification, bursitis, hypertension, scleroderma, emphysema, Parkinson's disease, and muscular dystrophy. Dr. Evers reported that 90 percent of his patients with these conditions experienced improvement, and 75 percent experienced virtually complete recovery.[369]

WARNING: Some authorities feel that intravenous chelation should not be done until all of the metals are out of the mouth. Otherwise, more metal will simply be pulled from the teeth into body tissues.

PRESCRIPTION ORAL CHELATORS

Several prescription drugs work as oral chelators. A 1997 study comparing the effectiveness of seven chelating agents in mobilizing mercury from renal tissue ranked their effectiveness as follows (from most to least): *DMPS, DMSA, penicillamine, 1,4-dithiothreitol, glutathione, lipoic acid,* and *EDTA.*[370] *DMPS (Dimaval)* and *DMSA (Chemet)* seem to be the safest and most promising. Dimaval is used in Europe for treating certain neurological disorders (ALS, MS). Both drugs are said to be safe even for young children. An oral DMSA dosage of 10 to 30 milligrams is recommended per kilogram of body weight. *NOTE: These chelators will also remove zinc, which should be supplemented during treatment. Glutathione, on the other hand, should* not *be taken during this treatment.*[371]

Autism and Hyperactivity Reversed with Oral Chelation

In *Turning Lead into Gold: How Heavy Metal Poisoning Can Affect Your Child and How to Prevent It* (Vancouver: New Star Books, 1995), Nancy Hallaway, R.N., and Zigurts Strauts, M.D., relate the remarkable saga of author Hallaway's two hyperactive, autistic children. Their conventional doctors had pronounced the condition hereditary and irreversible; but Dr. Zigurts ingeniously surmised that the problem was heavy metal poisoning resulting from a house remodeling and nearby freeway fumes. The children's symptoms were reversed simply by giving them an oral chelator called *Cuprimine (D-penicillamine).* A number of children in their neighborhood who were found to have the same condition were also helped by this prescription drug.

HERBAL CHELATORS

There are also natural oral chelators that are available over-the-counter and in the supermarket.

The *chlorophyll* in plants is a natural chelator. *Cilantro*, a leafy-green herb, is particularly effective.[372] The problem is finding a pure source. In the United States, most commercial cilantro has absorbed environmental toxins. An alternative option more likely to be uncontaminated is the freshwater algae *chlorella.* The recommended dose is ½ teaspoon a day, up to one-and-one-half teaspoons according to tolerance.

Other useful natural products are the *essential oils*, particularly *carvacrol oil* (essential oil of oregano). The "blood of the plant," essential oils are aromatic and volatile liquids extracted from plants through distillation. They help open deficient pathways in the electromagnetic network running through the body by oxygenating the tissues. A good mail-order source is Pacific Research Laboratories (310-320-1132).

Alpha-lipoic acid is a new and very powerful antioxidant that can bind to toxic metals, increasing the liver's detoxification and metabolic-enzyme production abilities. It is both water- and fat-soluble, so it can travel to and permeate all the cells of the body, including the brain. Present naturally in spinach, kidney, heart, skeletal muscle (beef), and broccoli, it can also be purchased in concentrated form as a supplement.[373]

HOMEOPATHIC CHELATION

Homeopathy is another chelating option. The chelating properties of homeopathic remedies were compellingly demonstrated in a laboratory study involving rats discussed in Chapter 3.[374]

A new line of combination homeopathic products has been designed specifically for neutralizing heavy metal poisoning, dental work, and environmental toxins. *Oratox* by Deseret is recommended for two or three weeks after dental work. Other Deseret combination homeopathics include *Enviroclenz* and *Metox*. A remedy by Apex called *Protomer* helps clear mercury from body tissues after its removal from the teeth. Other combination products are *Dental Detox* and *Amalgam* by PHP. For a case history demonstrating their effectiveness, see "Cholesterol, High." *Alumina* is good for metal detoxification and is particularly indicated in cases of senile dementia. Supplemental *zinc* is also good, to help counteract mercury and nickel absorption.

Hemorrhoids

Hemorrhoids are swollen blood vessels, or varicose veins, that form in the lower rectum or anus. They usually aren't painful, but they can bleed, itch, or protrude. Most adults get hemorrhoids at some time in their lives. They are aggravated by pregnancy, childbirth, and straining at stool. The typical American diet of refined foods, which lacks the fiber and bulk necessary for forming soft stools, contributes by causing constipation.[375]

DRUG TREATMENT

Preparation H has the $100-million-plus hemorrhoid market cornered, but both the FDA and the *Medical Letter* question its advertising claims. These authorities assert there is no acceptable evidence that Preparation H can shrink hemorrhoids, reduce inflammation, or heal injured tissue. Unfortunately, no other drugs seem to accomplish these feats any better. Not only do they not cure the condition; ointments and suppositories can make it worse, by aggravating the trouble and sensitizing the skin.[376]

The vasoconstrictors touted as shrinking hemorrhoids do constrict blood vessels. The problem is that the effect is only temporary. After a few days the drugs may produce a rebound effect, causing the blood vessels to become more dilated than before. Since these stimulant drugs are rapidly absorbed from the lining of the rectum, they can also cause significant side effects, including heart palpitations, sleeplessness, and paranoia.

Benzocaine, a local anesthetic found in products such as *Americaine* and *Lanacane,* can deaden feeling in the sensitive area. But again the relief is only temporary, and the drugs don't promote healing. In fact the anesthetic, which tends to be irritating, can actually prolong the healing process. It can also cause sensitization, rendering you allergic not only to benzocaine but to related anesthetics including the novocaine used by your dentist.[377]

Hemorrhoidal preparations often include agents for wound healing, but these too lack evidence of effectiveness and so do the hydrocortisone products widely marketed for rectal itch. The latter have the further drawback that if used for long, they can cause skin disorders.[378]

Your best pharmaceutical bets are old-fashioned *petroleum jelly* and *zinc oxide.* They don't treat the underlying problem, but they can ease anorectal pain and itch without significant side effects, and they can serve as a protective coating over the skin to prevent further irritation. Fortunately, uncomplicated external hemorrhoids usually go away by themselves in a couple of weeks without treatment.

If the problem persists—and particularly if you are bleeding from the rectum—see a doctor. Bleeding that is dark rather than bright red may be a symptom of colon cancer. Bleeding may also be related to ulcers.[379]

NATURAL REMEDIES

The Chinese have an effective patent remedy for hemorrhoids called *Fargelin for Piles.* The dosage is three pills three times a day. Users typically report that their pain and swelling have been relieved in a day and that hemorrhoids and symptoms are gone in three days. If the problem continues, it could be something more serious. In Chinese medicine, the Qi that holds the abdominal organs in place is weak, so everything falls. Organs prolapse, and the blood vessels bruise easily and bleed. To remedy this condition, it is best to see a homeopath or acupuncturist for individualized constitutional treatment.

Homeopathic remedies useful for hemorrhoids are *Hemorrhoid* by BHI, or *Hemorrhoids* by Boiron.

OTHER HELPFUL AIDS

Additional suggestions for easing hemorrhoidal discomfort include porous underwear that won't trap moisture, sitz baths, moist heat, rest, and cleanliness (though not with a harsh soap or antiseptic, which can be irritating). Most important is to correct the underlying problem, usually constipation. (See "Constipation.")

Hypertension (High Blood Pressure)

Nearly 50 million Americans, or one in four, have hypertension, a persistent elevation in blood pressure above the normal range (120/80). High blood pressure is a major risk factor for heart attacks, strokes, kidney failure, and blindness. Causes can include constricted arteries, a heart that's pumping too hard, or tired kidneys that are retaining fluid.

About half of all hypertensives take medication for it, and once hypertension is diagnosed, the drugs usually have to be taken two or three times a day for life. Since the average age at diagnosis is 50, that means the drugs are typically taken for 20 years or more. Bringing down the blood pressure is considered worth the sacrifice even if it means a loss of energy, loss of sex drive, and so forth, because high blood pressure has been found to be a major risk factor for heart disease and stroke. (See "Atherosclerosis.") The problem is that people with lower blood pressures in the studies reaching this result didn't get them from drugs. A careful review of studies in which these risk factors *have* been lowered with drugs indicates that *no* increase in survival has resulted, except in that limited group of high-risk patients who have already suffered a heart attack or stroke, or who have unusually high blood-pressure levels.[380] For the 75 percent of hypertensives who have only "mild" hypertension (defined as blood pressure above normal but below 160/90), drug treatment hasn't been proved to significantly increase survival. That category includes nearly 40 million Americans. Antihypertensive drugs have been prescribed for millions of them, although they felt fine before treatment and had no visible symptoms.

CONVENTIONAL TREATMENT

Drug treatment is aimed at bringing down the blood pressure by various means. Since all of these means involve disrupting natural functions, all of these drugs have side effects.

Diuretics work by causing the kidneys to increase the amount of water excreted. Different types of diuretics act on different parts of the kidney. Thiazide diuretics act on the kidney tubules. Loop diuretics act on the loop of Henle. Potassium-sparing diuretics act on the distal tubules. All of them pull water from the blood, decreasing blood volume and thus blood pressure. Diuretics have traditionally been considered the safest and most conservative first-choice treatment. However, they can cause weakness, dizziness, sexual dysfunction, impotence, gastrointestinal distress, rash, muscle cramps, and hearing impairment. In one major study, one out of three patients had to discontinue drug treatment because of intolerable side effects.[381] Diuretics can also increase blood sugar, uric-acid and serum-cholesterol levels, increasing the risk of diabetes, gout, and heart disease. Diabetes frequently develops during treatment with diuretics.[382]

Beta-blockers, the other first-line antihypertensives, cause the heart to beat more slowly by blocking nerve-receptor sites called "beta receptors," which are stimulated by adrenalin and adrenalin-like chemicals to work the heart. When these receptors are blocked, the brain can't signal the heart to beat faster or the arteries to constrict. Heart function is diminished, less blood is forced through the arteries, and blood pressure is reduced. Beta-blockers can cause drowsiness, dizziness, low blood pressure, nausea, weakness, diarrhea, numbness and coldness in fingers and toes, dry mouth and skin, impotence, insomnia, hallucinations, nightmares, headaches, bronchial asthma or difficult breathing, joint pains, confusion, depression, reduced alertness, and constipation.

These side effects are a direct result of the drugs' mode of action: beta-blockers slow the heart's pump. The brain tells the heart to beat faster and pump harder for a reason. In many people, it's because the arteries have become corroded with deposits of calcium and fat. These narrow the arterial openings, requiring a greater pressure to push enough blood through to keep the body running at normal levels. Any artificial reduction in this pressure will at least make you feel tired. At worst, it can weaken your heartbeat enough to cause heart failure. The depression caused by beta-blockers is also predictable: They kill the "adrenaline rush" that makes life exciting. They can trigger bronchial asthma by suppressing epinephrine, the natural chemical that opens up the bronchi or breathing tubes. (Epinephrine is often used to *treat* bronchial asthma.) Serious problems can also result if beta-blockers are withdrawn suddenly; so once you're on them, it's hard getting off. Beta-blockers may make sense for younger hypertensives whose condition is likely to be caused by a stress-induced stimulation of adrenalin, but they're not the ideal drug for the elderly, who comprise the majority of hypertensives. In older people, hypertension is more likely to be caused by calcified arteries. Blocking their adrenaline rush isn't going to calm them down. It's just going to slow them down. Older people are also more likely to suffer side effects from beta-blockers, since their drug clearance is slower; and the drugs aren't as effective in older as in younger people.[383]

The "second-line" drugs also have side effects. *Calcium channel blockers* or *calcium antagonists* work by interfering with the normal flow of calcium to the muscles and nerves, relaxing the arteries and reducing their resistance to blood flow. Although they are generally well tolerated, they can cause dizziness or lightheadedness. *Alpha blockers* block nerve receptors in the autonomic nervous system. They can cause a drop in blood pressure on standing suddenly. *Angiotensin-converting enzyme inhibitors (ACE inhibitors)* cause blood vessels to dilate by blocking the formation of a natural chemical called angiotensin II. Their most common side effect is a dry cough.

LONG-TERM EFFECTS OF DRUG TREATMENT

Drugs that make you feel better in the short term may be worth taking regardless of their effects over the long term, since they've relieved your pain in the meantime. But drugs that make you feel *worse* in the short term need to have some compelling and incontrovertible evidence behind them before reasonable people will risk their side effects. But convincing evidence of increased survival for mild hypertensives taking blood-pressure-lowering drugs has yet to be forthcoming.

Earlier studies did find an apparent survival benefit from drug treatment, but they were poorly controlled. The "treatment" group not only took drugs but modified their diets and lifestyles.[384] In later, better-controlled studies, the expected benefits have not been found. In some, it seems, antihypertensive drugs actually *decreased* overall survival. The Multiple Risk Factor Intervention Trial (MRFIT), reported in 1982, involved 12,866 men aged 35 to 57 considered to be at increased risk for CHD (coronary heart disease). Those in the treatment group received special care, involving both antihypertensive drugs and counseling to reduce smoking and alter their diets. The disturbing result was that deaths were actually *higher* in the *treatment* group. The difference wasn't statistically significant—it could have come about by chance—but the drugs clearly failed to save lives. And in men who weren't hypertensive at entry (and thus didn't get the drugs), the holistic changes in lifestyle *did* significantly reduce the CHD death rate—by 21 percent. It was only among the men who *were* hypertensive at entry (and thus got the drugs) that coronary heart disease deaths were greater than among the hypertensive controls. It seems the diuretics used to lower blood pressure also increased serum cholesterol and triglyceride levels. Thus they countered the effects of dietary change, which reduced these risk factors.[385]

The 1980 Oslo Study produced equally unsettling results. It involved nearly 800 mildly hypertensive but asymptomatic men aged 40 to 49 years. Half received drugs; half didn't. The patients were followed for five and a half years. Drug treatment reduced blood pressures an average of 17 mm Hg systolic and 10 mm Hg diastolic. Cerebrovascular events (strokes) occurred only in the control group, which received no drugs—an apparently good result, until it was observed that *CHD* incidence, including sudden death, was *50 percent higher* in the drug group than in the no-drug group. This was particularly disturbing, because *hypertensives are five times as likely to die of a heart attack as of a stroke.* The overall result, as in the 1982 MRFIT, was that there were 11 percent more deaths from all causes in the treated than the untreated group. Again, the difference wasn't statistically significant; but neither was the difference in the death rate from strokes. The drug-treated group simply traded the risk of a stroke for the risk of a heart attack—along with the unpleasant side effects of the drugs themselves.[386]

The Stockholm Metoprolol Post-Infarction Trial compared diuretics and beta-blockers. Patients who had already suffered a heart attack were found to be significantly more likely to have another one if they were on diuretics than if they were on beta-blockers, although both drugs lowered blood pressure to the same degree. In a second study involving 565 older hypertensive patients, the beta-blocker metoprolol also proved to be significantly safer and more effective than the diuretic hydrochlorothiazide.[387]

Why? One explanation may be that diuretics lower blood pressure by increasing fluid excretion. Valuable minerals are lost at the same time. Potassium is the most critical, since its loss can seriously affect the heart's electrical activity. Recent studies have shown that potassium actually helps *prevent* strokes, the dreaded scourge antihypertensive drugs are supposed to prevent. Drugs that deplete this mineral are therefore counterproductive, even if they do lower blood pressure. Diuretics also deplete magnesium, which is necessary to retain potassium in cells. If blood magnesium is low, cells become more permeable. Potassium leaks out, and sodium and calcium leak in. The cells become electrically unstable, producing irregular rhythms. In the worst case, this can mean sudden death.[388] In a 1980 Australian study, mortality among hypertensives treated with thiazide diuretics was found to be *twice* that in the other treatment groups, which included (1) the beta-blocker propanolol, (2) simple salt restriction, and (3) *a placebo*. In other words, *twice as many deaths occurred among hypertensives taking diuretics as among those receiving no treatment at all.*[389]

Concerns about the side effects of diuretics in the 1980s prompted the Joint National Committee on Detection, Evaluation and Treatment of High Blood Pressure to propose beta-blockers as the first step in stepped-care treatment.[390] But the ability of these drugs to increase survival hasn't been established either.

The British Medical Research Council study is considered the largest trial of its kind likely to be done in our time. It involved 17,354 mildly hypertensive patients (90–109 mm Hg diastolic) aged 35 to 64 years. They were treated either with a beta-blocker (propanolol), a diuretic (bendrofluazide), or a placebo. After five years, strokes were cut nearly in half by active treatment. However, the number of strokes in both groups was so low that this reduction was termed an "infrequent benefit." More troubling was the lack of an effect on CHD, the most serious and common complication of high blood pressure. Again, the overall result was that *no fewer patients died with drugs than without them.* It would have been a draw, except for the side effects of the drugs themselves. Both drugs caused impotence, lethargy, nausea, dizziness, and headache. The diuretic also caused impaired glucose tolerance (predisposing to diabetes), abnormally low potassium levels (predisposing to neuromuscular, kidney, and stomach disorders), gout, and constipation. The beta-blocker caused numbness and pain in the fingers and toes, rashes, and labored breathing.[391]

Problems with the old "first-line" drugs prompted the development of newer antihypertensives. By 1995, more prescriptions were written for calcium channel blockers, the current favorites, than for any other type of drug, including antibiotics. The manufacturer of a popular calcium channel blocker called isradipine was so confident of its product that it funded the Multicenter Isradipine Diuretic Atherosclerosis Study (MIDAS) to compare isradipine to the old-fashioned diuretic hydrochlorothiazide in treating hypertension and atherosclerosis. The results were published in the *Journal of the American Medical Association* in 1995. To the manufacturer's chagrin, the calcium channel blocker was associated with a *higher* incidence of angina, stroke, and other "major vascular events" than the diuretic, and the cheaper diuretic worked just as well as the calcium channel blocker for treating atherosclerosis. Before the end of the three-year study, several of the main investigators had quit, reportedly because the manufacturer had tried to control the presentation of results and had failed to highlight the negative clinical findings. This study, combined with others linking calcium channel blockers to an increase in heart disease and cancer, prompted the National Heart, Lung, and Blood Institute to issue a statement saying that beta-blockers and diuretics should continue to be the first-line treatment for high blood pressure and that calcium channel blockers should not be used unless the other two types proved ineffective.[392]

In September of 1995, a Dutch study published in the *Annals of Internal Medicine* again raised doubts about the wisdom of using beta-blockers and non-potassium-sparing diuretics. Compared to patients primarily treated with potassium-sparing diuretics, both of these drug types increased the risk of sudden cardiac death in hypertensive patients, reducing the drugs' projected survival benefits by as much as half. Patients on non-potassium-sparing diuretics had a 1.8 times greater risk of sudden cardiac death, while those receiving beta-blockers had a 1.7 times greater risk.[393]

THE CAUSE: TOO MUCH SALT—OR TOO LITTLE?

The problem with drugs that lower blood pressure is that they do it by blocking essential body functions. The ideal cure would eliminate the cause. But what causes high blood pressure has yet to be agreed upon. Nine out of ten people with the condition have what is called "essential hypertension." That means hypertension for which doctors don't know the cause. Sodium has long been a chief suspect. But a massive study called INTERSALT designed to substantiate the theory led researchers to conclude, "Salt has only small importance in hypertension."[394]

Dr. F. Batmanghelidj, M.D., in *Your Body's Many Cries for Water*, maintains that the body's tendency to retain salt is an effect rather than a cause of high blood pressure. The underlying problem, he says, is a lack of water. When the body lacks sufficient water, it compensates by reducing the openings of its main blood vessels and closing down its peripheral blood vessels, so the scant water that is left can service the whole system. The body retains salt in order to reduce water losses in urine and sweat. The result is an increase in blood pressure. Treating this condition with diuretics and a no-salt diet, says Dr. Batmanghelidj, "is wrong to the point of absurdity." The correct therapy is to drink *more water* (enough to equal half your body weight in ounces per day). You should also *increase* your intake of salt (preferably unheated salt), and get more exercise. (See Chapter 2.) Dr. Batmanghelidj has reproduced letters from a number of people in whom this therapy has produced dramatic cures, including the following:

Hypertension Cured with Water

Charles Ramsey, 58, was advised by his doctor to take antihypertensive medication when his blood pressure rose to 140–160/100–104. He increased his water intake instead. When his blood pressure was taken two weeks later, it had dropped to a remarkable 106/80 without medication.

Michael Peck reported that increasing his water intake to appropriate levels caused a 10-point drop in his blood pressure. He also lost 30 pounds, had fewer colds and flus, and was no longer bothered by asthma and allergies.

E. Michael Paturis lost 45 pounds and was able to abandon his blood pressure medication simply by increasing his water intake.

Walter F. Burmeister also got off his blood pressure medication by drinking more water. His pressure dropped without drugs from 150–160/95–98 to 130–135/75–80.[395]

DIETARY SOLUTIONS

Diet is another recognized factor in hypertension. Foods like fried fats, refined sugar and processed salt heated to high temperatures can contribute to a clogging of the arteries. Clogged arteries have narrower openings, requiring greater pressure to move blood through them. Deficiencies of *calcium, magnesium,* and *potassium*—nutrients found in fresh whole foods— have also been linked to high blood pressure.

In April of 1997, the *New England Journal of Medicine* reported the results of a landmark multicenter study sponsored by the National Institutes of Health. It found that blood pressure can be lowered as much by diet as by drugs, without side effects or risks. The antihypertensive diet used was rich in fruits, vegetables, and low-fat dairy products. Previous studies had demonstrated that reducing weight, salt, and alcohol can reduce blood pressure, but this study established that merely changing the diet can do it. The study was hailed as demonstrating the most significant improvement in life expectancy of any dietary intervention to date.[396]

For 11 weeks, the volunteers, who weren't on blood-pressure medication, ate standardized meals designed to stabilize their weight and salt intake. Daily servings were individualized but were along these lines: seven or eight servings of grain products; four or five of vegetables; four or five of fruits; two or three of low-fat or nonfat dairy foods; and one or two of meat, poultry and fish. The diet also included four or five weekly servings of nuts, seeds, and legumes and limited amounts of fat and sweets. The effects of the diet were apparent within one week and peaked within two weeks. For people with moderate hypertension, the average reduction in blood pressure was 11.4/5.5. More moderate reductions resulted when milk products were eliminated from the diet, suggesting an important role for calcium. Diuretics and calcium channel blockers work by increasing calcium retention. The researchers suggested that dairy products accomplish the same result naturally. This simple diet, if widely followed, they thought could reduce the risk of heart disease by 15 percent and the likelihood of stroke by 27 percent.[397]

This American study followed a more stringent Swedish study, in which hypertensive patients who were unhappy with the side effects of their drugs switched to a "vegan" diet, without animal products or salt. After one year, most of them had succeeded in abandoning their blood pressure medications entirely, while maintaining blood pressure levels that were lower than with drugs by a full 10 mm Hg diastolic.[398]

CAUTION: Consult your doctor before changing your current health plan. Don't abandon your antihypertensive medications without your doctor's advice.

HERBAL OPTIONS

Blood pressure can also be normalized without side effects by using medicinal herbs. One possibility is *hawthorn berry complex*. It has the advantage over drugs that it will lower blood pressure to normal but not below normal. Another possibility is *dandelion leaf,* an herb shown to have diuretic properties equivalent to those of Lasix, a popular diuretic drug.

CAUTION: Certain herbs including goldenseal, ginseng and licorice raise the blood pressure and should not be taken by people whose pressures are already high.

Blood Pressure Lowered with Herbs

A woman whose blood pressure hovered around 190/95 reported that after she started taking hawthorn berry extract, her blood pressure had dropped to a healthy 122/82 without drugs. It was checked weekly and remained consistently in that range—except once, when it shot back up. Questioned about what she had been doing, she said she was taking goldenseal root for a cold. She was switched to another herb (elderberry). Her blood pressure has remained normal ever since.

NUTRITIONAL SUPPLEMENTS

Nutritional supplements can also help lower blood pressure. One option is *coenzyme Q-10*. In a recent study from the University of Texas, Co Q-10 reduced blood pressure in about 85 percent of the 109 subjects studied. Nearly all of the participants were on antihypertensive medications at the beginning of the study, but by its conclusion, about 25 percent of them were able to control their blood pressures with Co Q-10 alone. The average dose given was 225 mg. The average blood pressure drop was from 159/94 to 147/85. Blood pressure fell within three to four months of beginning the supplement.

Another nutrient that can lower blood pressure is *magnesium,* called "Nature's calcium channel blocker." Hypertension is accompanied by low levels of magnesium, which seem to be a better predictor of disease risk than calcium or sodium levels.[399]

Other natural blood pressure regulators include *garlic* (for example, *Super Garlic 3x* by Metagenics) and *cayenne.*

OTHER FACTORS

Other factors linked to high blood pressure include obesity, stress, lack of exercise, smoking, alcohol, coffee, and tea.[400] Another link is with poisoning from heavy metals, including lead, cadmium, and mercury.

The major source of mercury in our bodies is the silver/mercury amalgam dental filling. A study comparing fifty 22-year-olds who had mercury amalgams to fifty-one 22-year-olds who did not have them found that blood pressures in the former group averaged six systolic points higher than in the latter group. The amalgamated subjects also had a greater incidence of chest pains, tachycardia (racing heart beat), anemia, fatigue, and loss of memory—and these were young adults. The difference undoubtedly gets greater over the half-century that it takes to develop "essential hypertension."[401]

Another cause of hypertension can be drugs. Potential culprits include diet pills, many cold remedies, and oral contraceptives.[402]

Exercise has been shown to lower blood pressure, and so has laughter.

RELAXATION TECHNIQUES

If your hypertension is the kind linked to tension, relaxation techniques may be your answer to beta-blockers. The sympathetic nervous system increases blood pressure as part of the fight-or-flight response to stress. Beta-blockers reduce blood pressure by blocking the activities of this regulatory system; but the same effect can be achieved without drugs, by simple techniques for letting go of tension.[403] Yoga, meditation, and biofeedback have all been shown to effectively lower blood pressure.[404]

Transcendental Meditation is a simplified Yoga technique that was popularized by the Beatles in the sixties. When meditators finally convinced researchers to study its effects, the technique was found to lower blood pressure from the borderline hypertensive range to normal.[405] Even better results have been reported for meditation reinforced by biofeedback, a technique that gives you continuous information about the state of your body. Electronic equipment tells you your blood pressure, your heart rate, your skin temperature, and the state of your brain-wave pattern. Just by knowing how these parameters vary, many people can learn to regulate them. In one study, 77 patients with high blood pressure were trained in biofeedback techniques for dilating the blood vessels in the hands and feet. Of those patients not on antihypertensive drugs, 70 percent were able to bring their blood pressures down to normal. Of those who were on drugs, over half were able to get off them and still reduce their blood pressures an average of 15/10 mm Hg. An additional 35 percent succeeded in cutting their prescriptions by half, while reducing their blood pressures an average of 18/10 mm Hg.[406]

In an Indian study, patients trained in biofeedback techniques showed average drops in blood pressure from 158 to 141 mm Hg systolic and from 99 to 87 mm Hg diastolic. These reductions were greater than those induced by drugs in other studies, and they were retained after six months of follow-up. The patients also reported that they felt better, slept better, and worked better.[407]

What about using drugs to induce relaxation? This doesn't seem to be effective. The artificial relaxation resulting from sedatives and tranquilizers not only hasn't been shown to lower blood pressure but, like the drugs that do lower it, they're troubled with side effects.[408]

The psychological factor in high blood pressure is reflected in the observation that for some people, blood pressure is high only in the doctor's office.[409] *You should always get several readings, preferably in the security of your own home, before starting any antihypertensive drug regimen.*

Hyperthyroidism

Hyperthyroidism, or an excess of thyroid hormone, is most commonly seen in a condition called *Graves' disease*. Symptoms include nervousness, irritability, sweating, and muscle weakness.

Postpartum thyroiditis is an overactivity of the thyroid gland occurring a few months after childbirth. The condition may be followed by underactivity of the thyroid a few weeks later.

PHARMACEUTICAL TREATMENT

Conventional treatment for Grave's disease consists of antithyroid drugs that cause hormone production to drop: *methimazole (Tapazole)* or *propylthiouracil (PTU)*. The drugs' side effects may include drowsiness and, in rare cases, a blood disease called agranulocytosis. If the drugs fail, a high-dose radioactive iodine capsule or beverage is given that slows the thyroid by permanently damaging overactive cells. But if too many cells are destroyed (as is often the case), the patient winds up on hormone supplements for life.[410]

For postpartum thyroiditis, some doctors prescribe drugs to relieve anxiety and nervousness. However, the condition generally goes away by itself.

NATURAL ALTERNATIVES

Hyperthyroidism can be a function of the same hormonal imbalance that produces an underactive thyroid. (See "Hypothyroidism.") Homeopathic remedies can rebalance the system, eliminating the need for synthetic thyroid.

Hyperthyroidism Corrected Naturally

Carey, 28, had a two-year history of thyroid problems. When her condition was first diagnosed, she was told she was hypothyroid and was put on *Synthroid.* At a later visit, however, her doctor found she was hyperthyroid. She vacillated from one extreme to the other for two years. Her frustrated doctor finally proposed surgically removing her thyroid and keeping her on permanent medication.

Carey avoided surgery by using a homeopathic product called *Thyroplus* by Deseret. She took it for one month to balance her thyroid function. Then she took CompliMed's homeopathic *Thyroid* for a further two months. Her thyroid function was subsequently checked by a thyroid endocrinology specialist. He said he couldn't understand it: All Carey's lab tests were perfectly normal. The tests were still normal a month later, although the homeopathic remedies had by then been discontinued.

Hypothyroidism

Estimates are that ten million Americans have severe thyroid disorders, and that nearly two million of them don't realize it. They think they are just getting old. Hypothyroidism (a deficiency of thyroid hormone) generally begins as unexplained fatigue and weakness. It can also cause weight gain, cold extremities, anemia, headaches, menstrual problems, and an increased susceptibility to infection, heart disease, cancer, and premature aging. Women, who are three to five times as likely to get the condition as men, have a one in eight chance of experiencing thyroid problems sometime in their lives.[411]

Hypothyroidism causes stomach acid and other digestive juices to be in short supply and intestinal movements to be weak, producing gas and constipation. The hypothyroid person can be malnourished even on a good diet, because she isn't properly assimilating her food. She can also gain substantial weight even when she is honestly (as she tells her friends) eating almost nothing, because she isn't burning her calories efficiently.

A simple home test is to check the body temperature on awakening. A temperature below 98 degrees and a slow pulse may be indicative of hypothyroidism. *If thyroid therapy is necessary, it should be prescribed by a competent professional.* Excess thyroid supplementation may be harmful, since it stimulates the osteoclasts, the cells that tear down or resorb bone. Bone resorption should be in balance with bone formation. An excess of resorption over formation results in bone loss.[412]

DRUG TREATMENT

The usual thyroid medication is synthetic *thyroxine* (*levothyroxine* or *Synthroid*). Ranked among the top ten prescription drugs in America, it is taken by millions of women every day. One drawback is that once you're on synthetic thyroid, you're liable to be on it for life. Another drawback is that the same stress that blocks the thyroid can block conversion of the synthetic hormone to T3 (triiodothyronine), the form in which thyroid hormone is most active in the body.[413] There may also be side effects, including heart palpitations, insomnia, nervousness, and diarrhea.

NATURAL THYROID SUPPLEMENTATION

A more natural and less habit-forming option than Synthroid is *Armour Thyroid*, a desiccated thyroid preparation extracted from pigs. Like Synthroid, Armour Thyroid is standardized to government specifications to allow proper monitoring.

THE HOMEOPATHIC ALTERNATIVE

Even more supportive of the body's own mechanisms are homeopathic remedies, which work to correct the problem at its source. Hormone levels go out of balance for a reason: stress, pregnancy, menopause. Homeopathy works to regulate the thyroid gland so the body can function normally without drugs.

Weaned Off Drugs with Natural Remedies

Kara, 25, had been on Synthroid since she was diagnosed as hypothyroid at the age of 16. Her doctor said she would have to take the drug for life. But after nine years of this course of treatment, she asked to be switched to Armour Thyroid, and he reluctantly agreed. After about three months on Armour Thyroid, Kara began taking homeopathic *Thyroid* by CompliMed. Over the next three months, she then slowly weened off Armour Thyroid and onto a product called *Raw Thyroid.* After that, she took only the CompliMed *Thyroid.* Throughout this treatment, she got repeated lab tests that showed her thyroid levels to be normal.

Kara is now in South America studying herbology. She reports that she has taken nothing for her thyroid for eight months, during which time her thyroid function has remained normal. Remarkably, she no longer needs thyroid remedies of any sort.

OTHER NATURAL ALTERNATIVES

Acupuncture can help stimulate thyroid function. Supplementing with trace minerals can also help. Thyroid function is dependent on a balance of two trace minerals, *manganese* and *iodine*. Hypothyroidism could be due to a shortage of either. Herbs are available that are thyroid stimulants, including dulse and kelp. A Dr. J. Christopher *Formula T,* made by Nature's Way, is also effective.

*I*ndigestion, Bloating, Gas

Minor stomach problems including indigestion, bloating, cramps, and gas pains are normally traceable to bad eating habits (too much or wrong types of food) or stress. They can also be caused by drugs, including birth-control pills, antihistamines, and Valium. Ulcers can also be caused by drugs, including steroids and NSAIDs.[414] (See "Gastritis," "Ulcers.")

OVER-THE-COUNTER DRUG TREATMENT

More over-the-counter drugs are sold for digestive ills than for any other complaint except pain and colds. *Antacids* are alkaline substances that are pro-moted as relieving a variety of stomach problems. They are advertised as achieving their effects by neutralizing "excess stomach acid." The problem is that stomach acid is necessary to the normal digestion of foods: Your diges-tive enzymes work properly only when the acidity of your stomach is proper-ly balanced. The amount of stomach acid you secrete is carefully regulated by the body according to the amounts and types of food you eat. The cause of your upset stomach may not be too much acid but too few digestive enzymes to handle an overload or improper mixture of foods. Antacids can also have unwanted side effects; and if taken regularly for long periods, these effects can be quite serious. Different brands of antacids contain different principal ingre-dients, but all of them are subject to negative effects of some kind.

   Calcium carbonate (the chief ingredient in *Tums*) used to be the antacid of choice, until prolonged use was found to raise the calcium in the blood. The result can be impaired kidney function and kidney stones. The problem is par-ticularly serious for people whose kidneys are already impaired, or for people who drink a lot of milk, since milk is already high in calcium. (Ulcer patients are liable to do just that, since milk has traditionally been recommended for their condition.) Calcium carbonate can also impair iron absorption, can cause constipation, and can produce an "acid rebound" in which its use is followed by significant *increases* in stomach acid. That means you can wind up with more acid in your stomach than before you started on the drug.[415]

   Sodium bicarbonate, or baking soda, is the major ingredient in *Alka Seltzer* and *Bromo Seltzer*. It is relatively harmless for occasional use, but if used repeatedly it can disturb the body's acid-base balance, especially in people with kidney problems; and it can lead to kidney stones and recurrent urinary tract infections. Sodium bicarbonate is high in sodium, so it's not good for people on low-sodium diets; and like calcium carbonate, it can impair iron absorption. *Alka Seltzer* combines sodium bicarbonate with aspirin. If your objective is to relieve a headache, this combination, dissolved in water, can relieve some of the stomach irritation produced by ordinary aspirin tablets; but if you have an upset stomach, the combination is calculated to make it worse, since the aspirin can further irritate your stomach, particularly if your problem is caused by ulcers. *Bromo-Seltzer,* which combines sodium bicarbonate with acetaminophen instead of aspirin, is easier on the stomach than Alka Seltzer. But it's harder on the liver, a hazard especially for alcoholics. Both antacids can have a rebound effect: the problem is worse when you stop them before you started.[416]

Pepto-Bismol is approved by the FDA both as an antacid and as a diarrhea and hangover remedy. Besides salicylate, which can have the same adverse effects as aspirin, it contains bismuth, a potentially lethal nerve poison. Bismuth hasn't been detected in the blood or urine of people taking recommended doses, but overdose can result in kidney failure and liver damage. In France and Australia, reports of bone and joint disorders and encephalopathy (a degenerative disease of the brain) from the use of bismuth salts even at recommended doses have led to restriction on their use.[417]

Magnesium salts (as in *Phillips Milk of Magnesia*) tend to cause diarrhea; and if used regularly for more than a week or two, the result can be severe. They can also exacerbate kidney problems and cause drowsiness in some people.

Aluminum salts (as in *Rolaids*) have the opposite drawback: they can obstruct the intestines and cause intractable constipation. The industry solution was to combine these two ingredients, as in *Maalox, Mylanta, Gelusil* and *Di-Gel Liquid.* The theory was that their opposing side effects would cancel each other out, but in practice, these combination products can cause the side effects of either ingredient.[418]

There is also evidence for a potential link between aluminum antacid preparations and more serious side effects, including bone disease and Alzheimer's disease.[418] (See "Alzheimer's Disease.") Aluminum displaces calcium from the bones, causing them to be brittle and to break easily. Antacids in general also inhibit calcium absorption by neutralizing stomach acid, raising the pH of the stomach. Calcium can be absorbed only in its soluble ionized form, which requires a low pH.[419] Aluminum-containing drugs are particularly dangerous when taken with orange juice, with any other citrus fruit or juice, or in drugs containing citrate, a combination that increases the absorption of aluminum into the bloodstream by as much as 50 times. The result can be both brain damage and thinning of the bones.[420]

As for the feeling of bloating and distention after eating, studies show that it is *not* caused by "excess gas." And the FDA has found no over-the-counter drugs that are safe or effective for alleviating it, TV ads notwithstanding.[421]

NATURAL REMEDIES FOR INDIGESTION

Rather than suppressing the digestive juices, the alternative approach to indigestion is to encourage digestion. One way is with *digestive enzymes.* A popular option is chewable papaya enzymes, which contain papain, a natural digestant.

CAUTION: Digestive enzymes should not be taken if the stomach is inflamed, as from ulcers or inflammation due to nonsteroidal anti-inflammatory drugs (aspirin, Advil, Motrin, and the like). (See "Ulcers.")

Herbal remedies are safe and effective alternatives. Herbs and herbal teas good for settling the stomach include *licorice, ginger, peppermint, chamomile,* and *St. John's-wort.*

The Chinese herbal formula *Pill Curing* is another effective remedy for settling the stomach, or for relieving what the Chinese call "food stagnation"—the feeling after a large meal that the food is stuck in your stomach.

An effective homeopathic remedy for simple indigestion with gas and bloating is *Carbo Veg 6c.* Take three tablets every 15 minutes. For severe upset, take up to six doses. Also good are a combination product called *Nux Vomica* and *Carbo Veg* (take as needed every 15 minutes after a meal, up to three doses) and *Gastrica* by CompliMed. Marco Pharma makes an effective remedy for gas, bloating, upset stomach, sluggish bowels and spastic colon called *Frangula.*

To stop the morning-after nausea and headache of a hangover, try *Nux Vomica 6c,* three tablets every 15 minutes, up to six doses. *Hangover* by Source Natural and *Vitamin-B Stress Tabs* are also good for hangovers.

For an upset stomach due to food poisoning, see "Food Poisoning."

NATURAL REMEDIES FOR GAS AND BLOATING

For intestinal gas, a remedy that goes back to Hippocrates is *charcoal.* One quart of charcoal will absorb *eighty* quarts of ammonia gas. Its downside is that chronic use can interfere with the absorption of nutrients and other drugs.

This side effect can be avoided with homeopathic remedies for gas and bloating. Try *Vermicin* by Complimed or *Gasalia* by Boiron.

An herbal remedy for gas, bloating, and overeating is peppermint tea.

Specific food sensitivities may also underly the feeling of bloating and distention after eating. Excess belching has been traced to air swallowing. Stomach gas consists primarily of oxygen and nitrogen, which come from swallowed air. Increased air swallowing can be caused by eating rapidly, gulping, stress, gum chewing, poorly fitting dentures, thumb-sucking, postnasal drip, dry mouth, or carbonated soft drinks.

DIETARY SOLUTIONS

For chronic stomach complaints, permanent relief depends on tracking down and eliminating the cause. It could be dietary: overeating in general, eating wrong combinations of foods, or food allergies or intolerances. Common offenders that can upset sensitive stomachs include the lactose (milk sugar) in milk, the gluten in wheat, and yeast, sugar, coffee, eggs, and soy products.

The theory of proper food combining lacks scientific evidence, but sensitive people swear by it. The theory is that different types of food require different digestive enzymes. If you mix your foods improperly, some will sit in the stomach and create havoc while others are being processed. If you're prone to indigestion after ordinary-sized meals, try eating fruits, proteins and carbohydrates in separate meals. Proteins or carbohydrates can be eaten with greens (salads or cooked vegetables), but proteins and carbohydrates should not be eaten together; and fruits should be eaten alone.

Dr. Peter J. D'Adamo has another theory that has produced dramatic recoveries from indigestion. In his book *Eat Right for Your Type*, he explains that as a result of heritage and ancestry, people with certain blood types don't make the appropriate enzymes to metabolize particular foods. The biggest problem seems to be for O blood types who indulge in excess carbohydrates: bread, cookies, cake, ice cream, and so forth. Heartburn, indigestion, and bloating result. Relief comes from avoiding these offenders.

Low Carbohydrate Diet Gives Digestive Relief

Within about two days of beginning the Atkins Diet (basically meat and vegetables), people have reported not only losing weight but getting dramatic relief from their severe chronic indigestion, which was apparently caused by the carbohydrates in their normal diet. However, the approach doesn't work for everyone. Differences in blood type may explain the differences in response.

AUGMENTING YOUR ENZYMES

If changing your eating habits doesn't resolve your digestive ills, you may need to look for a more fundamental cause. Sometimes the pancreas produces insufficient pancreatic enzymes. It needs to make amylase to break down starch, lipase to break down fat, cellulase to break down vegetable fiber, protease to break down protein, and insulin to break down sugars. Without these enzymes, food goes through the intestines undigested, where it ferments and decomposes in the colon, causing gas, bloating, and upset. Taking pancreatic enzymes can help (two to five with each meal). But unless you fix the underlying problem, you will be taking enzymes indefinitely.

A product called *Pancreas Total* by Futurplex helps to stimulate the pancreas to produce its own enzymes. Take ten drops three times daily between meals, while continuing to take digestive enzymes after meals. Used over about a three-month period, this remedy can effectively help the digestive system get back on track.

Liver cleansing can also help. The liver clears toxins from the blood. When the liver gets congested, toxins go to the pancreas and prevent its production of enzymes. Parasites can also stop the pancreas from making digestive enzymes. See "Environmental Illness, Liver Stagnation," "Parasites."

Infection, Immunity

Science has yet to find a cure for the common cold; and infections by *E. coli* and *Staphylococcus aureus* are becoming more common, despite everything medical science has to offer. The "wonder drugs" that were supposed to eradicate infectious disease—antibiotics, childhood immunizations, and cortisone—are now actually being been blamed for the spread of disease. An increasing incidence of staph infections, otitis media (middle-ear infection) among children, and sinusitis among adults is blamed on the overuse of broad-spectrum microbial drugs, creating widespread drug resistance and breeding "super bugs" that are immune to antibiotics. Between 1975 and 1990, office visits for otitis media went up a staggering 175 percent.[423] Childhood immunizations have been blamed for other modern diseases, including an alarming increase in asthma and childhood autism. (See "Asthma," "Communicable Diseases.") Steroids (for example, cortisone) are other suspects. Steroids act by suppressing the immune system, the converse of supporting the body's own efforts to heal itself.

CONVENTIONAL TREATMENT

Antibiotics are the conventional answer to bacterial infection. But bacteria have had more than half a century to adapt to these drugs and are finally becoming resistant to them. Predictions are that in a few more years, antibiotics won't be available to treat the serious diseases for which these medicines have earned their reputation as lifesaving "wonder drugs." Diseases that were once responsive to antibiotics either require stronger and stronger forms of the drug or no longer respond at all. In August of 1997, for the first time in the United States, scientists isolated a strain of common *Staphylococcus* that can survive treatment with vancomycin, the one antibiotic that until now has been 100 percent effective against that potentially deadly bacteria.[424]

Antibiotic resistance is attributed to overuse of the drugs, not only in humans but in animals. The livestock industry purchases an astounding one-half of all antibiotics sold. The drugs are incorporated into feed to kill bacteria that stunt the growth of the animals. Resistant bacteria then develop and multiply; and when you eat the animals, you can become infected with the resistant strains. Cooking the meat will kill the bacteria, but the antibiotic remains in the flesh and is absorbed into your bloodstream when the meat is eaten. The doses absorbed are low but are sufficient to allow the bacteria to develop a resistance to the drug. Your risk is increased if you've taken antibiotics recently yourself, since the normal bacterial population in your intestines will have been wiped out, allowing the invading strains to take over. Another suspected source of antibiotic resistance is the use of antibacterial soaps in the kitchen, giving the organisms an opportunity to adapt to the antibacterial agents in the soap.

Antibiotics also depress the immunological response to bacteria, preventing the development of natural antibodies and interfering with the development of natural immunity; and they permit overgrowths by resistant Candida microbes, which then produce toxins that can weaken the immune system and further reduce resistance.[425] (See "Candidiasis.")

Steroids like cortisone, which suppress the immune system, give infections even greater opportunity to spread. (See "Skin Problems.") Steroids are contained in drugs for asthma, arthritis, and other diseases that are progressively becoming more serious and widespread.

ELIMINATING "MAINTAINING CAUSES"

Many people, concerned that their resistance to infection is low, ask for "something to boost my immune system." Natural remedies are available that can help. However, supplements can't fully restore the immune system until it has been cleared of past illnesses that have been suppressed with antibiotics or steroids. The system must be cleaned out before it can be built up. "Maintaining causes" for poor resistance—the body's constant bombardment with allergens, toxins, stress, and so forth—need to be tracked down and, if possible, eliminated.

One maintaining cause may be reinfection by bacteria on the skin. You reinfect yourself by biting your nails, putting your hands in your mouth, and similar actions. In the *Total Body Cleansing System*, the face and hands are washed with an herbal combination product four or five times a day to eliminate these bacteria, which are said to run the immune system down. The concept is liable to raise eyebrows, but a number of people have reported that within a week or two on the program, their symptoms of chronic sinusitis and postnasal drip disappeared. Andreas Marx, developer of an effective antiparasite protocol, recommends the Total Body Cleansing System to his patients to prevent reinfection with parasites.

For eliminating other maintaining causes, see "Allergies," "Heavy-Metal Poisoning," "Stress."

NUTRITIONAL IMMUNE SYSTEM BOOSTERS

Vitamin and mineral supplements can also help boost the immune system. *Jarrow Pak Plus*, a high-dose vitamin, mineral, and herbal supplement originally developed to bolster the immune systems of AIDS patients, is particularly effective. Many people prone to continual colds and flus throughout the winter report that it is has kept them healthy through those precarious months. (See "Flu.")

The trace mineral zinc has been shown to reduce the duration and severity of a cold from seven to three days.

Cat's claw (una de gato) is an Amazon vine with immunity-restoring properties. It is also healing to the stomach.

N-acetylcysteine (NAC) has also been shown in a clinical trial to be effective in blocking flu symptoms in elderly and chronically ill people. (See "Flu.")

Another effective new immune-booster is colostrum. Derived from the first milk of cows, it is now available in pill form. In many reported cases, taking colostrum capsules every hour or two at the first sign of a cold has kept the cold from developing. A pure colostrom product is available by mail order from Pacific Research Laboratories (310-320-1132). The same company makes an essential oil called *Carvacrol* and a mineral supplement called *Coral Minerals,* both of which help to boost the immune system.

HERBAL REMEDIES

Olive leaf extract is a natural antibiotic and antiviral. It has also been shown to be valuable in treating degenerative disease.[426]

Echinacea helps strengthen the immune system so that it can ward off pathogens. This herb should be used, however, only when you are well. (See "Colds.") It is particularly good when others around you are getting sick and you want to avoid the contagion.

Other immune-building herbs recommended by Chinese doctors include *reishi* and *maitake* mushrooms and *astragalus.*

For kids, a cell salt called *Bioplasma* is particularly popular. It is easy to take, tastes like candy, and dissolves easily. The recommended dose is four pills three times a day.

HOMEOPATHIC REMEDIES

A homeopathic product called *Thymactive* by NF Formulas is quite effective.

A remarkable line of products by Sanum, newly approved by the FDA, is based on the theories of Dr. Guenther Enderlein of Germany. Dr. Enderlein maintained that antibiotics don't actually kill bacteria. Bacteria are pleomorphic; they can change forms from viruses to bacteria to fungi.

In reaction to antibiotics, they change to fungi, creating systemic candida infections. The Sanum products address not these pleomorphic life forms, but the "soil"—the internal environment of the body that allows them to thrive. Dr. Nancy Sacks, a Southern California homeopath, reports dramatic success using these remedies.

OZONE

An alternative for clearing the system of unwanted bacteria and viruses that is controversial but heavily supported by research is ozone therapy. Ozone treatments are popular in Europe for boosting the immune systems of AIDS patients and others with serious immune impairments. Ozone is O3—a free oxygen molecule with an extra oxygen added. Ozone is the strongest killer of viruses known to man, and it kills every virus known to man. It has been used for water and sewage treatment in Europe since the turn of the century, replacing chlorine, which produces carcinogenic compounds such as chloroform. Ozone leaves no toxic residues, and its disinfection is 5,000 times more rapid than chlorine's. In the body, it has the flora-friendly effect of killing anaerobic but not aerobic bacteria. Aerobic microbes are friendly, healthy bacteria that thrive in an oxygenated environment. Anaerobic microbes are unfriendly and unhealthy, and they cause the majority of human diseases. They gnaw at the joints, causing inflammatory arthritis; give off calcium waste matter, cementing the bones; lodge in the liver and kidneys, producing bile that forms stones; live in the lining of the arteries, leaving hardened deposits on the arterial walls; and attach to the lining of the nervous system. However, these anaerobic microbes can't live in an aerobic, or heavily oxygenated, environment.[427]

SUN THERAPY

Ultraviolet light from the sun helps not only in building strong bones but in killing infectious bacteria. Early in the twentieth century, sunbathing and UV therapy were considered the most effective treatments for many infectious diseases, including tuberculosis. Then in 1938, penicillin was discovered. Sun therapy was forgotten, as drugs became big business.[428] But antibiotics have now been so overused that they are losing their effectiveness and may soon be obsolete. Nature herself is forcing us to return to her own remedies, including prudent sunbathing.

Insect Bites and Stings

More people are killed in the United States each year by the stinging Hymenoptera—including bees, wasps, hornets, yellow jackets, and fire ants—than by any other poisonous animals, including rattlesnakes.

Normal reactions to insect stings include pain, redness, swelling, itching, and warmth at the site of the bite. These reactions can be quite painful and annoying, but so long as they're confined to the area of the sting, they're considered normal inflammatory responses. The reactions that require emergency treatment are those from multiple bites, which can produce toxic reactions in normal people; and allergic reactions in sensitive people to a single bite, which can be just as serious.

Symptoms to look for when determining whether to call a doctor if you or your child is stung are severe pain, redness or itching at the site of the sting; sudden, serious swelling of the lips, tongue, eyes, or body; itching all over the body; hives (itchy bumps on the skin); wheezing, sudden coughing or trouble breathing; dizziness and weakness; serious nausea; or collapse.

Drug Treatment

The conventional approach to treating ordinary bites is to suppress itching with oral antihistamines or calamine lotion applied to the skin. (See "Itching.") A serious allergic reaction is treated by epinephrine by injection, antihistamines by injection or mouth, and adrenal steroids. If you know you're allergic to insect stings, you should keep an emergency insect treatment kit containing these items on hand (available only by prescription).

Drugstore Prevention

There are no drugstore repellants effective against the stinging Hymenoptera. But most other biting insects, including mosquitos, chiggers, ticks, and biting flies, can be driven off by topical insect repellants. The active ingredient in *Off* and most other popular brands is DEET, short for N,N-diethyl-m-toluamide. Most brands contain only a little of it, but some, such as *Muskol,* are pure DEET. The problem with this chemical repellant is that it is toxic not only to bugs but to humans. DEET can cause a variety of health problems, from dizziness to death. In 1995,

6,745 poisonings from it were reported to the American Association of Poison Control Centers, including 4,332 for children under six and one fatality in an adult; and many more cases of DEET-related problems are thought to go unreported. The important thing to be aware of is that chemicals that are sprayed on the skin are absorbed into the circulation: About 10 to 15 percent of each dose of DEET can be recovered from the urine.

CAUTION: Toxic effects from DEET are particularly likely in infants and young children, in whom excessive or prolonged use of ordinary insect repellants has caused serious reactions. Only brief exposure to smaller amounts of the higher-concentration products has caused serious reactions in both children and adults, including anaphylactic shock and grand-mal seizures. Swallowing DEET can be fatal.

NATURAL ALTERNATIVES

These risks can be avoided by using one of the nontoxic insect repellants now available. Formulated from all-natural plant oils, they are quite effective. *Buzz Away* by Quantum (containing citronella oil, eucalyptus, lemongrass, cedarwood, and pepperment oils) has passed EPA safety and efficacy tests and is rated effective against mosquitoes for two and one half hours after application. *Green Ban* is another effective DEET-free bug repellant.

An insect repellant popular among campers is Avon's *Skin-So-Soft*, a concentrated bath oil containing di-isopropyl adipate, mineral oil, isopropyl palmitate, dioctyl sodium sulfosuccinate, fragrance, and the sunscreen benzophenone-11. In one study, Skin-So-Soft successfully repelled the mosquito that carries yellow fever. The *Medical Letter* cautions, however, that this remedy may be effective for as little as 10 to 30 minutes, compared to one to several hours for products containing DEET.

Another natural insect repellant is the B vitamin thiamine. Taken at the rate of 100 mg per day beginning a week before you're going to need it, it will come out in your skin, repelling bugs because they don't like the smell. Eating large portions of onions and garlic can also have this effect.

The natural product that gets the most rave reviews, however, is a homeopathic called Biting Insects by Molecular Biologicals. Taken orally a few hours before exposure, it is remarkably effective at discouraging insects.

Essential oils can also discourage bugs from bugging you.[429]

If you do get bitten, you can reduce inflammation by licking an aspirin and applying it to the bite. Also good for treating insect bites is homeopathic *Apis* 6x or 30x (three pills every fifteen minutes for one hour).

No More Flea Bites

A woman complained that fleas loved her—she was always the first to be bitten—but she was highly allergic to them. Her legs would swell and she would itch all night, keeping her from sleeping. She took *Biting Insects* and reported, to her amazement, that she hadn't gotten a flea bite since. Even when people around her were getting bitten, she remained impervious to the bugs.

OTHER PREVENTIVE MEASURES

Other measures you can take to avoid getting bitten include wearing clothes that are close-fitting, that cover as much of the body as possible and are boring to insects. Brightly colored clothes may be mistaken for flowers. Dark-colored clothing (brown or black) may also provoke an attack. The least interesting to bees are white or light khaki-colored materials. Scented soaps, perfumes, suntan lotions, and other cosmetics, as well as shiny jewelry or buckles can also attract stinging insects. Bees won't attack unless you threaten their hives or step on them. If stung, remove the stinger and attached venom sac, since these can continue to inject venom after being torn from the insect. Ice can help lessen pain and swelling.[430]

Insomnia

Sleep, nature's balm, eludes an estimated 60 percent of Americans at least occasionally. But "insomnia" is a state of mind. The number of hours you sleep doesn't matter so long as you feel well rested. If you habitually can't sleep and don't feel well rested, you might want to see a doctor to rule out possible underlying factors such as anemia, an infection, sleep-disturbing medications, or sleep apnea (in which sleep is disturbed by improper breathing). If no physical problem explains your insomnia, you may just need to retrain your body and mind. Sleeping well is a habit. Four out of ten insomniacs get a good night's sleep on placebos (sugar pills that they think are sleeping pills).

DRUG TREATMENT

For the desperate, there are prescription sleeping pills—*barbiturates* and *benzodiazepines*. But these drugs (discussed under "Anxiety") can depress brain function, have unwanted side effects, and can be addicting and cause crises on withdrawal. They also tend to lose their effectiveness after about two weeks of continuous use, so users must keep increasing the dose. That means increasing the buildup of metabolites (byproducts of the drug's active ingredients), along with their hangover-like side effects. Elderly people branded as senile may actually be suffering from the side effects of these drugs. The sleep they induce is druglike, with insufficient time spent dreaming; and withdrawal can lead to rebound insomnia and other side effects, including anxiety, restlessness, headache, tremors and visual disturbances. Prescription sleeping pills can be fatal in people with certain health problems, and you can't necessarily tell ahead of time if you're one of them. The drugs can also be fatal if mixed with other drugs, or with narcotics or alcohol.

These concerns have made doctors leery of scribbling prescriptions for sleeping pills, leaving inveterate insomniacs to their over-the-counter remedies. But in 1979, the FDA found that *no* over-the-counter drugs on the market were safe or effective for treating insomnia; and it banned the sale of all of them. Resourceful drug manufacturers then turned to antihistamines, which have the *negative side effect*, officially recognized by the FDA, of inducing drowsiness in some people. Originally marketed for the relief of allergies, antihistamines thus became the main ingredient in over-the-counter insomnia remedies such as *Nytol* and *Sominex*. The problem is that antihistamines can also have other side effects, including nausea and vomiting; dizziness; dryness in the mouth, throat, and nose; ringing in the ears; frequent urination; fatigue; and double vision. Dizziness and confusion are particularly likely in the elderly. In children, the drugs can produce restlessness and insomnia, the very problems they're supposed to prevent. In pregnant women, certain antihistamines can produce birth defects. And breastfed infants can experience adverse effects from the antihistamines taken by their mothers.

RESETTING YOUR BIOLOGICAL CLOCK

A safer, more natural alternative is *melatonin,* a hormone secreted by the pineal gland when darkness falls. In pill form, melatonin has been touted as a wonder nondrug that will soon make sleeping pills obsolete. The usual dose is 3 milligrams nightly. But dosage can vary from 0.5 to 10 milligrams, and researchers have given people up to 6,000 milligrams a day (600 to 3,000 times the usual dose) without causing toxicity. The FDA has recorded only four complaints about the hormone, all of them mild. Besides being effective in inducing sleep and combating jet lag, melatonin seems to have immune-stimulating and antiaging properties. (See "Aging.")

While melatonin is definitely an advance over the barbiturates, it does have limitations. Ten percent of insomniacs report no effects at all from its use, and another 10 percent complain of side effects including nightmares, headaches, morning grogginess, mild depression, and low sex drive.[431] Anecdotal evidence also suggests that melatonin works better for men than for women. And it isn't recommended for habitual use for people under forty. (See "Aging.")

HOMEOPATHIC OPTIONS

An alternative with absolutely no side effects is homeopathic *Melatonin 12x,* which works by stimulating the body to produce its own melatonin.

Another effective homeopathic remedy for insomnia is *Passiflora* 3x or 6x. Take two pills in the evening (around 8 or 9 P.M.), then two before going to bed. Leave two on your night stand, and take them if you awaken before morning. Users report that in a few days, they are sleeping through the night and waking feeling refreshed, not drowsy. This ritual also helps to reset your sleep patterns.

Homeopathic *chamomile* is good for inducing sleep in restless children.

There are also many effective combination homeopathic remedies, including *Quietude* by Boiron, *Noctura* by Nelson, and *Calms* by Hylands.

THE ORIENTAL APPROACH

Chinese doctors recognize different types of insomnia, with different causes and cures. The type of sleep and time you awaken in the night are considered important diagnostic indicators. Some people have restless sleep; some can't fall asleep; some fall asleep, then wake up and can't go back to sleep; some say they haven't slept through the night in years. In Chinese medicine, these are different ailments that require different remedies. For people who can't fall asleep in the first place, a Chinese patent formula called *Anmien Pien* can help by calming the mind. For other types of insomnia, other remedies are indicated.

Insomnia Cured at Last

John claimed he hadn't slept through the night in 17 years. He habitually awoke at 1 A.M., got up, and took a bath. He was desperate to break this cycle. After experimenting with a number of natural options, he finally tried the Chinese herbal formula *Suan Zao Ren*. He came back and bought a case of it. Six months later, he reported it was still working.

No More Nocturnal Waking

Ken, 54, said he could fall asleep, but he would awaken at 3 A.M. and couldn't get back to sleep. In Chinese medicine, 2 A.M. to 4 A.M. is the "time of the liver," when the liver meridian is the most energized. Awakening at that time indicates the liver is out of balance, congested, or "stagnant." Ken revealed that he had had extensive surgery eight months earlier. It seemed that either the anesthetic had damaged his liver energy, or his liver was overworked from breaking down the drugs he was given for his surgery. His liver needed a housecleaning. Within a week of beginning the Liver Cleanse Diet, he began to sleep through the night. (See "Environmental Illness, Liver Stagnation.")

WESTERN HERBS AND NUTRIENTS

Western herbs are also available that can help induce sound sleep. Studies have shown that the herb *kava* is as effective as drugs for treating mild cases of insomnia and anxiety, while avoiding the side effects of drugs. (See "Anxiety.") Recommended dosage is 150 to 200 mg of kavalactones (the active ingredients) 30 to 60 minutes before bedtime.[432]

Other effective sleep-inducing herbs include *valerian, passion flower,* and *skullcap.* Useful herbal combinations are listed in the accompanying chart.

Rescue Remedy is a Bach flower combination that can bring on the relaxation required to fall asleep. It is particularly effective for children after a stressful day. (See Chapter 3.)

Evening primrose oil helps promote production of the body's own hormones. Two capsules (totaling 2,600 mg) taken before bed (not earlier) promotes deep sleep. Evening primrose oil also softens the skin and improves hair and nails.

NOTE: Women should not take evening primrose oil during their menses, as it promotes bleeding. For the same reason, it should not be taken by people on coumadin or other anticoagulant therapy.

If you are prone to leg cramps that keep you awake at night, try taking supplements of *potassium, calcium* or *DMG (dimethylglycine)* before bed. A favorite remedy by Boiforce is *Calcium Absorption.*

OTHER HELPFUL TIPS

Insomnia can be caused by drugs. Drugs containing stimulants include analgesics like Anacin and Excedrin, which contain caffeine; over-the-counter diet aids, nasal decongestants, and asthma products; and many prescription drugs, including those for asthma, many cough and cold remedies, amphetamines, and thyroid preparations. Centrally acting adrenergic blockers, hypnotics, and diuretics taken late in the day are other drugs that can worsen sleep.[433] Sleeplessness can also result when you try to discontinue the drugs intended to counteract it. For that reason, it's best not to start on them if you can help it.

The traditional hot bath, good book and hot drink remain viable aids.

A good meditative habit, once in bed, is to stop thinking. As thoughts comes in, slow them down by categorizing and putting labels on them ("memory," "plan," and so forth). The act of analyzing the thought stops it from flowing.

Another simple home remedy is to walk barefoot in the grass before bed. Dr. John R. Christopher, a renowned herbalist, maintained that static electricity that has built up in the body prevents people from getting a good night's sleep. This is a problem particularly for men who wear rubber-soled shoes.

Cured by Walking Barefoot

An "incurable" insomniac was asked about his footwear. He said he habitually wore tennis shoes. He was advised to try going barefoot in the grass for 15 minutes before bed. He returned to report, to his frank amazement, that after this simple therapy he had slept through the night for the first time in years.

Itching (Pruritis), Rash, Poison Ivy, Poison Oak, Hives

Pruritis, or itching, is the most common skin complaint. It can be caused by insect bites and stings, poison ivy or oak, sunburn, or dry skin. (See "Allergies," "Insect Bites.") *Itching can also signal something more serious, including diabetes mellitus, hypothyroidism, gout, leukemia, lymphoma (cancer of the lymph nodes), infection by parasites, kidney failure, or liver disease. In an estimated 10 to 50 percent of cases, generalized itching over a large area of the body that lasts more than a week is a symptom of systemic disease requiring a doctor's attention.*

DRUG TREATMENT

For itching of the more mundane variety, there are nonprescription remedies. A skin rash typically represents the body's attempt to expel irritants. Histamine is released in furtherance of this process. Over-the-counter anti-itch products may contain antihistamines, corticosteroids, local anesthetics, or counterirritants.

Corticosteroids are by far the most effective option for relieving itching from simple rashes, hives, bug bites and poison ivy. They're the most effective, but not the safest. Corticosteroids are potent drugs that normally aren't sold without a prescription; but the FDA has allowed two of them, *hydrocortisone* and *hydrocortisone acetate,* to be sold in low dosages over-the-counter for the self-treatment of minor skin irritations. These steroid creams are effective because they inhibit the body's elimination of irritants and prevent the release of histamine.

One problem is that if the irritant itself isn't removed, the rash is liable to come back in full force when the drug is stopped, an example of the "rebound effect" plaguing many drugs. A worse problem is that when inflammation is reduced by suppressing the immune system, resistance to infection is lowered at the same time. The result can be secondary infection, including boils and thrush. If steroids are used to treat skin disorders caused by infection, much more severe infections can result, which can spread over large areas or produce ugly skin ulcers. When hydrocortisone cream is put on a rash caused by an infection such as ringworm, the rash is liable to clear up but reappear later. If hydrocortisone cream is reapplied to the area, the cream will suppress the immune system on the skin where it's used, and the infection will spread. Other stubborn rashes on which hydrocortisone is frequently misused are those that turn out to be skin cancer. *If the cream doesn't work after a week, or if the rash returns after you stop using it, you should see a doctor.*[434]

Other potential adverse effects of topical steroids include allergic reactions, irreversible marks on the skin, unwanted hair growth, and acne. If used on children's skin or in large amounts by adults, the drugs can also enter the general circulation and reach the pituitary, where they can have systemic effects such as those seen with systemic steroids.

Other over-the-counter itch remedies are *local anesthetics*—drugs with active ingredients ending in "-caine." Their main drawback is that they can cause sensitivity reactions in susceptible people. Unfortunately, the people who react most severely to poison ivy and poison oak are also those most likely to have an allergic reaction to local anesthetics. The result can be skin rash, hives, and eruptions, the very symptoms the drugs are intended to relieve. When large amounts of some of these drugs, including *lidocaine, dibucaine,* and *tetracaine,* are applied to large areas of damaged skin, much of the drug is absorbed. Life-threatening toxic reactions can result. This reaction is rare, however, and doesn't happen with the more popular benzocaine, which is insoluble in body fluids.

Antihistamines taken in liquid or chewable tablet form immediately after a sting, bite, or exposure to poison ivy or poison oak can block the histamine receptors before they have time to release their itch-provoking hormone. Antihistamines applied to the skin can also relieve itching.

Counterirritants such as *camphor, menthol,* and *phenol* seem to work by causing a mild irritation at other skin sites, diverting the pain receptors at the site of irritation.

CAUTION: Phenol can cause serious skin burns, and if swallowed can cause internal injury, even in very weak concentrations. It should be kept away from children and should never be used to treat diaper rash.[435]

The Natural Approach: Treating the Cause

An effective natural alternative that is much safer than steroids like hydrocortisone cream is a Chinese patent remedy called *Armadillo Pills.* It will take away a skin rash, hives, or itching in a couple of hours to a couple of days, depending on severity.

Armadillo Pills are safe, but they still treat only the symptom. Rashes often have a "maintaining cause": something in the environment, something you are eating, or something habitually coming in contact with your skin that provokes the body to react. In those cases, it's best to locate and remove the cause rather than merely suppressing the reaction.

Even if no maintaining cause can be found, the right homeopathic remedy can often eliminate the rash permanently.

Mysterious Rash Eliminated with Homeopathic Remedy

Allen, 38, had a rash on both legs that would not go away, although he had been seeing a doctor for it for a number of months. The doctor's approach was cortisone, which would temporarily suppress the problem; but the rash kept coming back. Questioning about Allen's detergent, socks, boots, and so forth, failed to turn up a maintaining cause. Homeopathic *Apis 6c* immediately caused the rash to disappear, but it came back. Homeopathic *Apis 30c* and *Armadillo Pills* then got rid of the rash, but again it came back. A very high potency of *Apis* finally eliminated the problem permanently.

Natural Remedies for Particular Conditions

For poison oak or poison ivy, good homeopathic combination products include *Contact Allergies* by Molecular Biologicals and *Nix Itch* by Quantum. A good single remedy is *Rhus tox.*

For hives, try Hyland's homeopathic combination *Hives.*

Good topical remedies for dry skin are *evening primrose oil* or *The Ultimate Oil* by Nature's Secret.

As drawing salves to pull out toxins and relieve pain, clays may be applied to the skin. Options include *Bentonite Clay, Kaolin Clay, French Green Clay,* and *Aztec Secret. Black Ointment* by Nature's Way also acts as a drawing salve, which works to pull out not only toxins but splinters, slivers of glass, and so forth.

Another effective treatment for itching and excess dryness of the skin (a major cause of itching) is the wet dressing. Wet dressings work because the water evaporating from them cools the skin. They also gently clean the skin. To apply a wet dressing, soak a layer of gauze or thin cloth in water. (Diluted Burow's solution is sometimes recommended, but it contains high amounts of aluminum that may be absorbed by broken or inflamed skin.) Apply the wet dressing to the irritated area. Soak and reapply the cloth every two or three minutes for 15 to 30 minutes. The procedure can be repeated several times a day. If itching covers an area too large for wet dressings, a cool bath can soothe irritation. Cool water constricts blood vessels. Avoid warm baths, which can increase vasodilation and itching.[436]

For taking the itch out of mosquito bites, try one or more of these nondrug suggestions.

1. Make a paste from unseasoned meat tenderizer and water and leave it on the bite for thirty minutes.
2. Coat the bite with fresh papaya, which contains an enzyme that neutralizes venom.
3. Squeeze the flowers and leaves of a honeysuckle vine and rub the juice into the bite.
4. Moisten the skin and sprinkle ordinary table salt on it.
5. Dab the bite with toothpaste.[437]

For natural ways to keep from getting bitten, see "Insect Bites."

*J*et Lag, Jet Travel

"Jet lag" is a syndrome of fatigue, weakness, sleepiness, and irritability caused by a disruption in the normal cycle of sleeping and waking, as when traveling across several time zones in a short time. Adapting to a time zone can take 5 to 15 days.

Jet-setting can throw off not only your sleep patterns but also your immune system. Air travelers are prone to getting ill from exposure to an onslaught of germs as a result of poor air circulation, jet stress, the low oxygen content of recycled air, and exposure to free radicals. Where planes once used 100 percent fresh air that was circulated every three minutes, newer model planes save fuel by using half recirculated air that is freshened every six or seven minutes or longer.[438]

DRUG TREATMENT FOR JET LAG

You can coerce your body into sleeping on cue by taking a sleeping pill, but the drug may leave you drowsy during the day. Taking the popular

Halcion before a flight can be quite dangerous, resulting in some cases in an incapacitating condition called "traveling amnesia."[439] (See "Anxiety.")

NATURAL SLEEP CAN BE YOURS

A popular natural alternative for correcting a disturbed sleep pattern is *melatonin*. A hormone secreted by the pineal gland in response to light hitting the eyes, melatonin determines when we sleep and when we wake up. Five milligrams taken nightly have been shown to help airline employees adjust to new time zones.

For other natural sleep inducers, see "Insomnia."

STAYING WELL IN THE AIR

For countering the onslaughts to the immune system wreaked by air travel, herbal and homeopathic remedies are available.

This recipe for immunity is particularly effective: Put one dropperful of a homeopathic formula called *Geopathic Stress* by Deseret in a bottle of water and add one tablet of *Cold and Flu Solution PLUS* by Dolisos. Sip this mixture the entire time you are aloft.

Traveler's Flus Forestalled

Janet, a writer for a major New York magazine, is under substantial pressure professionally and can't afford to be sick, but she spends a great deal of time on planes and is prone to getting colds and flus during her travels. She was pleased to report that she had gotten neither for more than a year, after learning the foregoing recipe for immunity.

NEUTRALIZING FREE RADICALS AND HARMFUL ELECTROMAGNETIC RADIATION

To counter the free radicals to which jet setters are exposed, heavy doses of antioxidants are recommended. For a list of antioxidants, see "Aging."

Another option is to wear a device called a *Diode* that counteracts harmful radiation emanating from low-frequency electromagnetic fields. New research shows that the body has an electrical field of its own, which protects the body's rhythms and keeps it functional.[440] When harmful electromagnetic radiation is passing through the body, the body's own electrical system is disturbed. The Diode is said to work by giving the body's electrical system the extra boost it needs to stay in balance. The device is a small, square, solid-state monopole piece of lightweight, non-toxic material projecting 47 different frequencies. When worn on the left side of the body, it balances the body's own electrical energies and counteracts conflicting energies (for example, microwaves) within the airplane. The *Dio-Pad*, a large pad on which you sit during flight, works on the same principle. The Diode can also be used to counteract harmful radiation emanating from computers, televisions, fluorescent lights, and X-ray machines. It may either be attached to the radiation-producing machine or worn directly on the body.

Flight Attendant's Leg Cramps Eliminated

T.J., a male flight attendant and long-distance runner, complained that he could not run well the days following his flights and that he had leg and muscle pains when flying. Taking antioxidants and wearing a Diode eliminated his pains and enabled him to run a 26-mile marathon immediately after a flight.

OTHER HELPFUL TIPS FOR JET SETTERS

1. Drink plenty of water to avoid dehydration. It's best to avoid alcohol and coffee; but if you can't, drink even more water to replenish the losses they precipitate. Carry your own bottled water that is fresh; airplane water isn't.

2. Reduce food intake.

3. Wear comfortable clothing.

4. Resist the urge to go to sleep immediately upon arrival in a country where it's still daylight, even if your own body clock says it's the middle of the night. Try to hold out until the locals are going to sleep. Go for a walk in the sun to stimulate your pineal gland and reset your internal clock.

5. For sleeping on the plane, bring eyeshades, earplugs, and an inflatable neck pillow. A great mental exercise for inducing sleep is to stop thinking. It takes some practice, but once you acquire this meditative habit you will be addicted to it, on an airplane or anywhere else you have the luxury of doing absolutely nothing. (See "Insomnia.")

Kidney Stones

Kidney stones form in the center of the kidney and are composed of crystallized calcium, uric acid, and other substances. The pain of passing a large stone can be excruciating and has been compared to childbirth. Stones too large to pass out through the bladder may get stuck in the kidney, where they can wreak serious havoc; but 90 percent of stones pass of their own accord, particularly if large amounts of water are drunk to move them along.

CONVENTIONAL TREATMENT

The usual conventional treatment is analgesics to suppress the pain and sometimes diuretics to forestall recurrences. A newer option called extracorporeal shock-wave lithotripsy (ESWL) breaks up the stones, but the stone fragments still need to be passed and there may still be discomfort. Patients say that passing the gravel can be as painful as passing the whole stone.

ALTERNATIVE TREATMENT

The ideal treatment would be one that not only dissolves but reabsorbs the stones. A Chinese patent formula called *Passwan* actually does this. It also stops the body from forming new stones. The classic Chinese patent formula is called *Te Xiao Pai Shi Wan* and is by Mai Yun Shan. Take six to eight pills three times daily. The Zand version is called *Passwan*. Take two droppersful in water three times daily.

An herbal formula, *berberis,* helps relieve pain when passing stones by relaxing the muscles. Take ten drops of herbal *Berberis Mother Tincture* in water three times daily.

Homeopathic *berberis 30c* is also effective. Take three pills hourly if needed for pain, or three to four times daily.

Recurring Kidney Stones Relieved

A 62-year-old man said he had suffered four times with kidney stones. He had tried everything—changing his diet, drinking lots of water, changing the pH of his body—but still the stones returned. He went to the doctor for a checkup, only to find that he was developing more stones. Completely discouraged, he tried *Passwan* and *berberis* out of sheer desperation. Four years later, he reports that he has not had another stone since. He takes *Passwan* preventatively six weeks out of the year—six pills three times daily for two weeks at a time, three times a year.

*L*iver Disease, Hepatitis, Jaundice

The liver's chief function is to detoxify the body. Besides the harmful byproducts of metabolism, the liver has to deal with pesticides, pollutants, drugs, and toxic chemicals. Alcohol contributes to the liver's load, precipitating *cirrhosis* (chronic inflammation) of the liver in the chronic alcoholic. Constipation and the habitual use of pharmaceuticals can also overburden the liver, leading to its degeneration over time. *Jaundice* is a yellow/orange discoloration of the skin and eyeballs resulting when toxins accumulate in the blood. *Hepatitis* is a viral infection that inflames the liver.

Hepatitis A, the least dangerous form of hepatitis, does not cause long-term liver damage. It is usually transmitted through fecal matter from food or water (for example, from restaurant workers who don't wash their hands). Symptoms include loss of appetite, fatigue, mild fever, muscle or joint aches, nausea, vomiting, abdominal pain, dark urine, and jaundice.

Hepatitis B is the most widespread of the hepatitis viruses, affecting 300,000 Americans annually. It can be passed from mother to child or through sexual contact, blood transfusions, or the shared needles of IV drug users. Most victims recover completely, but some develop chronic hepatitis and possibly cirrhosis of the liver.

Hepatitis C is the most frightening form. Usually spread through blood transfusions or contaminated needles, it can have no or only mild symptoms for 10 or 20 years, while the liver is insidiously being destroyed. The victim may feel exhausted, but the disease is detected only by a blood test showing that liver enzymes are abnormally high. A definitive diagnosis then requires a biopsy (a test in which a piece of the liver is cut out and analyzed).

CONVENTIONAL TREATMENT

Conventional medicine has little to offer for hepatitis. Certain drugs such as interferon have been tried experimentally, but none are clearly effective. Hepatitis B vaccines are available but are so controversial that doctors themselves often refuse to take them. Doctors usually say diet has nothing to do with recovery. The patient can eat whatever he wants.

THE ALTERNATIVE APPROACH

Alternative practitioners disagree. They maintain that diet is key to clearing liver disease. A diet heavy in greens can clean the liver and reduce recovery times dramatically. German homeopathic remedies by Staufen called *Hepatitis A, Hepatitis B,* and *Hepatitis C* are also highly effective. Herbal supplements useful for cleaning the liver include *milk thistle* and *yellow dock.* Also highly recommended is the "Liver Cleanse Diet," described in detail under "Environmental Illness, Liver Stagnation." The liver needs to be given a rest from proteins, which are hard for it to handle and should be eaten only in very small amounts if at all.

Back to Work in a Week on Greens

A 35-year-old male nurse who was diagnosed with hepatitis A was told he would be out of work for two to six months. He was quite concerned, since he couldn't afford that much time out of work. He was advised to start on the Liver Cleanse Diet and generous doses of green leafy vegetables and green drinks, and to take the German homeopathic remedy *Hepatitis A.* Within three days, all his symptoms were gone; and in a week he was back at work. He reports having had no problems since.

An actor with hepatitis A who wasn't able to obtain homeopathic and herbal remedies immediately was advised to begin on the green diet at home. When all his jaundice and other symptoms were gone in a week, he was quite impressed, particularly since his doctor had told him it didn't matter what he ate. He was later given the Staufen homeopathic *Hepatitis A* even though he was asymptomatic, just to circumvent further problems.

Hepatitis C Victims Stabilized with Simple Remedy

Two patients diagnosed with Hepatitis C report that their previously high liver enzymes have returned to normal and they are doing well after taking the Staufen homeopathic by that name. They aren't necessarily cured, but the drop in their liver-enzyme levels is unusual and is a positive indicator.

Lyme Disease

Lyme disease is a flulike bacterial infection induced by the bite of an infected black-legged tick. The cause is clearcut but diagnosis is difficult. The complaints of people with Lyme disease tend to change from day to day. The patient can feel great one day and wretched the next. The illness is liable to be misdiagnosed or to be branded as "psychological." In cases that come to the practitioner without a diagnosis, the major problem is determining the cause of an elusive set of symptoms. The clearest early sign, a bull's eye-shaped rash appearing within weeks of the tick bite, is often missed; and other symptoms of the condition imitate other diseases, including chronic fatigue syndrome and fibromyalgia. Early symptoms of Lyme disease include muscle and joint aches and swelling, headache, stiff neck, overwhelming fatigue, fever, facial paralysis (Bell's palsy), meningitis, and less commonly eye problems and heart abnormalities. Late-stage symptoms include intermittent or chronic arthritis and neurological conditions such as confusion and memory loss.[441]

DRUG TREATMENT

Standard drug treatment consists of a month-long course of intravenous antibiotics, which must sometimes be repeated. But IV antibiotic treatment can be quite disruptive and toxic to the body, so doctors caution that it should be used only when the case is advanced and the diagnosis is definitive. The problem is the difficulty of diagnosis. If you are misdiagnosed, you may be subjected to quite toxic drugs for the wrong underlying condition.

HOMEOPATHY WORKS WHERE ANTIBIOTICS DON'T

In hundreds of cases of Lyme disease received by referral from a medical office, homeopathy has proven to be remarkably effective. These cases were referred because the patients' symptoms had returned after treatment with antibiotics. The drugs simply had not worked; they had suppressed rather than cured the disease and had thrown off the natural balance of the body in the meantime. The remedy that resolved these patients' symptoms was a German formulation of homeopathic Borrelia. The recommended protocol was a single dose (in strengths varying from 200x to 5x) taken every three days for a month. As is typical of homeopathic treatment, the symptoms tended to get worse before they got better (the "healing crisis"). But then symptoms generally disappeared permanently.

Elusive Symptoms Relieved with Lyme Disease Remedy

David, 47, had been battling for three years with recurring hip and knee pains, abdominal discomfort, and other mysterious complaints. Homeopathic treatment succeeded in alleviating his pains for several weeks at a time, but then he would "overdo it" and his symptoms would return. The key to his case was establishing a proper diagnosis. His condition was presumed to be Lyme disease when the homeopathic remedy for that condition eliminated his symptoms. He took the German homeopathic *Borrelia* and was dramatically better the following day. He experienced some "healing crises" for the next two weeks, but reports being well ever since.

PREVENTIVE MEASURES

The ideal remedy is prevention. If tick-infested areas can't be avoided, you should:

1. Protect your arms and legs by wearing long sleeves and long pants tucked into socks or boots.

2. Use insect repellents. Permethrin-containing insect repellents can be applied to pants, socks and shoes. However, the conventionally recommended DEET-containing repellents aren't ideal for exposed skin, as DEET is very toxic. Effective DEET-free herbal bug repellents are now on the market. A homeopathic remedy called *Biting Insects* by Molecular Biologicals is also quite effective. See "Insect Bites."

*M*enopause

Menopause, or the cessation of monthly menstrual periods, occurs in Western women at around the age of 50. Hot flashes are suffered by more than two thirds of them and are the most common reason they seek medical attention for menopausal complaints. Other disturbing symptoms may include loss of interest in sex, depression, moodiness, crying, anger, irritability, shortness of breath or difficulty breathing, dizziness, fatigue, indigestion, constipation, diarrhea, gas, headaches, heart palpitations, night sweats, insomnia, muscle and bone aches and tingling, shoulder and hip pain, cramps in the legs and feet, numbness in the arms, painfully sensitive skin, urinary problems, memory loss and mental sluggishness, dryness of the skin and vaginal tissues, breast tenderness, and weight gain. The risks of osteoporosis (bone loss) and heart disease also go up significantly after menopause. All of these problems are blamed on the loss of female hormones.

Interestingly, women in other cultures eating natural diets and following holistic lifestyles seem to escape menopausal symptoms. Japanese and Mayan women rarely experience hot flushes and other menopausal complaints.[442] Nature seems to have intended "the Change" to be a gradual process of reduced hormone output by the ovaries. As ovarian function falls off and hormone levels drop, the pituitary sends signals to the adrenals to increase their hormone output. When this backup hormone system is working properly, menopause should come with few or no side effects. The reason it fails for Western women has been blamed on adrenal exhaustion caused by stress, low blood sugar, and poor diet.

CONVENTIONAL TREATMENT

The conventional answer to waning hormone levels is hormone replacement therapy (HRT). The prescription version consists of pharmaceutical estrogen and synthetic progesterone, most popularly *Premarin* (derived from mare's urine) and *Provera*. Premarin has now become one of the most widely prescribed drugs in the country, but accompanying its rising popularity has been an alarming rise in breast cancer. Long-held suspicions of a link were confirmed when Harvard researchers reported the preliminary results of the ongoing Nurses' Health Study, involving 121,700 women. In June of 1995, researchers reported that women in the study who took estrogen after menopause had a 32 percent higher risk of breast cancer than those who had not taken the hormone. Women who had been off the drugs for two years or more, however, showed no increased risk. The implication was that taking estrogen for a few years to relieve hot flashes and other acute symptoms of menopause is probably safe, but taking it for decades could be hazardous. Estrogen is increasingly being prescribed, however, to slow postmenopausal bone loss; and for that, it *must* be taken for decades. In women who stop taking it, bone loss eventually catches up to the level of women who have never taken it.[443] The Nurses' Health Study also dashed hopes that taking synthetic progestins with estrogen (the combination called HRT) would counteract estrogen's effects in stimulating tumors in the breast, as it does for tumors in the uterus. Women on HRT actually had a *greater* risk of developing breast cancer than did women on estrogen alone.[444]

Synthetic or mare's-urine estrogen and synthetic progestions can also have unwanted side effects. Adverse reactions to Premarin listed in the *Physician's Desk Reference* include PMS-like symptoms; breast tenderness, enlargement and secretion; nausea, vomiting, abdominal cramps and bloating; skin and eye sensitivities; headaches, dizziness and depression; weight gain and water retention; bleeding between periods or missed periods; changes in libido (sex drive); and enlargement of uterine fibroid tumors. Side effects listed for synthetic progesterone (Provera) include bloating, water retention, nausea, insomnia, jaundice, mental depression, fever, masculinization, weight changes, breast tenderness, abdominal cramping, anxiety, irritability, and allergic reactions. Fluid retention can exacerbate asthma, migraines, epilepsy, and heart and kidney problems.[445]

NATURAL HORMONE REPLACEMENT

For women who feel they need hormones but want to avoid the side effects and risks of the prescription versions, estrogen and progesterone are available in natural plant form. Both plants and animals produce hormones that regulate cell metabolism and growth. In fact the sterols of plants such as soybeans and yams are the basis from which many cheap, commercially available hormones are made.

For many women, *natural progesterone cream* (*Pro-Gest* and others) can control hot flashes, without the use of estrogen. Their bodies apparently synthesize estrogen from it as needed. Progesterone is a hormone precursor, from which other hormones are made in the body. Studies show natural progesterone to be as effective as synthetic progestins in protecting against uterine cancer.[446] (This is no surprise; the synthetics just got tested first, evidently because large pharmaceutical companies were funding the tests.) Substituting natural for synthetic progesterone also allows most women on HRT to reduce their estrogen dose by at least half. After six months, many women taking natural progesterone who are well past menopause can give up estrogen altogether.[447]

The recommended protocol is to rub one-eighth to one-quarter teaspoon of natural progesterone cream on the abdominal area each night of the month, except during the menses (or if menses have ceased, for 25 days out of the month). Relief from hot flashes can take as long as several months, since the hormone gets to the blood by way of the fat layer under the skin and builds up only gradually; but other natural remedies can be used to reduce hot flashes while the progesterone is kicking in.

Natural estrogen creams derived from plants can also be used (for example *Ostaderm* and *Ostaderm V*). Preliminary research suggests that unlike animal and synthetic estrogens, plant estrogens aren't associated with increased rates of cancer of the breast and uterus and may even afford protection against those diseases. Research also indicates that plant estrogens are as effective as pharmaceutical estrogen in increasing HDL (good cholesterol), lowering LDL (bad cholesterol), and causing arteries to constrict and dilate when they should.[448]

Hormone levels can also be boosted with the hormone precursors, DHEA, and pregnenolone. Natural forms are better than synthetics.

ORIENTAL HERBS

The components of the traditional Chinese formulas include hormones derived from plants. Plant estrogens are much weaker than prescription estrogens and are more easily absorbed and used by the body. They are quite effective, while avoiding the strong side effects of prescription estrogen.

Chinese doctors consider menopause to be a deficiency of blood and Yin (the fluids of the body). They say your flow should stop without symptoms at around the age of 56—the later the better, since menstruation is considered an internal cleansing process. When symptoms do occur, Oriental doctors treat them with natural remedies that strengthen and build the blood. The approach has the advantage over drugs that you don't have to take the remedies forever. You need them only until your Yin is built back up and your body is back in balance. (However, you may want to continue to take different Chinese herbs as your body's needs change.)

Dong quai or *Tang-Kwei* (*Angelica sinensis root*) is a highly effective remedy for hot flashes, although its estrogen content is only one four-hundredth that of drugstore estrogen. Clinical and laboratory studies have shown Dong quai to be effective in stimulating uterine contractions, resolving blood clots, increasing the metabolism of the body and the oxygen consumption of the liver, lowering blood pressure, protecting the cardiovascular system, fighting bacteria and viruses, and reducing water retention.[449] When used in combination with other herbs, Dong quai is an effective antidote for menopausal anxiety, depression, nervousness and insomnia. Results may take a week or two, but homeopathic remedies can be used in the meantime for relief of symptoms.

Another common Chinese herbal component is ginseng. (See "Aging.") In menopausal women, it naturally stimulates estrogen production without risk.

Bupleurum is used in Chinese herbal formulas to reduce liver inflammation and congestion. The liver is where female hormones are converted into usable compounds.

Paeony (*Radix paeoniae lactiflorae*) is a Chinese herb that nourishes the blood. It is used for deficient blood patterns including menstrual dysfunction, leukorrhea (vaginal discharge), and uterine bleeding. It is also used for spontaneous sweating and night sweats, caused in Chinese medical terminology by deficient Yin that allows the fiery Yang to surface.[450]

Classical Chinese formulas contain these and other herbs in traditional combinations that have been proven safe and effective over centuries. A patent formula that is particularly good for menopausal complaints is Relaxed Wanderer (Hsaio Yao Wan or Xiao Yao Tang in Chinese). It works particularly well for women with a tendency to be cold (for example, to have cold hands and feet). For restlessness and hot flashes, a formula called Zhi Bai Di Huang Tang is effective. The Zand version is called Anem-Phello and Rehmannia Formula. The K'an Herb version is called Temper Fire. For the Chinese patent and American brand names of some other popular Chinese formulas for women's complaints.

WESTERN HERBS

The European and Native American herbal traditions also include excellent botanicals for premenstrual and menopausal complaints.

Red raspberry leaf (*Rubus idaeus*) is one of the most popular Western herbs for correcting hormone imbalances. A member of the rose family, it is best taken in the form of a simple infusion or tea. It restores and harmonizes uterine functions and helps rebuild uterine tissue, making it one of the few herbs that can actually be recommended throughout pregnancy. It also arrests bleeding and discharge and is useful in the treatment of uterine prolapse and mild digestive complaints, including diarrhea and constipation.

Black cohosh (Cimicifuga racemosa or *black snake root)* is an estrogen stimulant traditionally used for quelling hot flashes. The mechanism for its observed benefits was confirmed in a controlled study in which the levels of luteinizing hormone (LH) of 110 menopausal women treated with extracts of the herb declined. An elevation of LH has been linked to hot flashes.[451]

Another useful Western herb is *chasteberry* or *monk's pepper (Vitex agnus castus root)*. Valued in the Middle Ages by celibate monks for its ability to suppress sexual desire, it was later found to have this effect only in people afflicted with an excess of sexual desire. In people with the opposite affliction, it had the opposite effect. This balancing feature is chasteberry's strength for women's complaints. It works whether hormones are deficient or in excess, by stimulating the pituitary gland to harmonize hormone imbalances and make its own progesterone. Unlike with pharmaceutical hormones, you can't overdose: The herb won't force production of more hormone than the body needs. German research has shown that the chasteberry plant increases luteinizing hormone (which stimulates progesterone synthesis and secretion). It can also increase prolactin (which encourages milk production). Other studies have shown that the herb can help regulate periods involving too frequent or too much bleeding, and that it's a good treatment for fibroids and for inflammation of the lining of the womb. *WARNING: Chasteberry shouldn't be used during pregnancy, since it's a strong uterine stimulant.*[452]

Wild yam (Dioscorea villosa) contains a substance that converts to the steroid hormones progesterone and cortisone. It is used to treat inflammation, menstrual problems and (in small amounts) morning sickness.[453] Mexican yams are the source of the progesterone in the available natural progesterone and estrogen creams.

HOMEOPATHIC REMEDIES

The effectiveness of a German homeopathic remedy called *Mulimen*, composed of homeopathic doses of *Agnus castus* (chasteberry), *Cimicifuga racemosa* (black cohosh or black snake-root), *Hypericum* (St. John's wort), and *Sepia* (cuttlefish ink), was confirmed in a 1992 study. Half the women who took the remedy were relieved of their hot flashes, an objective result unlikely to be the product of suggestion.[454]

Another effective product for hot flashes and night sweats is a homeopathic version of the herb red raspberry leaf. A "gemmo-therapy" product—a special form of homeopathic made from the plant's baby roots, which are believed to have more life force than other plant parts— it is called *Rubus Idaeus* (the Latin name for the plant) and is manufactured by Dolisos.

An alternative for women who can't or don't want to take conventional doses of estrogen may be to take it in homeopathic doses. Like all homeopathic versions of prescription drugs, the FDA has made homeopathic estrogen a prescription-only item. But it's without long-term risks, since (like other homeopathic remedies) it's so diluted as to contain virtually none of the estrogen it's made from. Little information is available on homeopathic estrogen because it's too inexpensive to be worth promoting; but practitioners who use it report that it's generally effective for women who need it.[455]

A calcium and silica homeopathic product called *Calcium Absorption* helps stabilize the bones and prevent calcium loss by signaling the body to stop pulling calcium off the bones. In combination with *evening primrose oil,* it also helps provide the substrate necessary to manufacture better quality hormones.

Other homeopathic remedies good for hormonal complaints and their accompanying symptoms are listed below.

Popular Homeopathic Remedies for Hormonal Complaints

HOMEOPATHIC REMEDY	SELECTED SYMPTOMS AND INDICATIONS
Aconite	Complaints begin after a fright or sudden shock; great thirst for cold drinks; anxiety states; panic attacks.
Apis	Marked aggravation from heat; flushes of heat, made better by cold applications; severe menstrual cramps
Belladonna	Affected by change of temperature; all symptoms worse around menstrual period; intense heat in affected parts
Calcarea carbonica	Heavy bleeding; uterine fibroids; sensation of inner trembling; perspiration on head or back of neck; craves sweets (pastries and ice cream)
Caulophyllum	Arthritis of fingers or toes, worse before menses; vaginitis; infertility; vaginal discharge; painful menstruation

HOMEOPATHIC REMEDY	SELECTED SYMPTOMS AND INDICATIONS
Chamomilla	Feet feel hot and must be put outside covers; oversensitive to pain; complaints of anger, great irritability, aversion to being touched
Cimicifuga racemosa	Hot flashes worse at the onset of menstrual flow; severe headaches; changeable mood; talkative; jumps from one subject to the next
Ignatia	Perspiration only on face; lump in throat; sighing; easily offended, defensive
Kali carbonicum	Waking at night, especially 2–4 A.M.; wakes four hours after falling asleep
Lachesis	Hot flashes better at onset of menstrual flow; suspicion, even paranoia; hot; aggravated by heat; irritable; jealous; depressed; flushes of heat
Phosphorus	Tremendous thirst for cold drinks; bleeding bright-red blood; ovarian cysts; uterine prolapse
Pulsatilla	Weeps easily; headaches that are worse with heat, exertion, or after emotional stress, better in open air
Sabina	Gushing flow of bright-red blood, worse with motion; back pain with bleeding; thigh pain
Sanguinara	Migraine headache on the right side; hot flashes; hay fever; heartburn
Sepia	Involuntary weeping; symptoms worse from 2 to 4 P.M. or from 3 to 5 P.M.; flushes of heat with perspiration, worse at night
Sulfur	Worse with heat; worse after bathing; craves sweets, chocolate, fats; insomnia

DIET AND LIFESTYLE FACTORS

Studies suggest that the lack of menopausal complaints in women in Japanese and other non-Western cultures may be due largely to the high amounts of plant sterols in their diets. In one study, Japanese women were found to excrete 1,000 times the amount of phytoestrogens (plant estrogens) as did women in Finland.[456] Another study found that menopausal symptoms were significantly reduced in British women eating a diet high in phytoestrogens (furnished in that study as soya flour, red clover sprouts, and linseed or flax-seed oil).[457] Plant sterols are easily converted to human estrogen and progesterone in the body. The difference between getting hormones from pills or hormone-fed meats and getting them from plants is that in the plant form, you're getting only the precursors. Your body can take from these building blocks and make whatever it needs. You don't have to worry about pushing your estrogen levels to dangerous heights.[458]

So far, some 300 plants with estrogen-like activity have been identified, including carrots, corn, apples, barley, and oats; but soybean products such as tofu seem to pack the strongest hormonal wallop. Ideally, you should eat one soy product a day. However, not everyone likes tofu, and not all concentrated soy products contain the requisite isoflavones. If the soy protein in your soy burger, for example, has been extracted using alcohol rather than water, the isoflavones will largely have been lost. Another problem with eating large amounts of soy is that they can impair iron absorption, leading to anemia and iron deficiency in women.[459] One way to avoid these problems is to get your phytoestrogens from one of the concentrated estrogen skin creams derived from plants (*Ostaderm, Ostraderm V*). Research results on these creams aren't yet available, but estrogens derived from plant foods have been shown to be safe and effective.

Citrus fruits, cherries, grapes, hawthorn berry, and red clover are good sources of estrogen-containing bioflavonoids. Bioflavonoids have been found to be effective in controlling hot flashes, anxiety, and irritability, even though they're only one fifty-thousandth as strong as drugstore estrogen. They also help in strengthening the capillaries and preventing heavy irregular menstrual bleeding.

Other foods high in plant hormones include yams, papayas, peas, cucumbers, bananas, bee pollen, raw nuts, seeds, sprouts, and certain herbs (alfalfa, licorice root, red clover, sage, sarsaparilla, sassafras).

Nature's Plus makes a nutritional product called *Isoflavone 100,* which combines Genistein, Daidzein, and Puerarin, the active components of the soybean.

Hormone Therapy Avoided with Tofu Shake

A 44-year-old woman whose hormone level was a low 28 said her doctor wanted her to start on pharmaceutical estrogen and progesterone. However, she was opposed to taking hormones so early with no real symptoms; so about four mornings each week she started drinking a tofu shake, consisting of tofu, soy milk, and fruit mixed in a blender. Her hormones rose from 28 to 154 over a four-month period. Even her doctor was impressed and agreed she no longer needed the drugs.

NUTRITIONAL SUPPLEMENTS

Vitamin E has been shown in medical studies to be effective in reducing hot flashes.[460] It also helps relieve other menopausal complaints, including breast tenderness and vaginal dryness. When buying vitamin E, look for the natural product (d-alpha tocopherol or d-alpha tocopheryl), which is absorbed better from the digestive system and retained in the body longer than synthetic vitamin E (dl-alpha tocopherol or dl-alpha tocopheryl).[461] Vitamin E is also absorbed better when taken with meals than on an empty stomach. It should not be taken with iron supplements, which destroy it. Iron-rich foods such as raisins and spinach, on the other hand, can be eaten without harm to the vitamin E. Vitamin E is one of those vitamins you can get too much of, but for hot flashes, 400 to 600 international units (IU) daily is considered safe.[462] For quelling intractable hot flashes, some MDs prescribe up to 1,600 IU per day.[463] *If you experience blurred vision, you should stop taking the vitamin.*

Other antistress vitamins involved in progesterone production include *vitamin A, vitamin C,* and *pantothenic acid.* Estrogen production can also be maintained and hot flashes relieved by taking *evening primrose oil* (two at bedtime, totaling 1,300 mg).

The oils of seeds and nuts can also help counteract the dry skin, dry hair, and dry vaginal tissues that plague menopausal women, symptoms that can indicate a lack of essential fatty acids (EFAs). To counteract dry skin, two teaspoons of *linseed* or *flaxseed oil* are recommended daily. Also good is Ultimate Oil by Nature's Secret (capsules containing a blend of oils).

Bovine glandular extracts help augment uterine and ovarian function. If the uterus is weak, you can supplement either with natural progesterone or with an extract to stimulate its function called *Utrophin* (by Standard Process). If the ovaries are weak, you can supplement either with estrogen or with *Ovex* to stimulate their function. In women who still have their ovaries, progesterone levels may also be raised by *Ovatrophin,* made from bovine corpus luteum (the part of the cow ovary that contains progesterone).

For some over-the-counter nutritional products beneficial for menopausal problems, see the Appendix.

Menstrual Problems, Cramps, Excess Bleeding, "Flooding"

Flooding, or prolonged menstrual bleeding, is particularly common near menopause. Bleeding can be so heavy and draining as to propel women to get hysterectomies. But while their doctors may have promised that their problems would then be over, many women say they wished they hadn't rushed into these surgeries. (See "Uterine Fibroids.") For younger women, the bane of their monthly periods is liable to be painful cramping. Other premenstrual complaints are discussed under "PMS."

CONVENTIONAL TREATMENT

For persistent hemorrhage-like flooding in an older woman, the gynecologist may recommend surgical removal of the uterus. "You don't need that organ anymore," he may say. "Let's just solve the problem by getting rid of it." But hysterectomies can lead to a host of other, unanticipated problems, including osteoporosis, bone and joint pain and immobility, loss of libido, chronic fatigue, urinary problems, emotional problems, depression, prolapse, and increased risk of heart disease. (See "Uterine Fibroids.")

For menstrual cramps, the conventional approach is painkillers such as *Midol, Ibuprofen,* and *Advil.* But these drugs merely mask the symptom without addressing the real problem, and women often find they need more and more to get the same results.

RELIEVING CRAMPS NATURALLY

Menstrual cramps vary in degree and type. When the blood is dark with clots, Chinese doctors say that last month's blood has stayed in the tubes. The more stagnation there is in the body and the darker and more clotted the blood, the worse the cramps. Relief requires "moving the blood." The Chinese patent formula to achieve this result is *Hsiao Yao Wan.* Take eight pills three times daily from ovulation to menstruation.

In the homeopathic line, *Cyclease* by Boiron has many satisfied users. *Mag Phos,* a cell salt, is also good. Take it from the day before until the second day of the menstrual period. If these don't work, consult a homeopath for an appropriate constitutional homeopathic remedy.

Severe Cramps Relieved

Indi had such severe cramps that she usually missed a day each month from work. *Cyclease* and *Mag Phos* helped, but she was still uncomfortable. A homeopathic remedy called *Veratrum*, for cramps that radiate to the back and up the thighs, did the trick. Not only was her pain immediately relieved, but the following month her cramps were much more tolerable than before. This is, in fact, how the right homeopathic remedy should work: not just symptomatically at the time but over the long term.

NATURAL REMEDIES FOR FLOODING

Women who experience flooding may have blood levels shown in lab tests to be in the low but normal range. In Chinese medical theory, however, what counts isn't the absolute level but the change from high to low. A woman used to having high blood levels will feel weak and experience palpitations and nightmares if her blood levels suddenly drop. Chinese herbal remedies are aimed at correcting the resulting blood deficiency. A three-step approach is necessary: (1) stop the immediate bleeding, (2) build the blood back up, and (3) correct the underlying hormone imbalance. For remedies to build the blood, see "Anemia."

NATURAL REMEDIES TO STOP BLEEDING

A good start for bleeding is a simple homeopathic by BHI called *Bleeding*. Take one tablet every 15 minutes until bleeding has slowed. Then take one pill four times daily until menstruation ends.

For more severe bleeding, try this herbal remedy: mix 20 drops of *Trilium* with one tablespoonful of *luvos*. Drink this mix three times daily.

For bleeding from fibroids, an effective herbal tincture is *Thaspi Bursa*. Drink 20 drops mixed in water every 15 minutes for the first hour, then 20 drops every hour until bleeding has stopped. This remedy can be taken over several months to help reduce fibroids.

The Chinese have an effective patent formula to stop bleeding called *yunan paiyao*, used either orally or topically. In an emergency, capsules of this formula can be taken by mouth. However, other natural remedies need to be used to help balance the body and stop the underlying cause of bleeding.

The herb *capsicum (cayenne pepper)* mixed in water also stops bleeding. Again, however, merely fixing the immediate problem doesn't reach the underlying cause, which is hormone imbalance.

Natural Remedies to Correct an Underlying Hormone Imbalance

Natural progesterone cream (Pro-Gest) smeared on the abdomen can halt heavy bleeding. (See "Menopause.") Effective herbal tonics are also available for this purpose. Good choices are *Female Tonic* by MarcoPharma and *Female Balancer* by Apex. To correct a hormone imbalance involving bleeding from fibroids, try *Fibrosolve* by Apex.

Severe Case of Flooding Corrected Naturally

Becky, 46, was desperate; she had been bleeding heavily for more than six weeks. She was weak, couldn't sleep, and was very tired, but she worked at a very high-stress job and couldn't take time off. Just having to rush to the bathroom every hour was stressing her out. *Bleeding* by BHI slowed her bleeding some, but not enough. What solved her immediate crisis was the herb *trilium* combined with *luvos*. In about four hours, her bleeding had stopped. But she still had problems. Blood loss had caused her to be severely anemic. Her hair was falling out, she was having nightmares, and her hormones were still out of balance. She faithfully took *Female Balance* by MarcoPharma and used *Pro-Gest* cream. By the time of her next period, she reported that her bleeding level was normal and she felt like her old self again.

Mononucleosis, Epstein-Barr Syndrome

Infectious mononucleosis has been attributed to the Epstein-Barr virus, but the whole syndrome remains a mystery. Although mono has been called "the kissing disease," researchers have been unable to successfully transmit it from one volunteer to another. Yet it does frequently occur in adolescents and young adults living together. Symptoms come on gradually, with fever, sore throat, general discomfort, loss of appetite, and headache that can be severe. The lymph glands gradually swell, and the spleen and liver are frequently enlarged. The disease can last from one to eight weeks, after which the patient may feel abnormally weak and tired for weeks or months.

Symptoms may then recur, or may develop into chronic-fatigue syndrome, which can persist for years. (See "Chronic Fatigue Syndrome.") At least 100,000 cases of mononucleosis occur in the United States each year.[464]

CONVENTIONAL TREATMENT

The cure for mononucleosis is conventionally considered to be as elusive as the disease. The usual recommendations are just to wait it out, with bed rest, a soft diet, fluids, and aspirin. Antibiotics don't affect the course of the disease, but they often get prescribed before the diagnosis has been certainly established. The result can be repeated courses of different and stronger antibiotics, with a corresponding weakening of the body's immune defenses.

Toxic Radiation Treatments Narrowly Avoided

Hannah got run down from "burning the candle at both ends." She contracted mono and wound up on one round of antibiotics after another. Despite the drugs, she continued to relapse. Eventually the infection caused a swelling in her throat that was thought to be non-Hodgkin's lymphoma. Radiation treatment was recommended. Fortunately, when the tumor was removed, it was found to be nonmalignant. Radiation, a toxic cancer treatment linked to secondary cancers later in life, was narrowly avoided; but Hannah continued to be susceptible to infections and bouts of weakness. She "got her strength back" only after a long, slow program of vitamin and nutritional therapy to rebuild her immune system.

ALTERNATIVE TREATMENT

Hannah's cancer scare may have been avoidable. A viable treatment is available for mononucleosis that knocks the condition out early and permanently. A German homeopathic by Staufen called *Mononucleosis,* is recommended even for people who have had mono years earlier, since the disease has a tendency to turn into chronic fatigue. People are amazed at how much better they feel after taking it, even when they thought they were well before.

Lingering Mono Kicked in Two Weeks

A 14-year-old girl who had contracted mono was still tired, pale, and missing school four months later. After two weeks' treatment with

Mononucleosis by Staufen, she was back in school and quite healthy. Her mother still drops in to express her gratitude for the girl's remarkable recovery.

Nail Health

The drugstore answer to fingernails that are brittle and weak is to paint them with nail hardener, but this cosmetic solution fails to address the underlying problem. Chinese doctors and homeopaths view fingernails that split, break, or are concave instead of convex as symptomatic of underlying deficiencies. According to Chinese medical theory, the condition of your nails reflects the condition of your body: The strength of your nails indicates the strength of your bones; moons showing at the base of all eight fingernails indicate overall health; the shape of your nails may indicate the condition of your heart. Homeopaths, too, consider nail problems to be a symptom of something else. Finding the right remedy for the underlying problem corrects the condition of the nails at the same time.

Concave Nails Cured with Heart Remedy

Brent sought a remedy for fingernails that he called "spooned." They were concave rather than convex. His real problem, however, turned out to be his heart. He revealed that he had had severe heart problems, for which he had twice undergone angioplastic surgeries. A homeopathic remedy called *Cactus* was recommended for his condition. (See "Heart Disease.") After he began taking this remedy, Brent immediately noticed a difference in his strength and stamina. He was soon walking several miles each day. He also changed his diet. But what he most needed to change was his job, which involved spraying toxic chemicals on potatoes. In the two years since he abandoned that employment, not only have his heart problems disappeared but his nails have returned to normal.

HOW TO STRENGTHEN NAILS FROM THE INSIDE OUT

A number of good natural remedies are available for strengthening nails, hair and bones from the inside out.

A homeopathic combination formula called *Calcium Absorption* by Bioforce helps increase the amount of calcium absorbed from food and alters how the body uses the calcium it has.

A mineral product that increases nail calcium is *BioSil* by Jarrow. Six drops are taken daily in juice, a very economical alternative, since one bottle contains 600 drops and lasts more than three months. By the time the bottle is gone, users report that their nails are longer and stronger than they have been in years.

With-in by Trace Minerals is a complete daily mineral supplement that emphasizes the growth of strong, healthy hair and nails.

Another natural recipe for strengthening nails comes from the Golden Door Spa in Southern California. A whole egg (shell and all) is allowed to sit for 25 minutes in the juice of one lemon, which dissolves the eggshell. The eggshell is then removed and the juice is drunk. Taken three times a week, this remedy can make nails remarkably hard.

A secret of Flamenco guitar players who use their nails as guitar picks is to dissolve a packet of *gelatin* (unflavored) in juice and drink it. The gelatin is taken twice daily. Capsules called *Beef Gelatin* are also available from NOW Foods.

The herb *horsetail*, which contains *silica*, is another natural nail strengthener. *Alta Silica* by Alta Health or *Vegesil* by Flora are both extracts of *horsetail*.

Nausea, Vomiting, Motion Sickness, Morning Sickness

Nausea is unpleasant, but vomiting isn't normally something that should be suppressed. It usually represents the body's attempt to get rid of harmful bacteria or other toxins. Other common causes of nausea include motion sickness, stress, pregnancy (morning sickness), migraine headache, and allergies. Nausea and vomiting can also be caused by drugs. Cancer chemotherapy is well known to cause severe nausea, but there are other less well-known suspects as well, including antibiotics, certain heart medications, narcotic painkillers such as codeine, birth control pills and other female hormones, and prescription asthma medications. Iron supplements and salt substitutes have also been implicated.

Nausea can indicate something more serious, including ulcers, colorectal cancer, diabetes, an impending heart attack, Crohn's disease, meningitis, mononucleosis, or gallstones. If you are vomiting up blood or have abdominal pain, headache, dizziness, fever, or a racing heartbeat, or if the vomiting lasts more than four hours, of if you are very old or debilitated, you should consult a doctor.

DRUG TREATMENT

No over-the-counter drugs are recommended by the FDA for treating nausea and vomiting. There are drugs that work, but they either require a prescription or the FDA permits their over-the-counter sale only to treat motion sickness.[465] Motion sickness isn't caused by something your body is trying to get rid of, so suppressing it with drugs doesn't involve retaining potential poisons. The downside of over-the-counter motion-sickness drugs is that they make you tired and drowsy.

NATURAL ALTERNATIVES

For nausea and vomiting caused by indigestion, effective homeopathic remedies are available. One is *Carbo Veg 6c*. Take three tablets every 15 minutes. For severe upset, up to six doses may be taken.

For cramps, nausea, vomiting, and pain caused by food poisoning, try *Arsenicum Alba 6x*. Take two pills every 15 minutes, up to six doses. Another option is *Salmonella 200x*. Often a single dose will relieve severe cramping and nausea.

In the herbal line, *ginger* may be taken for nausea, either as capsules or drunk as a tea.

Pill Curing is an excellent Chinese herbal remedy for settling the stomach after a large meal or when the food feels stuck in your midsection. This remedy can also effectively quell motion sickness without making you drowsy. Other effective motion-sickness remedies are a Chinese formula called *Bao Ji Wan* and *ginger*. A particularly good homeopathic remedy for motion sickness is *Travel Sickness* by Dolisos (two pills three to four times daily).

The *Sea Band* is a very effective and easy motion sickness alternative. An elastic band placed on the wrist, it puts pressure on one of the major acupuncture points of the body. It is particularly good for restless children who complain about getting sick in the car.

Luxury Cruise a Success After All

At 42, Steve had signed up for his first luxury cruise, but he was so prone to seasickness, he almost canceled the trip. Then he learned about the sea bands. He took the trip, and came back delighted to report that he had experienced no seasickness or nausea. He said he hadn't taken the bands off during the entire trip—not even in the shower!

SAFE, EFFECTIVE REMEDIES FOR MORNING SICKNESS

For nausea during pregnancy, homeopathic remedies are completely safe, since they work on a vibrational rather than a chemical level. (The official position of the FDA is that they consist of nothing but water. See Chapter 3.) A classic homeopathic remedy for morning sickness is *Symphoricarpus.* Another effective remedy that is safe to use during pregnancy is a homeopathic combination by Molecular Biologicals called *Nausea.*

Homeopathic remedies are the only remedies that can be recommended during pregnancy with absolute confidence in their safety. No herbs should be used during pregnancy, with the possible exception of red *raspberry leaf,* which can be sipped as a tea during morning sickness and is good for use during the last six weeks of pregnancy to strengthen and tonify the uterus and prepare it for giving birth.

OTHER HELPFUL TIPS

Contrary to popular belief, liquids—especially carbonated drinks—are hard to keep down on an upset stomach. A cracker or other dry food is better. You can drink colas or ginger ales, but they should be flat, at room temperature, and taken in small sips. Other good fluids are apple and grape juices drunk at room temperature. Citrus juices aren't as good, since their acidity can irritate the stomach and they often contain solid pulp that is hard to digest.[466]

*O*varian Cysts

Ovarian cysts are fluid-filled sacs that develop in or on the ovary. They come and go and are usually cyclic, getting worse around ovulation or before the period. A cyst found by ultrasound may be gone two weeks later. The pain of an ovarian cyst is usually limited to the left or right side and is often confused with appendicitis.

CONVENTIONAL TREATMENT

The conventional medical treatment is immediate abdominal surgery, on the theory that the cysts might rupture. There is also a remote chance that they may be cancerous. The problem with surgery is that new cysts are liable to continue to form, and the procedure leaves painful scar tissue and can result in infertility. A recent study from Italy found that more than one third of women with ovarian cysts don't need surgery or even a biopsy. The problem spontaneously regresses without any medical intervention.[467]

ALTERNATIVE TREATMENT

Those figures were for women who got no treatment at all. If they were to get alternative treatment to balance their hormone levels, many more would probably find that their cysts spontaneously regressed. The authors of this book were both advised to get hysterectomies for cysts on the ovaries and for fibroid tumors. Both sought natural remedies instead and both have had no problems since. Lynne's case is described here and Ellen's under "Uterine Fibroids" and "Uterine Prolapse."

Ovaries Saved Naturally

Lynne was diagnosed by ultrasound with a large fibroid tumor and cysts on the ovaries at the tender age of 33. Her first doctor recommended a hysterectomy. Then she went to an older, more conservative doctor for a second opinion. He frankly advised her that if she did nothing, she would probably be fine. Even if the cysts burst, which was unlikely, he said the fluid would merely be reabsorbed into her body. She decided to try alternative remedies before resorting to surgery. Homeopathy, acupuncture, and Chinese herbs caused both the fibroid and the cysts to be painlessly reabsorbed.

NATURAL REMEDIES

Alternative practitioners maintain that the problem to be attacked is not the cyst itself but an underlying hormone imbalance. Correcting this imbalance can make cysts go away for good. The natural approach is a two-step one: first relieving the pain of ovarian cysts, then balancing the hormones. *Homeopathic Phosphorus* works well for the pain. To balance the hormones, a product called *Female Tonic* by MarcoPharma is effective. Acupuncture and hormone-balancing herbs can also help. (See "Menopause.") For women who know which way their hormones are out of balance, *homeopathic progesterone* or *homeopathic estrogen* (by Deseret) may be used.

NOTE: Whether your hormone levels are right for you can't always be determined from a blood test. What is "normal" varies considerably. Women with obvious symptoms of hormone imbalance often report that their doctors drew blood and said their levels were in the normal range. If your body usually has high hormone levels and they suddenly drop, you will not "feel like yourself." The balance between estrogen and progesterone levels is more important than absolute numbers. Symptoms usually result when estrogen levels are too high relative to progesterone levels. Problems can also result when either hormone is given in synthetic pill form without the other. Natural progesterone can be converted to estrogen by the body as needed, but synthetic progesterone doesn't convert well and can throw the hormones out of balance.

For recurring cysts, a German homeopathic remedy by Staufen called *Ovarialcystom* is recommended. Herbal remedies may also help shrink cysts. A Latvian topical remedy developed from the *stinkhorn mushroom* can be used not only on ovarian cysts but on hemorrhoids, sores, wounds, and inflammations of various sorts. Available by mail from Josef Gurvich in New York (telephone 201-433-5620), it is very inexpensive.

Overweight, Obesity

Second only to smoking as the leading cause of preventable death in the United States, obesity is a major risk factor for hypertension, heart disease, and diabetes. A 1997 study found that 35 percent of Americans are overweight enough to be unhealthy, up from 25 percent in 1980, making us probably the most overweight nation in the world. Besides the clinically obese, millions of people keep binging, dieting, and binging again, in a vicious cycle that has made dieting a \$35 billion industry.[468]

DIET DRUGS

The medical trend is to view obesity as a disease that should be treated with drugs. But while one weight loss drug after another has hit the market with much fanfare, they usually wind up getting pulled off the shelves when their dangerous side effects have become known. In the thirties, when the weight-loss craze is said to have been ushered in with the bathroom scales, the drug of the day was a derivative of the industrial poison dinitrophenol. Besides weight loss, it could cause rashes, fever, blindness, and sometimes death.[469] In the sixties, if you wanted to lose a few pounds, you could readily get a prescription for *amphetamines*. But the psychotic-like side effects and addiction potential of these drugs, as well as their failure to take pounds off long-term, eventually made doctors very circumspect in their use.

The inadequacies of the available options contributed to the fanfare when, in April of 1996, the FDA approved *Redux (dexfenfluramine)*, the first prescription weight loss drug to be approved in 23 years. Redux was a variation of another diet drug, *fenfluramine (Pondimin)*, which had been on the market since the seventies. Pondimin created a stir only in the nineties, however, when a study showed weight loss benefits in combination with a third drug, *phenteramine (Ionamin, Fastin, Adipex-P)*, a combination popularly called *fen-phen*. Fen-phen is chemically similar to amphetamines; while Redux, a similar drug without the amphetamine, is chemically more like the antidepressant Prozac.

Redux and fen-phen were heavily promoted. By 1997, more than two million Americans had taken Redux, and more than six million had taken Pondimin. Then in September of 1997, the drugs were suddenly pulled from the shelves, after the FDA analyzed heart tests on 291 dieters using them. Although most had no symptoms, almost a third of these users had damaged heart valves. Whether this damage is reversible after giving up the drug remains to be determined.[470]

Over-the-counter diet aids, however, are still available. They typically contain combinations of *phenylpropanolamine (PPA)*, *ephedrine* derivatives, and *caffeine*. These ingredients are weaker than amphetamines, but they have similar chemical structures and reactions in the body. They stimulate the sympathetic nervous system, the fight-or-flight emergency system; and in high doses, they can produce psychotic-like side effects and hypertensive crises as amphetamines do. In one reported case, a 35-year-old woman developed an intracerebral hemorrhage after taking only one tablet of the popular diet aid *Dexatrim, Extra Strength.*[471]

"NATURAL" UPPERS

Though less hazardous than the pharmaceutical variety, some herbal diet pills also carry risks. The natural stimulant *ephedrine* (under the names *Ma huang, ephedra* or *epitonin*) has replaced amphetamines not only in "natural" diet aids, but in herbal combinations that are popular among young people and that are advertised as producing a "natural high." Overdosing on natural ephedra, like on synthetic ephedrine, however, has been linked to heart attack, stroke, and sudden death, leading the FDA to consider banning or limiting the use of all ephedrine products both as weight-loss and as body-building aids. New York and Florida have already banned their sale, after a 20-year-old college student died following an overdose of an ephedrine-containing herbal product called *Ultimate Xphoria.*[472]

Opponents counter that herbal ephedra is safer than the synthetic ephedrine and amphetamine products it has replaced, both as diet aids and as "street drugs." The key is simply moderation.

For weight loss, both *ephedra* and *caffeine* are natural thermogenic agents that stimulate the burning of fat and suppress the appetite. A Swedish study comparing obese women given caffeine and ephedrine three times daily with women given a placebo found that the caffeine/ephedrine group lost significantly more fat and maintained more lean body weight after eight weeks.[473]

Taking ephedra for long periods, however, isn't advised. Ephedra depletes certain chemicals in the brain, causing depression. As with amphetamines, the dieter initially feels enormously energetic; but when the brain chemicals have been depleted, she can crash overnight.

Diet-related Depression Relieved

For months, Sherry had been taking *E'ola*, a popular multilevel marketing product that contains ephedra. Her life was going well, yet she was so depressed she was thinking about suicide. When it was suggested that the ephedra was her problem, she said she was afraid to stop taking it for fear she would put on weight and become even more depressed. She was finally persuaded; and after two weeks without the drug, her depression went away as suddenly as it had appeared.

OTHER HERBAL OPTIONS

Other herbal dieting products that are safer and that users report to be effective include *herbal Fen-Phen*, consisting of amino acids; and *HCA*, a plant extract (*Garcinic Cambogia*) contained in a product called *Citrimax*. NOTE: Results on Citrimax require patience. Typically not much effect is noticed for the first three to four weeks. Then you suddenly start eating less and losing weight.

HOMEOPATHIC DIET AIDS

Homeopathic remedies can also help. One called *Weight OFF* suppresses the appetite. Another called *Metaboslim* is said to speed up metabolism and burn calories faster. To correct depressed thyroid function, which can be a cause of weight gain, Complimed recommends taking homeopathic *Thyroid* (which rebalances a thyroid that is either under- or overactive) in combination with Metaboslim.

"Spare Tire" Eliminated

Marta, 32, would not have been considered overweight. But she was carrying an extra ten pounds around her middle that made her feel uncomfortable and that she couldn't seem to lose. Weight Off in combination with Metaboslim helped to redistribute her weight. The difference on the scales was a mere ten pounds, but her whole body shape was different. She looked and felt so good that she sent many other women for Metaboslim. They, too, reported good results.

DIETARY SOLUTIONS

Weight can be lost without drugs or herbs, just by exercising your body and your willpower. Dieting is as popular as ever. However, many popular diets are of dubious merit. Current fads include some of the following:

LOW-CALORIE, LOW-FAT DIETS.   This is the most common diet plan. Ideally, it consists of cutting out junk foods and concentrating on fruits, vegetables, whole grains, and lean meats. Problems arise when dieters try to trick their taste buds with artificial sweeteners and fake fats *(Olestra)*. The Calorie Control Council reports that four out of five Americans now consume low-cal, sugar-free, or reduced-fat food and beverages containing these altered substances. Yet since artificial sweeteners became popular, Americans have gotten heavier, not lighter. Another problem is side effects. *Aspartame (NutraSweet)* has been linked to brain tumors in laboratory rats. Human brain tumors jumped by 10 percent the year after the FDA approved aspartame for widespread use.

Olestra was conditionally approved by the FDA for marketing as a "fat-free fat" in early 1996. Virtually identical to mineral oil, it is a laxative that depletes the body of fat-soluble vitamins and other essential nutrients if used habitually, and that can cause diarrhea and cramping, among other side effects. Fake fat isn't liable to work any better than fake sugar for producing weight loss. Low-fat foods often contain more calories than high-fat foods; the fat is simply replaced with sugar.[474] In any case, you need some fat in your diet. Hormones, including estrogen, progesterone, and testosterone, are all made from cholesterol.

Fat-free Diets Deprive the Body of Essential Hormones

Several women on fat-free diets who had had surgery for reproductive problems reported that their surgeons found that their reproductive organs were adhering abnormally to the abdominal wall. Their bodies simply weren't making sufficient hormones for the proper functioning of their femal organs, leaving their surgeons no choice but to remove those organs.

HIGH-PROTEIN DIETS. In the seventies, books such as *The Complete Scarsdale Medical Diet* and *Dr. Atkins' Diet Revolution* propounded high-protein diets, based on the theory that too many carbohydrates prevent the body from burning fat. These diets have been revived in the nineties with books such as *The Zone* and *Protein Power.* The original high-protein diet allowed unrestricted amounts of protein (meat, fish, shellfish, poultry, eggs, and cheese), while high-carbohydrate foods were restricted (bread, potatoes, sugary foods, pasta). The Zone Diet is a modification that varies the percentage of protein, carbohydrate, and fat based on body and lifestyle factors. High-protein foods keep blood-sugar levels steady, so appetite is easier to control, and weight loss occurs quickly. But when carbohydrates aren't available, fats are burned, releasing ketones that can cause headaches, dizziness, fatigue, nausea, and bad breath. The diet also creates huge amounts of acid in the body, requiring enormous quantities of minerals, especially calcium, to neutralize it. The result is demineralization and bone loss. The diet is also high in fat and cholesterol. This increases the risk of heart disease as well as the risk of kidney damage from excess protein.

THE GRAPEFRUIT DIET. This is a three-week diet composed principally of grapefruits, which are said to contain a certain fat-burning enzyme. The diet also includes specific vegetables and small amounts of protein and totals less than 800 calories a day. Initial weight loss can be dramatic, but monofood diets are unbalanced. Grapefruit is missing many essential nutrients, and when eaten in excess, it throws off the acid/base balance of the body. Grapefruit juice also markedly increases the potency of common prescription drugs, including sedatives and antihypertensives, resulting in reported cases of unwitting drug overdose.[475]

FOOD COMBINING. Books such as *The Beverly Hills Diet* and *Fit for Life* follow the food-combining theories of the earlier natural hygienists: Eat fruit alone for breakfast and don't eat protein and starch in the same meal. Researchers contend there is no scientific evidence for the theory, but many people seem to lose weight on it; and people with a tendency to have digestive problems swear by it. The plan at least is well balanced and includes ample portions, so it can be followed indefinitely. It's a lifestyle rather than a crash diet.[476]

EATING ACCORDING TO BLOOD TYPE. Another approach that is a lifestyle rather than a diet is recommended by Dr. Peter D'Adamo in *Eat 4 Your Blood Type*. Dr. D'Adamo maintains that the right diet for your body is determined by your blood type, which reflects hereditary factors. "A" blood types do better on vegetarian diets; "O" blood types need meat. "B" types are in between. Many enthusiastic women claim painless weight loss following this protocol.

ELIMINATING THE CAUSE OF FOOD CRAVINGS

You can force dietary restriction with drugs or grueling willpower, but if the cause of overeating is not addressed, the weight is liable to come right back when the "heat is off." A real cure requires eliminating the underlying cause. The question is, why do we crave food? One theory is that when we don't eat for a few hours, our bodies switch into cleansing mode and start dumping toxins into our bloodstreams. The result is a headache and feeling of weakness. To dispel these uncomfortable feelings, we reach for more food.

We may also keep reaching for food because we are malnourished, even while eating plentifully, because we aren't eating the *right* nutrients. Fake fats and sugars can fool the taste buds, but our bodies know they need real ("good") fats and carbohydrates and will continue to crave them. To be well nourished, we need essential fatty acids, complex carbohydrates, fiber, and a wide range of vitamins and minerals.

A more fundamental problem may be that we are not properly absorbing the nutrients we ingest. Absorption is prevented by the buildup of a slimy sludge of toxins that coats the intestines as a result of poor elimination. For some remarkable photos of the tissue-like intestinal sludge eliminated during supervised fasting, see Dr. Bernard Jensen's 1981 classic, *Tissue Cleansing Through Bowel Management.*[477]

THE FASTING ALTERNATIVE

The proposed solution of fasting proponents is a regime of detoxification to eliminate this toxic buildup. Dr. Jensen recommends fasting with coffee enemas to clean the colon so that it can make better use of nutrients. When the body has been scrubbed from the inside out, your taste buds are sharpened. Simple, whole foods suddenly become sufficient and delicious. Fasting expert and natural hygienist Dr. Herbert M. Shelton wrote that he found nothing so satisfying after a fast as half a head of plain lettuce. (Interestingly, recent research indicates that people who are overweight have *less* sensitive taste buds than do people who are thin. Apparently, the more sensitive or "clean" your taste buds are, the less food you require for satiation.)

Despite fasting's long history, it remains controversial as a method of weight control. Some authorities contend it makes you put on weight, because the body starts storing calories in anticipation of famine conditions; and there are concerns about how safe it is, and about fanatical teenagers fasting themselves into anorexia. But, it's another program enthusiasts swear by. For protocols and recommended reading, see "Aging, Longevity."

*P*ain, Inflammation

Pain, the body's alarm system, is the most common symptom of disease, making analgesics (painkillers) the most commonly used drugs world-wide. Pain produces inflammation, a buildup of body fluids that serves to destroy or wall off toxins and injured tissue and carry immune-system cells to the site of injury. Inflammation then produces more pain, by pressing on the nerves in the injured area. The buildup of free radicals at the pain site causes further discomfort. To reach the cause of pain, a pain reliever would need to reduce inflammation by reducing local fluid levels and removing free radicals and damaged cells. But that is not how most anal-gesics work. Instead, they merely suppress the awareness of pain.[478] This is equivalent to treating a fire by turning off the alarm, leaving the fire to burn down the barn. That doesn't mean pain-killers don't serve necessary functions. Sometimes you're just trying to get through the day or the night. But where natural alternatives are available that treat the *cause* of pain, they're obviously preferable to drugs that merely mask it.

Over-the-counter pain relief is discussed in this section. For pre-scription narcotics, see "Surgical Trauma."

PHARMACEUTICAL PAIN RELIEF

Analgesics account for one fourth of the over-the-counter drug market. This lucrative business is divided among *aspirin, acetaminophen,* and *ibuprofen.* Aspirin, the oldest analgesic, has been around in pill form since 1899. A naturally-occurring form of the drug found in willow bark was known to Hippocrates millennia before that. Americans now take about 80 million aspirin tablets a day, or 29 billion a year, not to mention what's contained in many combination drugs. That works out to 117 aspirin tablets per person annually. The statistic is actually misleading, however, since 20 percent of users consume 80 percent of the drug.[479]

Aspirin's most popular use is in the relief of simple tension headaches. Its ability to reduce inflammation makes it the leading drug recommend-ed for arthritis, in which pain comes from the movement and stress of inflamed joints. Aspirin also reduces fever, retards blood clotting, and "thins the blood," a property underlying its recently touted use as a pre-ventative for heart attacks. (See "Fever," "Headaches," "Heart Attacks.")

Aspirin was on the market for nearly a century before the mechanism for its effects was discovered in the 1970s. The mechanism involves natural substances called prostaglandins. One called PGE2 alerts the body to disturbances in normal function by increasing the awareness of pain. Other prostaglandins contribute to the heat and swelling of inflammation and promote the coagulation of blood. Released when cells are injured or stimulated, prostaglandins can cause tissue damage themselves. Aspirin interferes with the body's biosynthesis of these prostaglandins, suppressing inflammation and the awareness of pain.

Other drugs in the aspirin group work the same way. Called *nonsteroidal anti-inflammatory drugs* or *NSAIDs* (as opposed to the steroids, which also reduce inflammation but have more serious side effects), they include *ibuprofen (Motrin, Advil), indomethacin (Indocin), naproxen (Aleve, Naprosyn), piroxicam (Feldene),* and *sulindac (Clinoril),* among others.

The drawback of this approach, besides its failure to address the cause of pain, is that prostaglandins have normal body functions that are inhibited at the same time. Some help to regulate the flow of blood through the kidneys and the filtration and excretion of sodium and toxins. When aspirin and other NSAIDs inhibit these functions, the result can be fluid retention and the buildup of nitrogenous wastes in the blood.[480] Other prostaglandins have a direct action on stomach cells. They inhibit acid production and prevent acid damage to the lining of the stomach. When these prostaglandins are suppressed, acid can eat holes in your stomach and intestines. This unwanted side effect is the largest single cause of disease and death due to aspirin and other NSAIDs. Aspirin overdose can also cause dizziness, ringing in the ears, impaired hearing, nausea, vomiting, diarrhea, and confusion; and aspirin can increase the bleeding resulting from wounds, tooth extraction, surgery, and childbirth. *Because aspirin keeps blood platelets from sticking together normally, it should be avoided by pregnant women, newborns, and people with clotting disorders or ulcers.*

Some of aspirin's drawbacks are avoided by its competitor *acetaminophen (Tylenol, Datril, Anacin-3, Panadol, Liquiprin).* Tylenol has passed up aspirin to become the bestselling analgesic in America, outselling its closest competitor *Advil (ibuprofen)* by two to one. Acetaminophen won't reduce the pain associated with inflamed joints, but it's easier on the stomach lining than aspirins. It is therefore considered safer. However, the FDA warns there is no basis for the claim. Overdoses of aspirin are unlikely to be fatal to adults if treated in time, but this isn't true for aceta-minophen. Only ten Extra-Strength Tylenol can be fatal to a child, and even small overdoses of either painkiller can be life-threatening. In large doses, acetaminophen can cause irreversible liver damage and death even in adults; and normal doses can cause liver damage if given daily for long periods. In December of 1995, the *Journal of the American Medical Association* reported on 21 patients who exceeded the recommended dosage and wound up with major liver damage. Three died, and two needed liver transplants. The same month, the *New England Journal of Medicine* report-ed that people who regularly take acetaminophen have an increased risk of advanced kidney disease.[481]

The side effects of *ibuprofen* are similar to aspirin's, but their inci-dence may be lower. Adverse reactions with other drugs are less likely with ibuprofen, and overdosing is less likely to have serious consequences; but the drug still isn't harmless. According to a Vanderbilt University study, elderly people who take ibuprofen are four times as likely to die from ulcers and gastrointestinal bleeding as those who don't take it.[482] Like all NSAIDs, ibuprofen also tends to cause sodium retention and to inhibit kidney function. *Ibuprofen isn't recommended for women who are pregnant or nursing, for alcoholics, or for people who have stomach problems or are allergic to aspirin.*

NATURAL ALTERNATIVES

In Western medicine, one pain reliever is used for all types of pain. Alternative medical practitioners view pain differently, treating it accord-ing to its cause. Headache pain, pain from a trauma or muscle injury, or chronic pain from a disease such as cancer all have different causes and different treatments.

For arthritis, the nutrients *glucosamine* and *chrondoitin sulfate* have been shown to relieve pain without the side effects of aspirin. These nutri-ents are the building blocks of cartilage and are thought to work by stim-ulating the production of new cartilage cells and reducing the action of enzymes that harm cartilage. See "Arthritis."

For migraine headaches, the herb *feverfew* has been touted as a mir-acle cure that can eliminate the need for drugs and their concomitant side effects. British researchers have found that feverfew not only cuts the number and severity of headaches but reduces the nausea that goes with them. See "Headaches."

Other nutrients are natural anti-inflammatories, which reduce pain either by decreasing local fluid levels or because of diuretic properties that reduce inflammation. They include *vitamins C and B6, potassium, Boswellin,* and *Turmeric.* The herbal form of aspirin is willow bark. Used by Chinese physicians 2,500 years ago, it contains salicin, nearly the same pain reliever as in aspirin. Another herbal aspirin is *meadowsweet tea.* These herbal options can be just as effective as aspirin at much lower risk.

Magnesium is also a natural pain reliever. Low levels of magnesium increase nerve cell excitability and pain.

Still other nutrients reduce pain by reducing free-radical formation. These are the *antioxidants,* including *vitamins E and C, beta-carotene, selenium* (found in garlic and onions), *pycnogenol, bioflavonoids, coenzyme Q10,* and *alpha lipoic acid.* The herbs *ginkgo biloba* and *bilberry* have antioxidant properties as well.

Pain can also be relieved naturally by improving circulation to help eliminate pain-response chemicals and exhausted immune-system cells. Effective therapies include massage, acupressure, heat treatments, stretching, and exercise.[483]

In the homeopathic line, there are also natural pain relievers. *Hypericum 30c* can work as well as aspirin for reducing inflammation, without the risk of side effects. Take three pills four times daily.

See also "Gout" and other specific conditions.

PAIN AND THE MIND

Recent research suggests that the pain-killing abilities of analgesics may be largely in the mind. Pain-killing drugs are particularly subject to the "placebo effect," a trick of the mind by which an anticipated effect is produced although the drug contains no active properties known to produce it. A Mayo Clinic study found that for 21 percent of patients tested, as much pain relief resulted from a placebo—a fake pill without active pain-killing properties—as from either aspirin or a stronger drug. The study also found that for pain relief, aspirin was as good as or better than any other drug tested, over-the-counter or prescription, including *Darvon,* the prescription-drug favorite.[484]

Up to one third of prescription drugs, and a much higher percentage of nonprescription drugs, are thought to act primarily as placebos.[485] The patient gets better because he or she expects to. Placebos apparently work by triggering the release of "endorphins," the brain's own chemical pain-relievers, which function like opiates in the body. Pure placebos—pills that have no physiological effect at all—can be effective pain relievers, but drugs that have actual physiological effects work better. This is true although their physiological effects are unrelated to the patient's condition. Thus an anxious patient will feel more relaxed if given a placebo that causes him to be light-headed or dry-mouthed than if given one that does nothing at all. The patient feels the drug is "working" and, having been told it will work to relax him, feels more relaxed.[486]

The ideal analgesic would trigger this trick of the mind without pills and their side effects. Certain biofeedback and meditation techniques are reported to work by triggering the release of natural endorphins. Acupuncture is an effective analgesic that is thought to work the same way. In China, major surgeries are done with only acupuncture for an anesthetic. Exercise (the "runner's high") and yoga-type breathing also release endorphins. Even the pain of cancer has been reduced by nondrug analgesic therapies, including biofeedback, relaxation training, hypnosis and behavior modification. Simply laughing or staying calm and happy can produce natural pain-killing endorphins.[487]

Parasites (Amoebas, Intestinal Worms)

Amoebas and intestinal worms were once considered problems mainly in the underdeveloped world, but the Centers for Disease Control now documents 15 to 20 outbreaks of waterborne parasites each year in the United States. Experts speculate that the true number of outbreaks is in the hundreds, since parasitic illnesses are often mistaken for stomach flu and other intestinal disorders. A 1994 study put the hidden parasite epidemic at two million U.S. cases per year.[488] In *Guess What Came to Dinner: Parasites and Your Health* (Avery Publishing, 1993), Anne Louise Gittleman lists these potential uninvited guests: hookworms, pinworms, roundworms, tapeworms, heartworms, various flukes, *Amoeba, Entamoeba histolytica, Endolimax, Giardia, Blastocystis Trichomonas vaginalis, Toxoplasma gondii, Cryptosporidium muris, Pneumocystis carnii, Strongyloides Trichinella, Anisakine Larvae, Filaria, Cestoda,* and *Trematoda.* Symptoms of infestation include gas and bloating, irritable bowel syndrome, joint and muscle

aches and pains, skin conditions, granulomas, nervousness, sleep disturbances, anemia, allergy, constipation, diarrhea, teeth grinding, chronic
fatigue, and immune disfunction.

DRUG TREATMENT

The standard U.S. treatment for intestinal parasites is *metronidazole
(Flagyl)*, an expensive drug required by law to bear the warning,
"Carcinogenic in rodents. Avoid unnecessary use." The drug is of limited
effectiveness and can have troubling side effects. Those listed in the
Physician's Desk Reference include convulsive seizures, numbness in the
extremities, nausea and vomiting, headache, and intestinal distress.
WARNING: Metronidazole should not be combined with alcohol, even
the alcohol in cough syrup.

To avoid giving this toxic drug unnecessarily, testing for parasites is
routinely prescribed in the United States before the treatment is begun.
But stool tests are notoriously unreliable, so parasites often go undetected
and untreated. In Central America, this problem is avoided because the
available remedies are much less toxic and less expensive. As a result, people don't worry about stool tests. Mothers routinely give their children
over-the-counter deworming drugs preventatively, the way veterinarians
regularly deworm dogs and horses. Parasite-eliminating herbs are also
incorporated into the local diet. *Apasote (pigweed)* is made into a soup;
jacaranda is made into a tea.

Safe and effective parasite drugs available in Central America include
tinidazole (Fasigyn or Metrovan) and *teclozan (Fulmonox 500)* for amoebas,
and *levamisole (Ketrax)* and *mebendazol (Mebendamin)* for intestinal
worms. The remedies run around $2.50 to $12 for a full course of treatment, which generally consists of a single dose. These remedies aren't available in the United States evidently because demand for them is not great
enough to prompt their European manufacturers to leap the $100 million
hurdle to FDA approval. Levamisole is available in the United States as a
treatment for colon cancer, but the prescribed regimen costs $1,200 a year.
The drug is classified as a "biologic response modifier" that, like interfer-
ons and interleukins, potentiates the immune response.[489]

Hysterectomy Avoided with Simple Worm Remedy

An American foreign-service spouse in Guatemala was emotional,
agitated, depressed, and suffered from such severe abdominal pains that

her gynecologist, suspecting uterine problems, had scheduled a hysterectomy. The woman called off the surgery after she took the local worm remedy mebendazol and eliminated a bowl full of tiny worms. Her symptoms disappeared with the parasites.

HERBAL AND HOMEOPATHIC ALTERNATIVES

Although European-made over-the-counter parasite drugs aren't available in the United States, effective nontoxic treatments may be obtained in the United States in the herbal and homeopathic lines.

For *giardia*, the nondrug remedy that seems to be most effective is a Staufen homeopathic from Germany called *Lamblia*. The prescribed regimen is one ampule (containing varying potencies from 30x to 5x) every three days for one month. Also good is a remedy called *Giardia* by Hanna Kroeger, but it works on newly acquired giardia only. Take ten drops three times a day until the bottle is empty.

For prevention if you are traveling abroad, try taking a homeopathic remedy called *Vermicin* by Complimed (ten drop three times a day) throughout your trip. Another alternative is *Ver* by Deseret. These remedies can also be used if you get home with an upset stomach, diarrhea, or other parasite symptoms. If you've had the parasites awhile, the remedies will give only symptomatic relief, but they can be used for occasional stomach upset while you're waiting for other remedies to work.

To rout out parasites that have been in residence for some time, a four- to six-week course of treatment is generally necessary. The best seems to be an herbal parasite protocol developed by Marco Pharma, including an antiparasitic remedy called *Para A*, an antimicrobial remedy, Luvos (mineral earth) to heal lesions, and other remedial agents.

Another option is to mix *wormwood, black walnut, cloves,* and *valerian.* Take two droppersful three times daily in water mixed with one teaspoonful of *Luvos Earth.*

Herbs to the Rescue

Alex, 49, had suffered with parasites for an ominous 17 years. His complaints included continual stomach upset, nausea, fatigue, disturbed sleep, and grinding of teeth. He had spent literally hundreds of thousands of dollars on his health without relief, including a prescribed course of Flagyl that lasted three months, a quite hazardous period of time to stay on the drug. Alex finally tried the Marco Pharma herbal parasite proto-col. He said he couldn't believe the result. For the first time in many years, he felt great. A full eight weeks were required to eliminate his parasites, but then they were gone.

To Alex's dismay, however, about four months later his symptoms returned. When Dr. Andreas Marx of Marco Pharma was consulted, he suggested that Alex's wife should be treated as well. Dr. Marx observed that symptom-free mates can pass parasite eggs back to their spouses. After both husband and wife were treated for a further four weeks, Alex's symptoms disappeared for good. The full treatment took a year, due to the extensive damage the parasites had done to his system over the previous 17; they had traveled into his gallbladder and caused complications. But he has now remained symptom-free for a full 18 months.

Multiple Parasites Eliminated

A 29-year-old from Australia who had traveled around the world complained that he could eat only certain foods and that he had suffered for months with stomach distress, alternating diarrhea and constipation, and severe gas and bloating (the main symptom of *giardia*). He was given the German remedy *Lamblia*. When he had finished the course, he said he felt wonderful. He thought he was cured. Then he decided to go away for the weekend. About four days later his stomach pains returned, though without gas or bloating. As with most people who have had parasites for an extended period of time, it turned out he had other parasites as well as *giardia*. After a week on the MarcoPharma parasite protocol, he again reported feeling wonderful. He continued on it for the full four weeks and had no further problems.

Parasites from Family Cat Eliminated in Family and Cat

Connie's problem turned out to be toxoplasmosis—infestation of a parasite carried by cats. She said she'd had cats all her life. Her nine-year-old daughter, who had always had trouble in school, was found to have toxoplasmosis as well. Both were given the German homeopathic remedy *Toxoplasmosis*, including ampules in varying doses from 200x to 5x. When the daughter's grades went from F's and D's to A's, her teacher called Connie to find out what was going on. The child's ability to concentrate had substantially improved.

To avoid reinfecting the family, the family cat was also treated. Connie was impressed when the cat, within about five minutes of taking the remedy, began vomiting up roundworms.

CAUTION: To avoid acquiring and transmitting toxoplasmosis, pregnant women should not change cat litter boxes.

NATURAL TREATMENT FOR PINWORMS

A homeopathic remedy called *CINA* is used by homeopaths to treat pinworms. Take two pills three times a day of CINA 30x (or for more severe cases, CINA 200x) for four days.

To check for pinworms in children, try the Scotch-tape trick. Worms come out at night to lay their eggs. If tape is put over the opening in a child's buttocks, the worms will stick to the tape and can be seen.

Another indicator is the moon. Worms are most active when the moon is full. If a child's symptoms are most pronounced at that time, he or she may have pinworms.

THE IMPORTANCE OF PROPER DIAGNOSIS

Food poisoning is often confused with parasites or worms. (See "Food Poisoning.") Conditions diagnosed as more serious intestinal diseases, such as Crohn's disease or colitis, can also turn out to be simply parasitic infections. Stool tests are recommended before undergoing toxic drug or surgical treatments for these conditions. Reliable stool tests are available from the Institute of Parasitic Diseases Laboratory, 3530 E. Indian School Road, Suite 3, Phoenix, Arizona 85018; 602-955-4211. Collection Kits can be ordered from Urokeep, Inc., 602-545-9236

Pneumonia

Pneumonia is a disease category that includes a number of different diseases that infect or inflame the lungs, caused by a number of different agents. Bacteria and viruses are the most common, but fungi, mycoplasmas, and inhalants are other possibilities. More than four million cases of pneumonia are estimated to occur annually in the United States. People considered at high risk include the elderly, the very young, and those with chronic underlying health problems.

Viral pneumonia is the most common form in the very young, but it's less common in adults with normal immune systems. The symptoms of viral pneumonia mimic the flu and include fever, dry cough, headache, muscle pain, weakness, high fever, and breathlessness.

The more serious *bacterial pneumonia* accounts for an estimated 40,000 deaths yearly. Pneumococcus is the bacteria that usually causes it. Symptoms in severe cases include shaking, chills, chattering teeth, severe chest pains, sweats, cough that produces rust-colored or greenish mucus, increased breathing and pulse rate, and a bluish tint to the lips or nails caused by lack of oxygen.

Mycoplasms are responsible for another 20 percent of cases of pneumonia.

CONVENTIONAL TREATMENT

Early treatment with antibiotics can eliminate the serious symptoms of bacterial pneumonia and can speed recovery from mycoplasma pneumonia. For people in high-risk groups, a pneumococcal vaccine may also be given. However, there are no effective treatments for most types of viral pneumonia. Antibiotics don't work on viruses, and the vaccine is for a bacteria. Fortunately, viral pneumonia usually heals on its own.[490]

HERBAL SUPPORT

Herbs can help the body with this healing process. *Elecampe* and *lungwort* are particularly good. Another good herbal pneumonia remedy is the Chinese formula *Ping Chuan*, which dries up excess fluid in the chest.

THE HOMEOPATHIC APPROACH

Homeopaths maintain that even for bacterial pneumonia, antibiotics don't eliminate the organisms that cause it. The drugs merely push the invader further in. When the system is run down and under stress, the condition returns. Only when the disease has been brought to the surface and eliminated can it be cured for good. For the pneumonia victim who doesn't have a strong immune system, however, antibiotics may still be required. If you are very run down, recovery on herbs and homeopathic remedies will be slow, and you are likely to continue to get weaker in the meantime. Even if you resort to antibiotics, homeopathic remedies should be taken along with them, since otherwise the pneumonia is liable to return year after year.

An excellent homeopathic remedy for clearing pneumonia from the system is a German formula by Staufen called *Mixed Pneumonia*. There is also a special homeopathic called *Myco Pneumonia* for mycoplasma pneumonia. *Dulpulmon* by CompilMed is a good combination homeopathic product. Take 10 drops every 15 minutes to start, then four times daily as needed.

Rapid Healing Without Antibiotics

Leslie, a 46-year-old triathlete, developed pneumonia ten days before a big bicycle race. Her doctor said she would have to go on antibiotics and couldn't race, but Leslie had been working out regularly and was in great shape. Instead of antibiotics, she took the Staufen *Mixed Pneumonia* formula. She was on the mend the next day, and got progressively better each day after that. On the day of the race, she was not only able to race but actually came in first in her class.

Pneumonia Syndrome Broken

Richard, a 43-year-old building contractor, complained that he had not felt well since he had had pneumonia a year earlier. The disease was technically gone, and he felt better than when he had had it; but he was always short of breath, and he was very tired at night. He simply did not have the same vitality as before, and his work output had diminished significantly.

Richard was given the *Mixed Pneumonia* German homeopathic formulation. Fifteen days later, he returned in some alarm to say that he felt his pneumonia was coming back. His chest felt "full." Yet, strangely, his energy level was good and he did not feel "sick." He was assured that this was a positive sign: it was the "healing crisis" that indicated the remedy was working. The pneumonia had been suppressed and was coming out. Thus reassured, Richard managed to avoid the trap of resorting to more antibiotics, which would have pushed the pneumonia back down and returned him to his former weakened state. By the end of a month, his energy had been restored as predicted and he was back at work in full swing. A year and a half later, he reports that he has not had even a cold since.

Lungs Cleared with Simple Remedy

One of the authors had a similar experience, after contracting pneumonia several years ago in Kenya. Having just written about how hazardous antibiotics were, she resolved to tough it out without them, although by hindsight this may have been the wrong decision. She survived but had a distressing tight feeling in her chest for months afterwards. Then she took the German *Mixed Pneumonia* homeopathic ampules. The night after taking the first vial she coughed up blood—an alarming development, until she remembered the homeopathic remedy. A day later she could breathe better than she had for months; and after she finished the series of ten ampules (at one a week), she could breathe better than she had for years. She didn't catch even a cold for the next four years. The connection was reinforced when a friend mentioned his own experience: he said he no longer catches cold, ever since he went through a case of pneumonia in Africa without antibiotics.

Premenstrual Syndrome (PMS)

Premenstrual syndrome (PMS) is a cluster of uncomfortable symptoms that sets in seven to ten days before a woman starts her period. They can include headaches, abdominal bloating, breast swelling, fluid retention, increased thirst, increased appetite, cravings for sweet or salty foods, and emotional symptoms including anxiety, irritability, mood swings, depression, hostility, crying, and loss of self-confidence. The condition normally begins sometime when a woman is in the thirties, when hormone production is slowing down. Once thought to be merely psychological, PMS gained recognition as a true physical syndrome when British gynecologist Katharina Dalton found that nearly half the women admitted to a hospital for accidents or psychological illnesses were in their premenstrual week. Other studies showed that about half the crimes for which women were responsible were committed during this period. PMS is now thought to plague from 25 to 90 percent of all women, depending on how it's defined.

Dr. Dalton was personally interested because she was a chronic sufferer of premenstrual migraine headaches herself. She noticed that her symptoms went away, however, during the last six months of her pregnancy. Knowing that progesterone levels are 20 to 30 times higher then than at other times, she proceeded to treat herself with daily injections of progesterone after her baby was born. Her migraines did not come back. Since then, the link with progesterone levels has been verified in thousands of other women.

PMS symptoms are now thought to be due to a hormone imbalance before menstruation. During the normal menstrual cycle, immediately after ovulation, levels of both estrogen and progesterone rise, and they continue to rise until menstruation. The progesterone acts as an estrogen antagonist, keeping estrogen levels from going too high. But progesterone stores can be depleted by stress (emotional, dietary, or environmental), causing progesterone to be converted to the stress hormone cortisol. Without enough progesterone, estrogen levels get too high. Excess estrogen can then produce salt and fluid retention, low blood sugar, blood clotting, breast tenderness, thyroid problems, and weight gain. These physical imbalances produce the mood swings and other psychological effects associated with PMS.[491] An imbalance of estrogen over progesterone has also been linked to cancer. Estrogen stimulates the proliferation of cells. Progesterone checks this growth.

DRUG TREATMENT

In theory, progesterone supplementation should correct estrogen imbalances by normalizing estrogen levels. But doctors have been slow to credit progesterone therapy with helping PMS, because controlled trials of several different synthetic progestins have failed to show a significant benefit on PMS symptoms.[492] Critics point out that these studies were flawed, since they used synthetic copies of the hormone. *Provera* (medroxyprogesterone acetate) and other chemically altered forms of progesterone not only don't work on PMS but can make it worse, by inhibiting natural progesterone production and lowering its concentration in the blood. Synthetic progesterone performs some but not all of the natural hormone's functions. It can't be converted in the body to other hormones as needed, and it comes with a long list of unwanted side effects. (See "Menopause.") Although these synthetic compounds are allowed to go under the name of progesterone, some are actually 2,000 times more potent than the form found in the body. Some are made strictly from chemicals. Others are made from the male hormone testosterone. Androgenic (male-type) progestins react like male hormones and can give you masculine characteristics. Others have estrogenic effects. They can bring on fluid retention and edema (swelling), symptoms related to an excess of estrogen.[493] Both pharmaceutical estrogens and pharmaceutical progestins increase the uptake of sodium and water by cells.

Diuretics, or water pills, are often recommended to relieve edema in PMS sufferers.[494] But the drugs work by forcing the kidneys to release body fluid; and with the excess water go important minerals and chemicals, throwing off electrolyte and mineral balance. That's why most diuretics are prescription-only drugs. In fact, PMS is the *only* condition for which their over-the-counter use is approved, and that's only because the pills are intended for use only a few days each month.

Natural Hormone Alternatives

Although synthetic progesterone has not tested out well for treating PMS, *natural* progesterone has. Only one controlled trial has reported significant improvements in PMS symptoms, and it used natural progesterone in oral micronized form.[495] Many doctors claim a high rate of success with the natural hormone, either in micronized pill form or as a transdermal cream derived from a type of Mexican yam (*Pro-Gest* and others). Dr. Ray Peat, who pioneered the transdermal form of natural progesterone, states that in the approximately 400 women he has observed, nearly all have found the appropriate amount to control their PMS symptoms.[496] Transdermal natural progesterone has the advantage over the pill form that much lower amounts are required to get an effect. A full two-ounce jar of the cream is recommended per month to start, or about one-half teaspoon per day. However, requirements are very individual. For menstruating women, progesterone should be begun on day 10 or 12 of the cycle (counting the first day of menstruation as day 1), finishing on day 25 or 26. For more detailed information, see Brown and Walker, *Menopause and Estrogen* (1996).

CHINESE AND WESTERN HERBAL AND HOMEOPATHIC REMEDIES

The approach of Chinese and homeopathic doctors is to aid the body in producing and balancing its own hormones.

Relaxed Wanderer, the brand name for a Chinese patent formula called *Hsaio Yao Wan* (or *Xiao Yao Tang*), is an excellent remedy not only for menopausal complaints but for PMS. The remedy works particularly well for women with a tendency to be cold (for example, to have cold hands and feet). For women who are approaching menopause and tend to be hot, the Chinese remedy *Bupleurum and Peony Formula* is likely to be more effective.

The European and native American Indian herbal traditions also include excellent botanicals for premenstrual and menopausal complaints. One is an American-made *red raspberry leaf* combination formula by Zand. It should be taken beginning a week before menstruation. For other hormone-balancing herbs, see "Menopause."

Homeopathic remedies are also available for treating PMS. One shown to be effective in a 1992 study was the German remedy *Mulimen*. (See "Menopause.") Good homeopathic formulas for PMS are *PMS* by Nelson's and *Natural Phases* by Boiron.

NUTRITIONAL SOLUTIONS

The high levels of estrogen on which PMS has been blamed may be the result of nutritional imbalances. One way to keep estrogen levels from going too high is by increasing your intake of *dietary fiber*. Fiber binds with the deactivated estrogen and moves it through the intestines. Studies show that women on high-fiber, low-fat diets have less PMS, less breast cancer, less premenstrual breast pain, and less trouble with their menstrual periods.[497]

Calcium can also help relieve PMS symptoms. A 1991 USDA study found that women with PMS had lower blood-calcium levels than other women and that their calcium levels were particularly low during their PMS phases. Symptoms were noticeably relieved in nine out of ten women when calcium intake was boosted to 1,300 mg per day. A 1989 study reached the same result using 1,000 mg of calcium, with 73 percent of 33 women reporting fewer symptoms during calcium treatment.[498]

Other nutritional supplements shown to relieve PMS symptoms include *vitamin B6, vitamin E,* and *essential fatty acids (evening primrose oil, black currant oil, borage).* Avoidance of caffeine and allergenic foods may also help.[499]

Multiple-vitamin products are also available that are specifically prepared for PMS sufferers. See Appendix.

Natural Remedies for Edema (Bloating)

To relieve edema or bloating, a clinical study showed that *dandelion leaf* works as well as Lasix, a popular diuretic. *Natural progesterone* can also relieve water retention and bloating without side effects, and so can the amino acid *L-arginine.* Unlike diuretics, which release fluid prematurely from the kidneys, these nutrients put the whole system back in balance, causing the release of built-up fluid at the cellular level all over the body. Other suggestions include drinking less and avoiding salt and salt-rich foods that cause you to retain water.

Prostate Enlargement and Inflammation, Benign Prostatic Hypertrophy (BPH), Prostatitis, Prostate Cancer

The prostate is a walnut-sized gland just below the bladder that surrounds the urethra, the tube through which urine and semen exit the body. The prostate supplies part of a man's seminal fluid, which it squeezes into the urethra just before orgasm. Virtually all prostates enlarge with age, because their old cells don't die off as fast as new cells grow. When the prostate grows, it narrows the urethral opening so that urine has trouble getting through. The result is a nonmalignant condition called *benign prostatic hyperplasia (BPH).* Some ten million American men now have clinical signs of BPH. Half of all men over 50 eventually get symptoms, but only a quarter of older males are bothered enough to see a doctor for them. Early symptoms include problems getting urine to flow, a weak stream, and dribbling at the end of urination. The bladder compensates by pushing harder, strengthening and thickening the bladder wall. This makes the bladder smaller and urination even more frequent. Retained urine can also irritate the bladder, creating a strong sudden urge to urinate. It can also cause bladder infections, bladder stones and kidney damage.[500]

BPH is linked to hormonal changes with age. Testosterone levels decrease after age 50, while prolactin and other hormones increase. The result is an increased concentration in the prostate of dihydrotestosterone, a potent testosterone derivative responsible for the overproduction of prostate cells causing prostate enlargement.

BPH incidence has increased dramatically in the last few decades. One theory is that this phenomenon reflects an increase in toxic chemicals in the environment. Pesticides and other contaminants (for example, dioxin, polyhalogenated biphenyls, hexachlorobenzene, and dibenzofurans) can increase the formation of dihydrotestosterone in the prostate. Diethylstilboestrol (DES) has also been shown to produce BPH-like changes in the prostates of rats.[501]

Other prostate conditions involving difficulties with urination include *prostatitis*, an acute inflammation of the prostate caused by a bacterial infection that can strike at any age, and *prostate cancer*, in which the proliferating cells enlarging the prostate are cancerous rather than benign. Prostate cancer is the most prevalent male malignancy and the second leading cause of cancer deaths in men. *Medical consultation is required to eliminate these possibilities.*

CONVENTIONAL TREATMENT

At one time, the medical approach to BPH consisted of "watchful waiting" followed by surgery when symptoms got too distressing. But surgery is a daunting undertaking, that can result not only in bleeding and damage to the bladder but in impotence. The development of drug treatments that avoided surgery were therefore considered a major breakthrough. The first of these drugs was the alpha-blocker *Hytrin*, an antihypertensive medicine that works by relaxing the smooth muscle in the prostate gland. Then came the alpha-reductase inhibitor *Proscar*, which shrinks the prostate by blocking a hormone in the chain of events that triggers prostate-cell growth.

Both drugs have side effects. Alpha-blockers can cause dizziness, headaches, fatigue, and nasal congestion in 5 to 10 percent of users. On Proscar, about 5 percent of men report loss of sexual potency and desire; birth defects can result; and the drug may take up to six months to work. Proscar is also expensive, costing around $2.17 per day. But the general consensus was that it worked—until the makers of these two drugs agreed to a comparative study. The surprising result, reported in 1996, was that while Hytrin significantly relieved BPH symptoms, Proscar worked no better than a placebo. The drug still has supporters, however, who say it works for very large prostates. The argument is that if your prostate isn't greatly enlarged, shrinking it isn't going to do much.[502]

HERBAL REMEDIES

Proscar is a synthetic drug that works in the same way as the active ingredient in the *saw palmetto* plant. Saw palmetto has been widely used in Europe to treat prostate and bladder conditions since the 1930s. No side effects except rare stomach upset have been associated with it, and it's much cheaper than Proscar. Saw palmetto has become so popular among BPH sufferers that it is now the sixth-bestselling herb in the United States. A study published in the *British Journal of Clinical Pharmacology* in 1984 found that saw palmetto extract (at dosages of 320 mg per day) increased urinary flow rate by over 50 percent, reduced urine residue by nearly 42 percent, and significantly reduced the subjective symptoms of BPH.[503] Another report, written in the *British Journal of Pharmacology* in 1993, found that saw palmetto berry was much more effective than a leading prostate drug in impacting urine flow in men with BPH.[504]

Another herb that is widely used in Europe for prostate problems is *Pygeum africanum*, a large African evergreen with active ingredients that reduce prostate enlargement and inflammation. A number of controlled, double-blind studies in European medical journals have verified its effectiveness in treating BPH.[505]

Ginseng, another popular herb, has been shown to increase testosterone levels and decrease the size of the prostate.

In a 1967 study, *bee pollen* was shown to give effective relief from prostatitis and other prostate discomforts.[506]

Chinese doctors have an effective herbal remedy for prostate enlargement called *Kat Kit Wan Prostate Gland Pills*.

Painful Urination Relieved

A 50-year-old professor revealed that he had had trouble with his prostate ever since he was 35. His symptoms were typical: painful urination and frequent trips to the bathroom at night. They worsened when he stood on his feet all day or had sex too often. When the Kat Kit Wan pills eliminated all his prostate symptoms within a couple of weeks, he was thrilled.

HOMEOPATHIC AND HERBAL COMBINATIONS

Effective homeopathic and herbal combination products are also available for prostate problems. They include *Sabal Serrulatum* by Nestmann, consisting of Sabal 1x, Lycopodium 4x, Pareira Brava 4x; and *Saw Palmetto Pygeum* by Jarrow.

Here is a combination approach that has been found to be effective for men who have to get up several times at night to urinate: Begin with the Kat Kit Wan pills, taking them for two or three weeks. Usually, the frequent nocturnal need to urinate stops within the first week, indicating that prostate swelling has lessened. Then take one of the herbal or homeopathic combination products for maintenance thereafter (15 drops in water three times a day).

Prostate swelling can also be reduced with *Prosta Kit* by Flora. It should be used for a month.

Homeopathic medorrhinum, a remedy for gonorrhea, may also help. Many homeopaths feel that prostate problems can be the result of suppressed gonorrhea infection (a "miasm"), even if it occurred 50 years earlier. Miasms are latent vibrational defects that can be acquired from a partner or forebear although you never had an active case of the disease. *DHEA is not recommended for men with prostate cancer.*

NUTRITIONAL SUPPORT

Zinc is important for the prostate, which uses ten times more of that mineral than does any other organ. Zinc does naturally what drugs try to do: It reduces levels of prolactin and blocks the body's production of dihydrotestosterone. Zinc is found in oysters, wheat germ, pumpkin and sunflower seeds, nutritional yeast, onions, and beans; but getting enough zinc from your diet is difficult, due to nutrient-poor soils and mineral losses from food processing. Supplementation is therefore recommended. It should be done in moderation, however, since *excess* zinc levels may be linked to Alzheimer's disease. The RDA is 15 mg. Zinc should be taken with *vitamin B6*, which aids its absorption.

Other food supplements useful for relieving BPH symptoms are *evening primrose* and *flax oil*. Amino acids may also help. In one study, an amino-acid mixture of *glycine, l-alanine*, and *glutamic acid* reduced prostate swelling in over 90 percent of patients, and most reported relief of their symptoms. Supplementation with *methionine, phenylalanine, arginine, GABA, niacin (vitamin B3), folic acid, vitamin E, magnesium, selenium*, and *calcium* is also recommended.[507]

To reduce the risk of prostate cancer, studies have also shown that certain nutrients can help. They include *vitamin E* (a potent antioxidant), *tomatoes* (which contain the carotenoid pigment lycopene, another well-known antioxidant), and *selenium* (an antioxidant found in seafood, certain organ meats, and grain). A laboratory study reported in 1997 also found that a compound derived from *aged garlic* dramatically diminishes the growth of human prostate cancer cells.[508]

PRESSURE-RELIEVING MEASURES

The following simple home measures can help relieve prostate symptoms:

- Cut down on coffee, tea, and cola, which contain caffeine, a diuretic that increases urination.
- Eat dinner early and minimize fluid intake thereafter. Avoid antihistamines (which reduce the force of bladder contractions) and colds remedies containing pseudoephedrine (which can aggravate symptoms by causing contractions of the smooth muscle tissue in the prostate).
- Avoid spicy foods and constipation (which may aggravate the urinary tract) and prolonged sitting (which can aggravate the prostate).
- Hot baths can help relax the smooth muscle tissue of the prostate.
- Sex can help by easing fluid congestion in the prostate.[509]

A resource is the book *Prostate Health in Ninety Days* by Larry Klapp.

Sexual Dysfunction:
Impotence, Lack of Libido, Infertility

As many as ten million Americans are affected by infertility problems. Sexual performance is another common concern, although it is rarely asked about except in whispers. Men sometimes ask for help for "a friend." They often ask for *yohimbe*, an herb that causes vasodilation, opening the blood vessels and causing the blood to rush into the penis to make it erect. Women ask for help to save their marriages. They commonly experience a lack of sexual desire during times of hormonal change or emotional stress.

While about 15 percent of all couples are infertile (unable to conceive after a year's effort), in only 1 or 2 percent is conception physically ruled out.[510] Sexual dysfunction can be caused not only by physiological but by emotional or lifestyle factors. Many drugs can cause or contribute to it, including amphetamines, antihistamines, barbiturates, beta-blockers and other blood-pressure medications, cimetidine (Tagamet), ketoconazole, sedatives, tricyclic antidepressants, cocaine, alcohol, marijuana, methadone, and Prozac. Prozac is so effective at numbing sexual feeling and drive, in fact, that it is often prescribed as a remedy for premature ejaculation.

CONVENTIONAL TREATMENT

For men, the synthetic version of yohimbe is a drug called *Yocon* or *Yohimex*. The main problem with both the herb and the drugs is that they can cause serious headaches. The man is liable to end up with a huge erection accompanied by a crippling headache. Other potential side effects of the drugs are elevated blood pressure and heart rate, increased motor activity, nervousness, irritability, tremor, dizziness, and skin flushing.

The latest impotence drug, *Viagra*, had the fastest takeoff ever seen for a new drug. Three weeks after it went on sale in April of 1998, 10,000 prescriptions a day were being written for it. Like with the synthetic yohimbe drugs, however, the erection it produces can come with a headache; and it takes an hour to work. Other side effects include flushed skin, upset stomach, and visual distortion.

For decreased libido in premenopausal women, *estrogen* or low doses of *testosterone* are conventionally prescribed. The treatment generally works but can have side effects. (See "Menopause.")

For infertility, ovulation may be induced with hormones or fertility drugs. But the drugs increase the chance of multiple births and can have other unwanted side effects.

NATURAL ALTERNATIVES FOR WOMEN

For infertility in women, effective Chinese herbal remedies are available. Chinese doctors believe that the Yin must be nourished for conception to occur. Most women are so Yang in their jobs—they have to be so aggressive and assertive—that their Yin gets out of balance so that the womb can't support a baby. Chinese remedies called *Infertility Pills* help rebalance the hormones. Chinese midwives also recommend spending some time at home: become soft and feminine, bake cookies, avoid violent movies that stir up the adrenaline.

Liver congestion can be another cause of infertility. The Liver Cleanse Diet is recommended for this problem. (See "Liver Disease.")

To stimulate sexual interest in women, several effective herbal and homeopathic remedies are available. *Natural progesterone cream (Pro-Gest)* is absorbed topically and increases the body's natural hormone levels. Progesterone is the hormone that kicks in during puberty in young girls and that makes women feel younger, sexier, and more interested in having sex.

In the homeopathic line, *Sexual Stimulation Drops* by PHP effectively increase interest in sex. Another product reported to work is *homeopathic testosterone*. It contains no actual testosterone but stimulates the body to produce its own.

Jasmine by Botanical Alchemy is an herbal and gem elixir formula that heals and increases sexual feelings toward a partner.

Marriage Saved with Herbal Remedy

At 44, Betsy had lost interest in sex, a distressing development that was jeopardizing her marriage. Her doctor had given her pharmaceutical testosterone, but it had caused her to have an offensive body odor and had made her facial hair thicken. Her doctor's response was to increase the dose. He insisted that the amount was too low to cause side effects.

Betsy, desperate, then sought alternative relief. She went home with *Jasmine* and took it faithfully, ten drops three times daily. Two weeks later, she returned to report that the herb had transformed her life. She and her husband were having the best sexual relationship of their marriage. Her drive was up, her sleep was better, and she felt less stressed.

Joys of Sex Rekindled

For over eight years, Kathleen had had a very active sex life with her husband. Then at 44, she suddenly found she had no sex drive at all. After four months in this state, she wondered if her interest in sex would ever return.

She was using natural progesterone cream, but it didn't seem to be enough. She began taking homeopathic testosterone drops, ten drops three times daily. After a week, she reported that her sex drive was not only back but was higher than it had been in years. Her husband was delighted. She was advised to decrease the dose to once a day, then decrease it further to ten drops two to three times per week. This seemed to be the right balance for her body.

NATURAL REMEDIES FOR MEN

For a man concerned about sexual performance, the first issue to be determined is whether he is capable of having an erection. Most men get one in the early morning hours. A popular test is to put a roll of postage stamps around the penis at bedtime. If the postage stamps have torn when the man wakes up, he is capable of this function. If not, he needs to see a doctor to find out why.

For men who have erections in the morning but not "on demand," there are natural remedies. One is the herb *ginseng*. It is not a quick fix but works over a period of time, perhaps several months. There are various ginsengs at various prices. A good formula containing four different varieties of ginseng is made by Natrol. A Chinese patent formula called *Look Bien Yuen* is another male tonic used to increase virility. A third ancient Chinese formula used as a male tonic is *deer antler*.

Homeopathic testosterone has successfully revived the flagging sex drives of both men and women. Men have also reported good results with *homeopathic aveno sativa*. This remedy works in just a few days. Once you have started to respond to it, it needs to be used only on those days when sex is anticipated.

For infertility, *homeopathic ginseng* increases sperm mobility. *Raw carrots* can also increase the sperm count. Other recommended measures include wearing loose underwear and avoiding hot tubs.

Shingles

Shingles is an adult viral infection caused by *herpes zoster*, the same virus that causes chicken pox. But shingles is a much more serious form of the disease. The virus hides in the nerve endings and can cause very painful, lingering symptoms called postherpetic neuralgia for years after the initial adult attack. Herpes zoster is also the virus that causes cold sores, and it was linked in a recent study to Alzheimer's disease.[511]

CONVENTIONAL TREATMENT

Shingles is treated conventionally with the antiviral drug *acyclovir*. The drug isn't very effective, however, and it's very expensive. If it doesn't work, it seems to cause painful postherpetic pain (numbness and tingling) long afterwards; so patients are generally better off without it unless they can start taking it at the first stage of the disease.

ALTERNATIVE TREATMENT

Homeopathy provides effective alternatives. The best is a German Staufen remedy called *Herpes Zoster*. It has the best chance of working if given early to patients who have not had prior steroids or other drugs. Taking the remedy at the first sign of shingles can boost the immune system so that the patient avoids the horrible suffering of postherpetic neuralgia. Often the remedy doesn't work immediately, so patients quit taking it; but if they continue until the last ampule is taken, the pain generally disappears.

The second choice of homeopathics is *Cliniskin H* by CompliMed. Other helpful homeopathic remedies are *Rhus tox* and *Aconite*. Acupuncture is also highly recommend.

Postherpetic Nightmare Relieved with Natural Remedies

For eight months, a woman in her sixties had had such terrible postherpetic pain that she couldn't wear clothes. She walked around naked and said she wanted to die. She was given *Aconite* and acupuncture around the stomach. The sensitive area went down from the size of a beach ball to the size of a half dollar, then disappeared completely.

Another woman, 83, had had shingles only a few months. She was quite uncomfortable with it but had taken no drugs. A single dose of *Herpes Zoster 200* by Staufen made all her symptoms completely disappear.

Sinusitis, Rhinitis

The sinuses are air-filled cavities lined with mucus membranes above and below the eyes. *Sinusitis* is a bacterial infection that causes the sinuses to be inflamed. The condition is characterized by persistent nasal congestion, cold or flulike symptoms that go beyond the usual seven to ten days, and pain and headache in the sinus area. A study of American veterans with sinusitis identified these symptoms: toothache, congested sinus cavities (as determined by transillumination, a diagnostic technique involving projecting light through the sinus cavities), poor response to nasal decongestants or antihistamines, and nasal discharge containing pus.[512] People who are particularly susceptible to sinusitis are those with allergies or deformities of the nose (for example, a deviated septum), those habitually exposed to bacteria (health-care workers, schoolteachers), and smokers.

Sinusitis is often confused with *allergic rhinitis*, which has similar symptoms but is not caused by bacteria. Rhinitis may be caused by a virus, an environmental allergen, extreme temperature change, or overuse of nasal sprays.

DRUG AND SURGICAL TREATMENT

Because it's caused by bacteria, sinusitis should respond to antibiotics. But an increasing number of cases are resistant to standard forms such as *amoxicillin*, causing doctors to resort to other, more powerful and expensive antibiotics, or to a four to six week course of treatment with amoxicillin combined with *Flagyl (metronidazole)*, a drug with substantial side effects of its own. (See "Parasites.") Sinusitis that doesn't respond after several weeks of antibiotic treatment is termed "chronic sinusitis" and is referred to a specialist, since if left untreated it can cause serious illness.

When antibiotics don't work, surgery may be resorted to. The development of endoscopic surgery, along with a substantial increase in antibiotic-resistant cases of sinusitis, has led to a dramatic increase in these surgeries. Endoscopic surgery uses pencil-thin telescopes and can be done without an incision. But while it's a relatively painless outpatient procedure, the pain after surgery is considerable; and its safety and effectiveness have not yet been established in controlled studies. There is some evidence that the incidence of disabling or life-threatening complications, including hemorrhage and toxic shock syndrome, may be as high as 5 to 18 percent.[513]

For allergic rhinitis, which isn't caused by bacteria, antibiotics aren't effective. The condition is treated conventionally with *antihistamines* and *decongestants*. If those drugs don't work, *corticosteroids* are generally prescribed. (See "Allergies.")

CAUTION: If over-the-counter decongestant nose drops or sprays containing phenylephrine (Neo-Synephrine) are used, they should not be continued for more than three days, since they can cause addiction.

HOMEOPATHIC TREATMENT

Homeopaths take a different approach. Rather than trying to prevent the nose from running, they use remedies that actually encourage that result and clear out old infections permanently. In fact homeopaths consider drugs that stop the nose from running to be a principle *cause* of sinus infections. When drainage is stopped, bacteria are trapped in the nose, where they fester and produce infection. Homeopaths also maintain that antibiotics taken for a sinus infection do not actually "kill" these bacteria but merely push the germs further into the sinuses. The symptoms go away temporarily, but they recur when the body tries to push the bacteria out again.

A German homeopathic remedy called *Peptostrep*, taken in strengths ranging from 200x to 5x over a period of a month, is remarkably effective in clearing sinusitis for good. It makes the nose run and old infection come out. Problems generally occur only if the sufferer, being unable to bear her runny nose any longer, resorts to drugs, which stop the cleansing and put her back where she started.

For nasal polyps, homeopathic *Polyps and Adhesions* by New Vista is effective. Also good is the Chinese patent remedy *Be Yen Lin.*

Sinusitis Cured with German Homeopathic Remedy

Robert, a 54-year-old real-estate broker, complained that he had had severe sinus infections several times a year for the past six years. Each infection would last about six weeks. Then a few weeks after it was over, a new one would start. At first, antibiotics seemed to work, but they got less and less effective with repeated infections. Meanwhile, the constant inflammation of his sinuses had led to continuous headaches. To suppress his symptoms, his doctor had prescribed Flonase, a commonly used steroid nasal spray that suppresses the immune system and stops the sinuses from becoming inflamed. But the conventional approach didn't seem to be doing much good, so Robert decided to try homeopathy. Told that the Flonase was merely aggravating his symptoms, he switched to Hydrastis, a natural nasal spray made by Nestmann. Then he started taking the German homeopathic Peptostrep. The arresting result was that huge chunks of dark, old mucus began issuing from his nose. After a month, his nose had stopped running and his condition had cleared. He reports having had no sinus problems in the 16 months since.

Hundreds of people have reported similar results with Peptostrep.

DRAINING THE LYMPH GLANDS

If homeopathic treatment is accompanied at the first sign of a sinus problem by procedures to drain the lymphs, infection can usually be stopped before it starts. Lymph-draining procedures include:

1. Massage to stimulate the lymph glands.
2. Drink substantial amounts of water (a large glass every hour).
3. Use lymphatic and bouncing exercises to move the lymph.
4. Take lymph-draining homeopathic remedies. Particularly good are *Lymphonest* (by Nestmann) and *Lymphomyosot* (by Heel). For others, see Chart.
5. Seawater can also be used to flush the sinuses.

Herbal Remedies

Chinese patent herbal remedies that are effective in treating sinusitis include *Pe Min Kan Wan* and *Be Yin Lin*. For both, take two to three pills two to three times daily.

Western herbal products good for treating the condition include *Sinuplex* by Metagenics and *Decongest Herbal* by Zand.

Home Treatment

The Care Wise Handbook adds these simple home measures to help relieve symptoms:

1. Lie down on your back and apply alternating hot and cold compresses to your forehead and cheeks to stimulate the flow of mucus.
2. Thin the mucus by drinking extra liquids, and clear the throat of mucus by gargling with warm water.
3. Increase humidity, especially in bedrooms.

Dental Treatment

Another possibility is to have a progressive dentist check your teeth. Toothache was identified in the veterans' study as a persistent symptom of chronic sinusitis.

Sinus Problems Relieved by Dental Overhaul

Robert Olson, D.D.S., a dentist in Fullerton, California, relates the case of one of his patients, who said she had developed sinus problems immediately after insertion of a dental bridge 22 years ago. She called it her "22-year-old headache." She had undergone six allergy tests and three surgeries to open the sinuses to drain them. Dr. Olson examined the bridge and observed that it seemed to be torquing her maxillary bone. He recommended that it be replaced. When it was cut off, The woman's first words were, "My God, I can breathe!" Her mouth was reconstructed using a removable partial denture. She reports having had no head or sinus pain since.

Skin Cancer, Melanoma

Skin cancer is by far the most common cancer in the world. Even with the increasing use of sunblock, one out of six Americans can now expect to contract it. Fortunately, most cases are easily curable. At one time, in fact, these conditions weren't classified as cancers for statistical purposes. Skeptical statisticians have suggested that the classification was changed to improve the cancer "cure rate" from conventional treatment.

The dangerous skin cancers are the 10 percent that are *melanomas.* They progress much faster than other skin cancers, can spread beyond the skin and are life-threatening. They are easily recognizable and are curable too, but they need to be detected early. *Suspicious growths should be examined by a dermatologist.*

THE CONVENTIONAL APPROACH

Skin tumors are removed with electric current, frozen with liquid nitrogen, killed with low-dose radiation, treated with chemotherapeutic agents, or removed surgically.

For prevention, some dermatologists have gone so far as to recommend lathering up with sunscreen every morning, no matter what the weather, just to make sure the skin is protected from any sunshine that might chance to befall it. But other experts maintain there is insufficient scientific data to support the belief that sunscreens prevent skin cancer. Dr. Samuel Berne asserts that studies linking sunlight and ultraviolet light to skin cancer were flawed. Massive doses of UV exposure were used on animals to create skin cancers and cataracts. The data were then extrapolated to apply to the more normal exposures of humans to sunlight.[514]

A 1982 British and Australian study found that the incidence of malignant melanomas was significantly higher in office workers than in people whose lifestyles or occupations regularly exposed them to sunlight. Office workers who worked all day under fluorescent lighting had twice the risk of melanomas as other people. Surprisingly, the *lowest* risk of developing skin cancer was actually in people whose main outdoor activity was *sunbathing.* These results were confirmed in two controlled studies conducted at the New York School of Medicine.[515]

Dr. David Williams points out that most sunscreens, regardless of advertising claims, block out only UVB wavelengths, not the deeper-penetrating UVA wavelengths. The use of sunscreens may therefore actually be *contributing* to skin cancer by encouraging people to stay out in the sun longer than they otherwise would. The fact that your skin's surface doesn't burn doesn't mean you aren't being exposed to harmful rays. The melanin produced on the skin by unblocked sunshine (the suntan) is actually what protects the tissues beneath.[516]

Another downside of sunscreens is that they interfere with the synthesis of vitamin D. The sun is our primary source of that vitamin, which is essential for the utilization of calcium and to make strong bones.

Sunscreens also contain harmful chemicals such as titanium. Contrary to popular belief, drugs applied to the skin can actually be *more* toxic than those that are ingested because they go straight into the bloodstream without being processed in the stomach. (See "Skin Problems.")

NATURAL PREVENTION AND TREATMENT

Zane Kime, M.D., in a groundbreaking book called *Sunlight*, demonstrates that the sun creates free-radical damage only in the absence of protective antioxidants and the presence of harmful fats. The antioxidants he discussed were *vitamins A, C, and E* and the trace mineral *selenium*, but there are many others. Harmful fats include hydrogenated oils, refined oils, and saturated fat; that is, the fats in the standard American high-fat diet.[517]

That antioxidants help prevent non-melanoma skin cancers has been confirmed in several recent studies. In 1992, Berkeley researchers found that exposure of rats to ultraviolet rays depleted the animals' skins of vitamins C and E.[518] In other research, people who took 200 mcg of selenium daily had a reduced incidence of skin cancer. Good food sources of selenium include garlic, grains, sunflower seeds, sea food, and Brazil nuts.

The herb *milk thistle (silymarin)* has also been shown to curb skin cancer. Applying it to the skin of mice exposed to UVB light caused a 75 percent reduction in the total number of resulting tumors. *Ginger* is another herb that has dramatically reduced the incidence and size of tumors when applied to the skin of mice exposed to a cancer-causing chemical.[519]

Zinc has been shown to improve healing time from sunburn. For other sunburn remedies, see "First Aid."

For skin cancers that have already formed, Mary Buckley, a Colorado Springs nutritionist, swears by *camphor* and *baking soda* applied directly to the tumors and covered with a Band-Aid. Two days later, she says, the skin cancers generally fall off.

Skin Problems: Dermatitis, Eczema, Psoriasis, Dry or Aging Skin, Scars, Stretch Marks

Dermatitis, or skin inflammation, is a term that includes a range of skin conditions characterized by dry, red, itchy skin. *Eczema* is chronically itchy, inflamed skin that is variously linked to allergies, asthma, stress, and heredity. *Psoriasis* is an unsightly and baffling skin disorder in which skin cells multiply much faster than normal, producing raised, white-scaled patches. Other common skin problems include dry and aging skin, scars, and stretch marks.

CONVENTIONAL TREATMENT

For serious skin conditions such as psoriasis, corticosteroids are sometimes prescribed. However, these drugs are not only counterproductive but can *cause* psoriasis to spread. Serious cases of that disease have been traced to the suppression of a simple skin infection with cortisone. Cortisone suppresses the immune system, so the body can no longer heal itself. In the typical case, hydrocortisone cream is applied to a minor rash on the skin, which turns out to be ringworm or some other infection. The cortisone suppresses the immune system at that spot, so the infection is allowed to grow. When the rash comes back, it covers a much larger area of skin because the infection has spread. If hydrocortisone cream is then used on this rash, worse problems can result.

For minor skin problems, a variety of drugstore topical remedies is available. But these, too, require caution, since many contain hazardous chemicals. We tend to think of drugs applied to the skin as being relatively harmless, since they're not taken into the body like those that are swallowed, but this is a misconception. Drugs taken by mouth go through the normal detoxification processes for which the stomach, kidneys, and liver were designed. Drugs applied to the skin, although less well absorbed, go directly into the bloodstream without metabolic intervention. In fact topical painkillers have been found to produce adverse reactions more frequently when applied to the skin than when swallowed. People who are allergic to foods or other substances should be especially careful with them. Babies' skin is particularly absorbent. *Topical painkillers should not be used on children under two without a doctor's advice.*[520]

THE NATURAL APPROACH

Many topical ointments are available for dry and aging skin that are made from all-natural, nontoxic components. Two effective restorative products that contain small amounts of natural plant hormones are *Nasturtium Restorative Moisturing Cream* and *Glace Formula Ki Overnight Conditioning Cream* by Prima Facie Ltd. (800-900-9265).

Diet is an important factor in preserving the skin. *Antioxidants* and *calcium* help prevent wrinkled, sagging skin. Essential fatty acids are in short supply in the normal American diet and also need to be supplemented. Omega-3 fatty acids help build more efficient cell membranes that exclude allergy-provoking proteins. Shark liver oil can be applied directly to the skin. *Evening primrose oil, fish oil,* and *essential fatty acids* can also be taken orally. An excellent combination product called *The Missing Link* contains omega-3 and mega-6 essential fatty acids, lignans, plant nutrients, enzymes, antioxidants, vitamins, minerals, friendly bacteria, fiber and protein.

For cracks and splits in the fingers during winter, try *homeopathic petroleum 6x* taken orally, two pills two to three times daily.

For cracks in the heel, use *lycopodium 6x*, two pills orally three times daily.

Green tea not only fights viral and bacterial infections but, applied topically, can prevent or even reverse sun and age damage to the skin.[521]

For scars, a remedy called *Scargo* has produced dramatic results. Another remarkable therapy for scars, stretch marks, rosacea, and other skin blemishes involves a Swiss-made hand-held device called a *Bioptron* machine, which emits polarized light that intensively stimulates the skin. Researched for 20 years in Europe, it has been found to be particularly effective on skin problems and for the healing of wounds.

Fifteen-year-old Scars Fade in a Few Weeks

Mary still had scars on her nose and face from a dog bite she had gotten 15 years earlier. She applied the Bioptron light to her face for four minutes per spot each day. In a few weeks, not only had the scars faded but her rosacea disappeared. At 60, her skin looks beautiful.

TREATING THE CAUSE

For chronic skin conditions, the underlying cause needs to be found. Often, it turns out to be food allergies. The "nightshades"—potatoes, green peppers, eggplant, and chillies—are frequently related to skin rashes.

Psoriasis Traced to Pizza and Potato Chips

Zach, 14, had small itchy bumps covering his body that had been diagnosed by a medical doctor as psoriasis. Zach would scratch them until they bled. When asked about his intake of nightshades, his mother said, "Zach never eats any of that." But further questioning revealed that he loved pizza and spaghetti and often had potato chips. When he stopped eating those foods, he improved, although not dramatically. He was then given a homeopathic remedy called *Nightshades Antigen* by Molecular Biologicals (ten drops three times daily). He also took *shark oil* as capsules (three times daily) and topically (applied once or twice daily). Within a month, the improvement in his skin was much more noticeable. The itching and scratching stopped and the dry patches cleared. He admits to still having a pizza now and again.

Sports Injuries, Muscle Aches, Endurance

Serious sports injuries such as compound fractures are the specialty of orthopedists. But most sports injuries are ordinary strains, sprains, and bruises. Good natural remedies are available to relieve muscle soreness and overcome arthritic pains. Other remedies improve endurance, stamina, and breathing.

NATURAL REMEDIES

To stop arthritic pains in the knees and joints, runners report that the regular use of *Arth-X* or *Arth-X-Plus*, composed of a combination of herbs and trace minerals, is quite effective. Take two tablets a day for maintenance therapy.

For breathing problems, shortness of breath, or asthma, *black currant seed oil* can open the lungs and increase breathing capacity. Many athletes take two capsules before a run or match to make breathing easier.

Endurox is an excellent natural workout supplement that augments endurance and increases fat metabolism by up to 43 percent while working out. It contains *Ciwujia*, a type of ginseng sometimes used in treating diabetes. Studies have shown that this supplement shifts the body's workout energy source from carbohydrate to fat, significantly increasing fat metabolism and slowing the lactic acid buildup that causes muscle soreness and fatigue.

Sportenine by Boiron is another good athletic aid that stops lactic acid buildup and reduces recovery time. Another option is *Redimax* by BHI.

Creatine is a nutrient that improves anaerobic capacity. It is found in food (mainly meat), but the amount necessary to influence athletic ability would be difficult to get from the diet. Supplementation is therefore recommended. Some experts suggest 20 grams per day for five days, then a maintenance dose of five to ten grams a day.[522]

For remedies for muscle cramps and spasms, see Appendix.

For remedies for muscle aches and the pain of sports injuries, see "Trauma." For athlete's foot and jock itch, see "Fungal Infections."

Stage Fright, Nervousness

Nervousness can ruin an artistic performance or a business presentation. But what can be done about it?

DRUG OPTIONS

You could take *Valium* for your nerves, but the drug would inhibit your performance and has side effects. Some speakers and performers take the blood-pressure-lowering drug *propranolol* before going on stage and report that it works; but it, too, is a prescription drug with side effects.

Natural Alternatives

Homeopathic remedies can overcome stage fright without side effects. *Gelsenium* re-tunes the emotions on a vibrational level. Another effective product is a combination homeopathic by Natra-Bio called *Nervousness*. *Rescue Remedy*, a Bach-flower remedy, is also excellent for calming the nerves. For people who blush or embarrass easily, *Ambra Grisea* can be a face saver.

Flawless Performance with Homeopathics

Sixteen-year-old Jamie was so nervous at her piano recital rehearsal that she couldn't hold her hands steady on the keys. She took *Nervousness*, 15 drops hourly for several hours before the performance, and played her complicated piece flawlessly at the recital.

Salesman Emboldened to Speak in Public

A man who couldn't talk in front of an audience because he would turn bright red swears *Ambra Grisea* changed his life. He can now speak before groups and has taken a job as a salesman.

Animals' Nervousness Calmed

Believe it or not, there is even a homeopathic for stage fright for performing animals. A trainer whose dogs recently won a grand championship maintains that this remedy, called *Show-Well*, made an amazing difference in her animals. Horse trainers also use it.

"Strep" Throat, Rheumatic Fever

"Strep" throat is a sore throat due to streptococcal infection. It is usually a self-limited disease, which means it will go away by itself without treatment.[523] But in the rare case, if left untreated it can turn into rheumatic fever, which can lead to serious heart disease. This threat was once a serious one, but deaths from rheumatic fever are now very rare in the United States. By 1970, they had plunged to about one per million. The decline is generally attributed to the widespread use of penicillin to treat sore throats, but rheumatic fever was actually well on its way to oblivion before the introduction of the drugs. Deaths due to rheumatic fever had already dropped a full 90 percent by the time antibiotics came on the scene. They have dropped another 90 percent in the last 20 years, even though antibiotic use hasn't increased during that time. Research suggests that improved nutrition and living standards are more important reasons for the decline. Rheumatic fever is known to be prevalent in areas where crowded and unsanitary living conditions prevail.[524] A five-year Rhode Island study found only ten cases of rheumatic fever (including some cases in which the diagnosis was uncertain) in a population of nearly a million.[525]

DRUG TREATMENT

Despite the dramatic decline in rheumatic fever, antibiotics are still used routinely in the treatment of strep throat to prevent the development of this threatening disease. But antibiotics themselves can be hazardous, resulting in allergic and toxic reactions, and in "superinfections" by antibiotic-resistant organisms; and they are becoming less and less effective. Of the ten people found with rheumatic fever in the Rhode Island study, more than half had developed the disease even though they had already been treated with antibiotics.

Given these risks and limited benefits, the prudent doctor should in theory wait for a positive throat culture before initiating drug treatment. But throat-culture results can take two or three days, and it's not always practical to wait that long. Kits are now available for rapid diagnosis, but they aren't as reliable as the old cultures. Antibiotics are therefore prescribed routinely, "just in case." As a result, while the odds that your painfully sore throat is caused by strep are less than one in five and the odds that you'll contract rheumatic fever from it are about two in a million, your odds of getting a prescription for antibiotics from your doctor for this symptom are about nine out of ten.

CAUTION: Once starting on antibiotics, you need to finish the full course even if your test results later come back negative, to prevent breeding antibiotic-resistant "superbugs."

THE ALTERNATIVE APPROACH

The problem with taking antibiotics is that they prevent the development of antibodies that defend against the disease. You're therefore liable to go through the winter with one sore throat after another. Homeopaths maintain that antibiotics merely suppress the strep bacteria, which resurface later when the immune system is in a weakened state.

Fortunately, effective herbal and homeopathic remedies are available. The most effective of the homeopathics is a German Staufen remedy called *Strep.*

Chinese patent formulas are also effective for treating strep throat and ordinary sore throats. *Lieu Shen Wan,* when given for a very sore throat with fever, has been known to cure the condition in a single day. (See "Colds.") *Zhong Gan Ling* is effective for strep throat and sore throat with high fever and body aches. Fever is the distinguishing trait for this remedy.

Strep Throat Cycle Broken

Eric, age 8, had had strep throat several times a year since he was five. The condition was so routine that his mother would simply telephone the doctor, who would then telephone the pharmacy with a prescription for another round of antibiotics. The mother was concerned, however, that the drugs weren't doing much good. She wanted to break this cycle.

Eric was given the German *Strep* homeopathic formulation. He was also given *acidophilus* (two pills three times daily) to reverse the harmful effects of repeated courses of antibiotics on his beneficial intestinal flora. Other remedies were used to build up his immune system. (See "Immunity.")

It took some time for Eric to fully recover from his three years of being ill. First the suppressed bacteria had to be brought to the surface, then the negative effects of the antibiotics had to be reversed, then his immune system had to be built back up. When the suppressed germs started coming out, Eric seemed to be getting sicker. But his mother, who understood this healing crisis, persisted. After a few days of homeopathic treatment, Eric was clearly getting better; and after three months, he was quite well. His mother happily reports he has not been sick in the two years since.

Stress, "Burn-Out"

Stress goes farther than mere emotional upsets. It is a mental, emotional, or physical stimulus that upsets the balance of the body and overwhelms it. Drugs, insecticides, synthetic fabrics, chemicals on and in our bodies, imported foods carrying parasites, and electronic pollution (electric lines, computer screens, TVs, cellular phones, hair dryers) all contribute to the stress levels borne by our bodies. So do crowds, noise, traffic, pain, travel, a new job, moving, a new baby, overwork, lack of sleep, illness, alcohol, and worry. A recent study showed that half the patients who visit general physicians have conditions triggered or aggravated by stressful situations.

The body responds with a number of physiological changes. All body functions and organs are now known to react to stress. Blood pressure, heart rate, and muscle tension increase. Digestion slows. Cholesterol levels rise to meet an increased need for cortisone. A rise in cortisol levels suppresses the immune system and inhibits the ability of white blood cells to help fight disease. Stress also increases the formation of free radicals, which damage and age the body.

DRUG TREATMENT

The approach of conventional medicine is to suppress the symptoms of stress with drugs. Anxiety is suppressed with sedatives and tranquilizers, elevated blood pressure with antihypertensive medication, elevated cholesterol with cholesterol-lowering drugs, a racing or erratic heartbeat with antiarrhythmia drugs, an upset stomach with antacids or H2-blockers. For a detailed discussion of these drugs and their downsides, see each of those ailments. Besides side effects, the problem with the drug approach is that the remedies merely suppress symptoms without reaching the cause of stress or building up the defenses that the body needs to deal with it.

NATURAL ALTERNATIVES

Nutritional and herbal remedies can boost the immune system and ease tension without side effects. See "Anxiety," "Hypertension," "Immunity."

One remedy that can give you a lift and boost your stressed-out adrenals is *Adrenal/Spleen* by CompliMed. Take 10 drops 3 to 4 times a day.

Homeopathic remedies address the cause of stress. To be effective, however, the right remedy must be selected based on circumstances and personality traits.

Stress Cycle Broken

A few days after Debbie broke up with her boyfriend of three years, the man she had thought she was going to marry was dating her best friend. Debbie was devastated. She couldn't sleep. She couldn't eat. She cried so much that she was sent home from work. She stayed in bed, not showering or even getting dressed. She dragged herself around without putting on makeup or fixing her hair. She kept repeating, "How could he do this to me?"

That statement was key to choosing a homeopathic remedy. *Ignatia* is a remedy for grief and emotional upset that is especially good for "disappointed love," which Debbie certainly had. Three days after she began taking it, she was a different woman. She was dressed to the teeth, her hair and nails were done, her makeup was perfect, and she was smiling. She joked and laughed. Asked if she had gotten back with her boyfriend, she said she hadn't. She had simply come to realize that she had made a bad choice. This man was not for her. Their breakup still hurt, but she was moving on.

Stomach Problems Relieved

Doug, a 35-year-old single father of three who was starting his own business, sought relief for his constant stomach ailments. Investigation revealed, however, that his real problem was stress. Doug wanted to be perfect in everything he did. He habitually arose at 4:30 a.m. because there were never enough hours in the day. He began by making breakfast and healthful lunches for all three children. Then there was cleaning the kitchen and making all the beds before going to work. The children could make their own beds, of course, but not well enough to satisfy their father. He vacuumed daily; yet no matter how hard he worked, the house never seemed clean enough. Doug's business involved masses of paperwork and deadlines, which he constantly worried he wouldn't meet, although somehow he always did. The remedy that relieved Doug's symptoms was *Arsenicum Album*, a homeopathic medicine for the stress of trying to be perfect. It works for people who create their own stress by worrying—the "type A" personality who never feels he has done quite enough.

CHOOSING A REMEDY

Here are some other homeopathic possibilities for different types of stress:

- *Adrenalinum* is for the person who "keeps on going" through a crisis, no matter how tired she is, no matter what else comes up. A few weeks after it's over, she comes in seeking help. "I'm so tired," she says, "and I'm not sure why. I was fine during the crisis. Why should I be so tired now, when it's all over?" The reason, of course, is that she has "burned out her adrenals." The Chinese say she has used up her excess Qi energy. For this personality type, a combination of homeopathic remedies containing Adrenalinum *in low potencies* is quite effective.

- *Magnesia Phosphorica* is for the person who is depressed, drowsy, dull, unable to study or think clearly, on edge, irritable, oversensitive.

- *Calcarea Phoshorica* is for more serious depression; for example, after the death of a loved one. The person is slow to comprehend, disappointed, moaning, irritable, hard to please, peevish, discontented, complaining, never satisfied, easily bored.

- *Phosphoricum Acidum* is for the person so overwhelmed with grief or physical illness that she is emotionally drained. She seems fatigued, slow to answer, flat, indifferent, even lifeless.

- *Cocculus* is for the stress of nursing a sick loved one; the ill effects of grief or anger; exhaustion from stress and anxiety over a loved one, sadness, grief, ailments from loss of sleep; the person who is sensitive to fear, anger, grief, noise, or touch; one who is easily startled.

- *Kali Phosphoricum* is for the person at the breaking point, the worn-out business or professional person, one very despondent about business, one for whom the slightest labor seems a heavy task; for weakened mental and physical states resulting from stress; for anxiety with nervous dread; for lassitude and depression.

- *Nux Vomica* is for the person who has stressed his body by overeating or with too much alcohol; the person who loves to party.

LIFESTYLE MODIFICATION

Stressed people tend to eat poorly. They say they don't have time. But proper nutrition and essential fatty acids are necessary to aid resistance to stress, and nutrients can detoxify and rebuild an overwhelmed system.

Relaxation, sleep, and exercise are also important for reducing stress. Meditation can help as well. You may not be able to control the crises in your life, but you can control how you deal with them. Stress is a state of mind. Some people thrive on it.

Stroke

Strokes result from a clot or rupture that interrupts blood flow to the brain, causing brain cells to die. The location of the clot or rupture determines the effects of the stroke; those bodily functions controlled by the oxygen-deprived cells deteriorate along with the brain cells. Right brain damage results in paralysis on the left side of the body and vice versa.

About one third of strokes end in death, and another third result in a permanent physical or mental disability. From the remaining third, however, the patients escape unscathed. Full recovery depends on recognizing the symptoms early and getting prompt treatment, which is more effective within the first few hours. Symptoms include numbness or paralysis of the face, arm, or leg; dizziness; sudden visual problems; speaking difficulties or incoherence; and sudden headache or nausea.[526]

Major risk factors for stroke include high blood pressure, obesity, smoking, and diabetes.

CONVENTIONAL DRUG TREATMENT

For strokes in progress, drugs can be lifesavers. The drug *TPA (tissue-plasminogen activator)* can break up a blood clot in the brain and stop its progression. But TPA must be used within three hours of a stroke to be effective.

For preventing strokes, *blood-pressure-lowering drugs* are widely prescribed. Recently, cholesterol-lowering drugs called *statins (Mevacor, Pravachol, Zocar)* were added to the conventional arsenal, following research showing that they can reduce the incidence of stroke by 15 to 30 percent.[527] Lowering blood pressure and serum cholesterol in this way, however, can have unwanted side effects. See "Hypertension," "Cholesterol, high."

THE NUTRITIONAL APPROACH

Better results can be achieved without side effects simply by changing the diet. In a study reported in the *New England Journal of Medicine* in 1987, adding only a single serving of fruit or vegetables to the daily diet was found to lower the risk of stroke by a full 40 percent, more than with cholesterol-lowering drugs and about the same as with a full course of antihypertensive drugs. Stroke deaths varied inversely with *potassium* intake: as potassium went up, deaths went down. Interestingly, the intake of sodium, the dietary variable most often associated with high blood pressure, was not significantly related to stroke deaths.[528] Other studies suggest it is the ratio of sodium to potassium that is important. Whole cereals, all fruits, and most vegetables contain 10 to 100 times as much potassium as sodium, but the modern diet contains more sodium than potassium, mainly because potassium is removed and sodium is added during processing and cooking.

Sodium and Potassium Contents of Some Common Foods—Processed vs. Unprocessed [529]

	[MG/100G]	
	SODIUM	POTASSIUM
Flour, wholemeal	3	360
White bread	540	100
Rice, polished	6	110
Rice, boiled	2	38
Beef, uncooked	55	280
Beef, corned	950	140
Haddock, uncooked	120	300
Haddock, smoked	790	190
Cabbage, uncooked	7	390
Cabbage, boiled	4	160
Peas, uncooked	1	340
Peas, canned	230	130
Pears, uncooked	2	130
Pears, canned	1	90

Besides potassium-rich foods, antioxidants can protect against strokes. The effect has been demonstrated for *vitamin C* and *vitamin A* in clinical studies.[530] The latest and greatest of the antioxidants for this purpose, however, seems to be *alpha lipoic acid (ALA)*. In recent research, rats given ALA were almost four times more likely to survive a stroke than was a control group. ALA is particularly valuable in fighting strokes because it's the only antioxidant that can easily get into the brain.

OTHER NATURAL ALTERNATIVES

Studies from China indicate that acupuncture can actually help revive the paralyzed extremities of stroke victims—a remarkable finding. Acupuncture works by stimulating the meridians, or lines of energy, that extend to the affected body parts. A review of nine recent Chinese studies found an approximately 90-percent effectiveness rate in treating strokes. Some methods produced a greater than 50-percent cure rate, with the remainder significantly improved.[531]

Constitutional homeopathic treatment can also help victims of stroke and stroke-like numbness.

Wayne Martin, writing in the January 1998 *Townsend Letter for Doctors*, states that three intravenous chelation treatments a year keep him from having spells associated with the cerebral ischemia preceding a stroke.

Stroke-like Symptoms Relieved

A 75-year-old woman had gotten in a fight with her daughter while jackpot gambling. When she awoke the next morning, she had no feeling on her left side and had become incontinent. The right side of her brain had gotten insufficient oxygen, shutting down the left side of her body. A complete medical examination, however, revealed no physical reason for the condition. Her baffled doctors said there was nothing to be done and no improvement could be expected. Within a week of taking constitutional homeopathic treatment with *Costicum* (a remedy specific to her condition), she could move the left side of her body, could use her left hand, and was no longer incontinent.

Surgical Trauma, Recovery from Cosmetic Surgery

Surgery became a feasible approach to attacking disease with the development of anesthesia in the nineteenth century. Before that, doctors had to proceed gently in support of the body's own efforts at healing; but anesthetics deadened the nerves that would have objected to destructive invasions. As with many medical innovations, the concept at first met with stiff resistance by conventional interests. Promoters of anesthesia were damned even from the pulpit, for daring to eliminate "the pain ordained by God."[532] But by the late nineteenth century, anesthesia was not only accepted but had transformed medical practice. Doctors began recommending major operations that required the development of expensive and lucrative hospital systems. At the end of the twentieth century, surgery and anesthesia are mainstays of conventional treatment.

Surgeries are becoming increasingly popular not only in life-threatening situations but for merely cosmetic purposes. In 1994, approximately 1.2 million cosmetic surgical procedures were performed in the United States, including face-lifts, liposuctions, collagen treatments, chemical peels, and eyelid lifts. Procedural innovations, including the use of lasers and endoscopy, have made cosmetic surgeries cheaper, easier and less traumatic. But surgery still represents a major stress to the body, and anesthetics and painkillers impose a sluggish drain on nerve and circulatory energy.

CONVENTIONAL POST-SURGICAL TREATMENT

For post-surgical trauma, narcotic analgesics are conventionally prescribed. They work by drugging the nerves. Morphine, codeine, and opium are narcotics that are natural plant derivatives. Synthetic or semi-synthetic narcotics include *propoxyphene (Darvon), meperidine (Demerol), pentazocine (Talwin), oxycodone* (contained in *Percodan with aspirin* and in *Percocet with acetaminophen*), and *codeine* (also used in cough medicines and for diarrhea). All narcotics can be addicting, and a virtually universal side effect is constipation.

A less well-known side effect is a weakening of the body's immune defenses. In research reported in 1997, mice regularly receiving morphine died from bacterial infections that would not have been lethal to normal mice. The researcher conducting the study warned that patients receiving morphine for postsurgical pain may face an increased risk of sepsis, a massive, often fatal bacterial infection.[533]

Aiding Recovery with Homeopathic Remedies

Homeopathic remedies can cut the amount of narcotic analgesics needed after surgery. Plastic surgery is particularly appropriate for homeopathic treatment, since it's an elective surgery for which people have time to prepare in advance. Patients have been impressed with how fast they healed, how little their surgery and recovery hurt, how little pain medication they required, how little bruising they experienced, and how quickly they were able to return to work as a result of using these simple remedies.

The best time to begin taking homeopathic remedies for surgical trauma is when you are being wheeled into the operating room. Since they are taken sublingually, they won't create nausea or vomiting (as food will if taken immediately before anesthesia). The remedies may all be mixed and taken at once.

Choosing and Taking the Remedies

Homeopathic remedies recommended in conjunction with surgery include:

- *Arnica*, to stop the body from overreacting to trauma. Arnica at a potency of 200c should be taken immediately before surgery and every hour for the first four hours afterwards. Then Arnica 30c should be taken three times daily until well. For cosmetic surgery, most of the doses need to be given right at the time of the surgical trauma, decreasing as time goes on. Ideally, have a friend come with you and give you a couple of pellets when you're being wheeled in, then immediately or soon after the trauma to your face, then every fifteen minutes for an hour or so, then every hour for the rest of the day. The following day, take the remedy in divided doses five times a day. Then reduce to three times a day. After the Arnica has done its job—once you're out of pain—you don't need it anymore.

- *Ledum* helps in the treatment of injuries that result in bruising and puffy skin, as first aid to prevent infection, and for eye injuries. After facial surgery, it's particularly useful for helping to relieve black eyes. It should be taken in the same way as homeopathic Arnica is, but after the second or third day it can usually be discontinued.

- *Bellis* is used to relieve blunt pain or trauma (the feeling of being hit in the face or of breaking the nose), to speed recovery after surgery, to help prevent infection, to treat abscesses, and to reduce swelling.

- *Calendula* is recommended for wounds that are slow to heal.

- *Hypericum* is used as a tonic for the nervous system and kidneys and to treat puncture wounds and pain after dental work. After surgery, it's particularly useful for treating pain caused by injury to the nerve endings.

- *Phosphorus* is used to treat anxiety, nervous and digestive ills, respiratory problems, and circulatory problems. In conjunction with surgical procedures, Phosphorus 6 or Phosphorus 30 helps relieve bleeding, nausea, and the lingering effects of anesthetics.

- *Staphysagria* aids in relieving the pain of incision. Staphysagria 30 may be taken four times a day following surgery until pain-free.

- *Cantharis* is most often used for bladder and reproductive problems, particularly when there is inflammation in those regions; but it's also useful in conjunction with surgery, for reducing the redness and swelling of burns. It should not be taken before a laser or face peel, however, since it neutralizes burns so well that it can reduce the effectiveness of the peel.

Cosmetic Surgery Without Pain Medication

A prominent woman in Sun Valley who was preparing to have extensive facial surgery and liposuction was skeptical of the homeopathic approach; but she was willing to try it because her sister, who had had the same surgery, had had a very difficult time with it. The sister had suffered substantial pain, bruising, and swelling; and she couldn't go out in public but had to stay "under cover" for a long time. The Sun Valley woman used the homeopathic remedies and was thrilled with the results. *She took no pain medications at all*, something her doctor said he had never seen. His patients typically required pain medication for two or three days after plastic surgery, which involves a great deal of trauma to the body. The woman experienced much less bruising, redness, and trauma to her face than in the usual case; her body healed nicely; and she was comfortable through it all, although she had liposuction at the same time.

ALLEVIATING THE PHYSICAL EFFECTS OF SHOCK

Surgical shock can be responsible for unanticipated and unwanted side effects. *Aconitum* is a common remedy for ailments involving sudden and violent onset of shock or trauma, and for fear and anxiety; for example, before surgery. In one double-blind randomized trial involving 50 children undergoing surgery, a significant reduction in postoperative pain and agitation was experienced by those given homeopathic Aconitum.[534] Take Aconitum 6 or Aconitum 30 the night before the operation and again in the morning before the operation on awakening, to help keep the body from going into shock. If anxiety continues after surgery, take one to three more doses.

Menopause Precipitated by Surgical Shock

A woman complained that her doctor had assured her that her hormone levels would not be affected by her hysterectomy, since he wasn't removing the ovaries; but her ovaries had quit working anyway. The shock of the surgery had evidently shut them down, bringing on hot flashes, night sweats, and memory loss. Eight months later, she was still having problems. *Contessa*, a combination homeopathic remedy made by MarcoPharma, brought her periods back; but she probably could have avoided this problem if she had taken *Aconitum* before and after her surgery.

PREPARING FOR SURGERY: NUTRITIONAL AND PSYCHOLOGICAL SUPPORT

The body's attempt to heal itself should be supported with nutritional and herbal supplements, proper diet, and toning exercises. Additional *vitamin C, vitamin B6,* and *magnesium* are particularly important to counteract the stress of surgery on the body.

A week before surgery, avoid taking anything that encourages bleeding, including aspirin, vitamin E, evening primrose oil, some Chinese herbs (for example, *Hsiao Yao Wan*) and certain prescription medications. Consult your doctor.

You should also try to enter surgery in a relaxed state of mind. Stress can exhaust nutritional stores and weaken the body's ability to recover. Use any technique at your disposal to maintain a positive and relaxed state of mind prior to your surgery: meditation, prayer, guided imagery, biofeedback, and so forth. (For a case in which agitation before surgery led to a dire outcome, see "Heart Attack.")

RECOVERING FROM SURGERY

A fundamental principle of Chinese medicine is that the body is crisscrossed with "meridians," or lines of energy, which provide the vitality necessary not only for healing but to maintain the workings of the body. Surgery inevitably cuts through these meridians, blocking both healing and bodily function. To reconnect them, Chinese doctors use acupuncture, a technique involving stimulating particular points on the body with very fine needles. Acupuncture treatments are helpful not only after surgery but before it, to increase energy flow and insure that it's moving properly.

For patients who say they have never been well since their surgeries, *homeopathic Phosphorus* can help eliminate the effects of the anesthetics. Homeopathic remedies give the best results for patients who are armed with them in the operating room, but they can also aid recovery after surgery or from the drugs used with it. If your system can't eliminate the anesthetics, you will continue to feel dragged out, tired, and sluggish.

Complete recovery, however, requires resolving the patient's underlying physical problems. Surgeries attack symptoms, but they often fail to address the real cause of disease.

Surgery Precipitated by Parasites

A case in point was that of a 35-year-old woman who had had serious pain in her gallbladder. Her surgeon, finding that her gallbladder had shriveled to the size of a walnut, had surgically removed it. The woman thought the surgery would eliminate her pain, but she had the same pain after the operation as when she went in; and now she couldn't get her vitality back. Homeopathic Phosphorus brought back her energy, but she continued to suffer from the pain. Further testing indicated that she was heavily infested with parasites. This was, in fact, likely to have been why she had had the gallbladder problem to begin with. She improved only after correcting this underlying problem.

Recovery from Surgical Scars

For speeding the healing of surgical scars, a remedy called *Scargo*, containing olive oil, peanut oil, lanolin, camphor, and yellow beeswax, does a remarkable job. Also quite effective for reducing redness and swelling (for example, of burns after laser surgery) is the *Bioptron* light machine. (See "Skin Problems.")

Scars Dissolved

A woman revealed that she had had a breast reduction a year and a half earlier. When she took off her shirt for acupuncture, huge angry purple/red scars were still evident on her chest. A month after the scars were treated with *Scargo* and the *Bioptron* light machine, they had completely faded.

Syphilis

Approximately 113,000 people are infected with syphilis each year. More than 70 percent are men, nearly 40 percent of them homosexual. A painless sore on the genitals may signal the condition, although carriers can have no symptoms at all. Untreated syphilis can cause serious heart problems, blindness, paralysis, mental disorders or death; and it can be passed from mother to child, causing stillbirth, active infection, or birth defects.

Drug Treatment

The syphilis bacterium is one that hasn't yet developed resistance to antibiotics, so the disease usually responds to penicillin. Drug treatment is often accompanied by fever, chills, headaches, worsening of lesions, and a general feeling of ill health. However, this complication is not an allergic response to the drug but is the result of the rapid release of antigens from the suddenly killed syphilis bacteria.[535]

HOMEOPATHIC TREATMENT

Syphilis victims are required by law to see a doctor, who must report each case to the health department. As a result, patients diagnosed with the disease generally wind up on antibiotics. But even if antibiotics are used, homeopaths maintain that homeopathic treatment should be sought from a qualified practitioner, to resolve not just the infection but any inherited "miasms" contributing to it. Children of a syphilitic parent often have underlying health problems. Homeopathic remedies clear the miasms along with the disease. A qualified homeopath can determine the appropriate remedies, based on a detailed patient history, to resolve not just syphilis but its inherited miasms.

PREVENTION

Condoms can protect against the disease but are not foolproof protection, particularly if open sores are present in the carrier. Your best defenses remain abstention or careful choosing of partners and regular checkups.

*T*innitus (Ringing in the Ears), Hearing Impairment

Tinnitus, or ringing in the ears, can have a variety of causes, but the most common seems to be prolonged exposure to loud sounds. Musicians, pilots, and heavy-machinery operators are prone to it. Another common cause of ringing in the ears and hearing impairment is blockage in the ear due to infection or wax buildup. Temporomandibular joint (TMJ) dysfunction can also lead to ringing in the ears. A less common cause is a medical condition such as a tumor.

CONVENTIONAL TREATMENT

If the cause is an underlying medical condition, that illness is treated first. For wax buildup, the doctor will mechanically clean the ears. But this approach isn't very effective, and it can leave water in the ears and create other problems. For bacterial infection, the doctor will usually prescribe hydrocortisone eardrops or antibiotics. For the downsides of these drugs, see "Infection, Immunity." For TMJ problems, referral is generally made to a dentist. See "Toothache."

NATURAL ALTERNATIVES

Chinese doctors say tinnitus is often an indication that the kidney energy is weak. When the Chinese talk about weak kidneys, however, they are talking about the adrenals. The adrenal glands sit on top of the kidneys and secrete adrenaline. The Chinese believe that the vital life force (Jing) is stored in the kidneys, and that there is a limited supply. When too much Jing (adrenaline) is used in a short period of time, the kidneys are weakened. Jing can be exhausted by poor diet, too much sex, too much alcohol, drugs, insufficient sleep, stress, or overwork. The remedy is to reverse these lifestyle factors: eat right, get enough sleep, cut out drugs and alcohol, reduce or cut out sexual activity, meditate.

The kidneys can also be strengthened with acupuncture or with Chinese herbs. Ginkgo biloba is an herb said by some people to help.

NATURAL EAR CLEANING

For ear cleaning, ear candles are a controversial but effective alternative to medical procedures. The ear candle is a waxed paper cyclinder that is placed in the ear, then burned at the protruding end. The flame creates a vacuum that draws out wax and infection. As a result, fluid moves and the sinuses drain. The FDA hasn't approved ear candles as medical devices, but many people claim remarkable success with their use. Ear candles not only can relieve ear pain but can improve hearing.

WARNING: Not all ear candles are the same. Some burn too hot, and with some the wax tends to melt into the ear, causing burning and other potential damage. Seek professional advice.

Deafness Cured

One dramatic case involved an 83-year-old woman who was deaf when she came for treatment. Ear candles were the only remedy used. Normally, ears come clean with one or two candles, but in her case four were required in each ear. An incredible amount of wax came out. When her ears were clean, to everyone's amazement, she could hear.

Toothache, TMJ Pain, Trigeminal Neuralgia

At one time, serious dental pain was cured by pulling the tooth. Then the "root canal" was developed. The procedure eliminates pain while preserving the tooth by killing the nerve. Root canals, however, have been suspected of causing insidious systemic infections, leading to a host of ills including heart and circulatory problems; kidney, liver and gallbladder problems; back, neck and shoulder pains; neuritis; neuralgia; appendicitis; pneumonia; rheumatism; shingles; arthritis; eye, ear and skin conditions; stomach ulcers; ovarian cysts; and intestinal disturbances. Cases are on record in which these symptoms have resolved just from pulling the offending teeth.[536] For a fuller discussion, see E. Brown, R. Hansen, D.M.D., *The Key to Ultimate Health* (1998). Root canals may be done just because the dentist, whose job it is to relieve dental pain, can find no other solution to a painful dental situation. In those cases, finding and eliminating the cause is obviously the preferable approach.

Trigeminal neuralgia is inflammation of the trigeminal nerve, causing severe, constant pain running down the side of the face. The cause is uncertain, but Richard Hansen, D.M.D., states that cases he has seen on x-ray generally involved osteoporosis. The degenerated jaw bones evidently collapse in on themselves, pinching the nerve.

Temporomandibular joint (TMJ) dysfunction is pain arising in the jaw joint.

A *dental abscess* is an infection in the tissue surrounding the tooth root, which can jeopardize the health of the entire body.

TMJ DYSFUNCTION: TREATING THE CAUSE

One cause of tooth pain can be a *faulty bite*. When the bite is "off," so is the temporomandibular joint (TMJ), which has an energetic relationship with areas all over the body. X-rays have verified that when missing or short back teeth cause the bite to be overclosed, the many nerves that leave the neck get pinched through the cervical plexus. Neurological symptoms follow, including pain, headaches, backaches, and fatigue. Harold Gelb, D.M.D., a professor of dentistry and founder of the Gelb Craniomandibular Pain Center at Tufts University School of Dental

Medicine, lists a host of other apparently unrelated symptoms, including chronic sore throat, asthma, upset stomach, diarrhea, arthritis, lowered thyroid activity, depression, and forgetfulness.[537] Symptoms have been relieved simply by correcting the bite, either with Gelb-type acrylic splints or with orthodontia.

Another cause of TMJ problems can simply be *tension*. Relaxing the TMJ muscle can realign the jaw. Chiropractic can also help.

NATURAL PAIN-RELIEVING REMEDIES FOR TOOTHACHE AND DENTAL TRAUMA

For temporary relief from toothache, a simple home remedy is to apply a few drops of a liquid extract of *echinacea* and *goldenseal* directly to the painful tooth. For particularly serious toothache, absorption can be enhanced by soaking a piece of cotton with a couple of drops of *DMSO* along with the echinacea/goldenseal extract. Leave it on the tooth for a few hours or overnight, freshening it periodically. *Oil of clove* applied directly to the tooth can also give temporary relief.

Excellent homeopathic remedies for toothache include *Gun Powder 6x* (3 pills 4 times daily) and *Bacticin* (10 drops every hour). *Pyrogenium* (2 every couple of hours as needed) expels pus. If you start getting pus or a bad taste in your mouth, don't panic; it means the remedy is working.

For dental pain due to inflammation, users report that *Hypericum 30c* works as well as aspirin, without its side effects or risks. Take 3 pills 4 times daily.

For relief from the swelling and pain of dental abscess, a German Staufen homeopathic remedy called *Corynebacterium Anaerobius Nosode* is excellent. Also remarkably effective is a new line of homeopathics called *Sanum remedies*.

For trigeminal neuralgia, *Hypericum* (for sharp or throbbing pain) and *Arsenicum album* (for burning pain) are quite effective. *Acupuncture* also helps relieve nerve pain, not only from trigeminal neuralgia but from other forms of neuralgia and neuritis.

Elusive Symptoms Relieved

Before she developed lupus, Shirley was told she had trigeminal neuralgia and was put on a prescription drug for it. She was surprised when she was informed that that particular drug has been linked to lupus, since her doctor had never mentioned the possibility. After talking to her doctor, she stopped the drug and took homeopathic remedies for the pain, which is now much relieved.

Audrey, 92, also has trigeminal neuralgia. She is able to tolerate the pain so long as she takes the homeopathic remedy *Arsenicum*.

Toxic Shock Syndrome

An estimated 5,000 to 10,000 cases of staphylococcal toxic shock syndrome now occur in the United States. The majority involve women, and estimates are that about half involve tampons or menstruation. Incidence of the condition declined in the 1980s, when certain highly absorbent tampons were taken off the market after a rash of cases was linked to them. But there has now been a sudden increase in the more dangerous streptococcal toxic shock, which has a death rate of up to 50 percent. Other precipitating causes besides tampons and menstruation include the use of contraceptive sponges, cervical caps, or diaphragms; childbirth; surgery; wounds; and influenza. Symptoms include sudden high fever, vomiting, diarrhea, a sunburn-like rash, low blood pressure, and shock.[538]

CONVENTIONAL TREATMENT

Conventional treatment is with antibiotics specific to staph infection, along with blood transfusions and other emergency treatment. The critical factor, however, is prompt diagnosis. Though potentially fatal, the disease is rare, so doctors may not recognize it. Family members need to be alert to the possibility of toxic shock and to seek immediate treatment.

ALTERNATIVE TREATMENT

Effective German homeopathic remedies are available for toxic shock syndrome, but they're little known and hard to find. In this case, it's best simply to seek prompt conventional treatment.

Trichomoniasis

This common protozoan infection affects about a quarter of all sexually active women, or about 2.5 million yearly. Its symptoms include vaginal itching and burning and a yellow or creamy-white vaginal discharge with a strong odor.

DRUG TREATMENT

The usual treatment is with the anti-parasitic *metronidazole (Flagyl)*. But the infection is liable to recur, and the drug can have substantial side effects (see "Parasites"). *Metronidazole is carcinogenic to rodents and should not be taken by pregnant women. Metronidazole taken with alcohol can result in nausea, vomiting, flushing, and difficult breathing.*

HOMEOPATHIC TREATMENT

Staufen, a German company, makes a safe, effective, nontoxic homeopathic remedy called *Trichomonas Vaginitis* specifically for trichomonas. It should be taken even if conventional treatment is used to prevent future recurrences.

Ulcers

A peptic ulcer is a hole or wound, usually less than half an inch wide, in the part of the lining of the digestive tract exposed to gastric juice (usually the stomach or first part of the small intestine). Gastric juice contains pepsin (an enzyme for breaking down protein) along with hydrochloric acid (an extremely powerful acid that activates pepsin). Not long ago, more than 10 percent of Americans suffered from peptic ulcers, although the condition has now become less common. Symptoms include a sharp searing pain, usually in the upper abdomen just below the breastbone, typically when the stomach is empty. The pain typically strikes at 1 or 2 A.M., is immediately relieved by food or drugs, and is gone in the morning. Serious complications can include bleeding that shows up in vomited blood or black bowel movements, peritonitis (inflammation of the membrane lining the abdominal cavity), and obstruction of the stomach outlet as a result of the formation of scar tissue.[539]

CONVENTIONAL TREATMENT

For half a century, peptic ulcers were blamed on diet and lifestyle factors (stress, spicy or greasy foods, alcohol, smoking). Standard treatment involved a bland diet and *antacids*. The drugs provided temporary relief by neutralizing the excess stomach acid that was thought to be the problem. But antacids can also exacerbate the condition, by promoting the production of more stomach acid through a rebound effect. A class of drugs called anticholinergics was also used to inhibit stomach acid secretion. Use of *belladonna*, the most popular of these drugs, was limited by its unpleasant side effects, including blurred vision, dry mouth, urine retention, constipation, and rapid heartbeat.

In the extreme case, surgeries involving the removal of three quarters of the stomach were done to prevent fatalities from deep ulcers.

This dire state of affairs set the stage for the H_2-blockers, drugs destined to become the best-selling pharmaceuticals on earth. In 1976, Smith Kline & French got FDA approval for treating ulcers with *Tagamet*, which blocks the secretion of stomach acid through inhibiting the release of a histamine called H_2. Tagamet topped the charts until 1988, when *Zantac*, a competitor H_2-blocker, passed it up. Zantac then became the world's best-selling drug, netting twice the income even of the drug in the number two slot. Other H_2-blockers, including *Pepcid* and *Axid*, have also joined in the boon.

Ironically, the reason these drugs have remained international bestsellers is that they don't cure ulcers. They merely mask symptoms; so to maintain their effects, you have to take them indefinitely. The drugs have been called "annuity medicines," since treatment can cost several dollars a day. Within two years of discontinuing the drugs, 86 percent to 93 percent of ulcer patients find that their ulcers have come back depending on the drug.[540]

Besides the cost, H_2-blockers can have side effects. Tagamet can cause a hormonal imbalance that results in breast enlargement and impotence in men; joint and muscle pains, sensitivity to light, and mental confusion; and in rare cases, depression of the bone marrow. Zantac is heavily promoted as giving you the benefits of Tagamet without its adverse effects, but the FDA is dubious, since Zantac has now been shown to cause some of the same problems as its competitor. One established advantage Zantac has over Tagamet is that it's less likely to interfere with the absorption of other drugs. Tagamet slows down the metabolism of many drugs, which can build up and produce serious toxic reactions. Antacids, too, can interfere with the absorption of many drugs, and one of them is Tagamet.[541]

More ponderous than the immediate and obvious side effects of H_2-blockers are their subtle and long-term effects. Whenever you tamper with the body's natural secretory mechanisms, you risk upsetting beneficial functions. Histamine receptors are found not only in the stomach but in the heart and blood vessels. Blockage of these receptors has caused fatal heart attacks in patients receiving H_2-blockers by injection. Stomach acid also has beneficial functions that can be suppressed by H_2-blockers. One is to aid in the absorption of iron from plant foods. H_2-blockers used long-term have been shown to block this absorption by 28 to 65 percent.[542] Another function of stomach acid is to kill bacteria and keep your stomach from being colonized by undesirables. Without the acid, you run the risk of infection by a number of organisms, including those causing typhoid, salmonella, cholera, dysentery, and giardia. One study found that patients with bleeding ulcers who were on acid-suppressing drugs (H_2- blockers or antacids or both) got pneumonia twice as often as did patients not on them.[543]

TREATING THE CAUSE

To eliminate ulcers permanently requires eliminating the cause. Fortunately, the cause seems finally to have been found. In a landmark 1982 discovery, it was determined to be a common bacterium called *H. pylori*. Also implicated as a leading cause of stomach cancer worldwide, this organism can be eradicated with antibiotics. That means most ulcers are now curable. The exceptions are the 15 percent that are caused by analgesic drugs (aspirin, ibuprofen, and the like), which can eat a hole in the stomach if taken repeatedly.

For reasons apparently related to market forces, however, acceptance of this revolutionary new cure has been slow. In January of 1993, the *Journal of the American Medical Association* finally published a paper asserting that there is now conclusive evidence that if you eradicate *H. pylori* you can cure ulcers. In 1994, the National Institutes of Health officially proclaimed that ulcers are caused by *H. pylori* and that people with these bacteria and an ulcer should have the bacteria treated. Yet the H_2-blockers remain the best-selling drugs on earth, ulcers remain rampant, and antibiotic treatment of ulcers remains rare. The reason seems to be that busy doctors get their information not from medical journals but from drug-company detail people, who aren't encouraged by their employers to spread the news that their blockbuster drugs are now obsolete. Neither drug companies nor gastroenterologists (for whom ulcers and other stomach-acid problems make up 25 percent of their practice) have much incentive to recognize a cure for this condition.

Currently, the most effective treatment for eradicating *H. pylori* is a course of the powerful antibiotic *Biaxin* taken with a new type of acid blocker called *Prilosec* that stops acid production almost entirely. Earlier attempts at antibiotic treatment were foiled because stomach acid destroyed the drugs before they could work; but Prilosec keeps Biaxin intact long enough to do its job. Other regimens used for eradicating *H. pylori* include a two-week course of a combination of *bismuth* (the active ingredient in *Pepto-Bismol*) and antibiotics; for example, *tetracycline* and *metronidazole (Flagyl)*. Even these treatments probably won't eliminate ulcers entirely. In Peru, most patients in whom the bacteria were killed had been reinfected by the following year. The treatment is nevertheless predicted to catch on, since a two-week course of antibiotics remains cheaper than a year's treatment with Zantac.[544]

Before getting antibiotic treatment, you should check with a physician to establish that you have both an ulcer and H. pylori.

HOMEOPATHIC AND HERBAL ALTERNATIVES

While antibiotics are the best of the conventional options, homeopathic doctors maintain that they still aren't the ideal solution. Antibiotics kill not just harmful bacteria but all the normal flora in the stomach, throwing it off balance for months afterwards. A German homeopathic remedy by Staufen called *Campylobacter pylori*, taken over a 30-day period, boosts the immune system to eliminate *H. pylori* without side effects or relapses.

The homeopathic remedy takes care of the bacteria, but to heal the wound in the stomach, other natural remedies may be needed. A simple Chinese formula called *Fare You*, consisting of vitamin U complex, can heal an ulcer wound in just a few days. Take two pills three times daily. Other options include homeopathic *Nux Vomica 30c* (three pills three times daily) or *Gastrica* by Complimed (ten drops three times daily).

British homeopath Dr. Jan De Vries uses *raw potato juice* to heal ulcer wounds. Drink one glass twice daily for three days. Eating *cabbage* is also beneficial for this purpose.

DIET AND LIFESTYLE SUGGESTIONS

The bland diet heavy in milk fats that used to be recommended for ulcer sufferers is now thought to have done more harm than good. The "Sippy Diet" of milk products actually increased stomach acid-secretion. The latest recommendation is just the reverse: a diet heavy in plant foods that are high in fiber and essential fatty acids. Research now suggests that these foods actually help heal ulcers. Vitamin C, found in fruits and vegetables, is also necessary for healing and tissue repair. Current thinking is that most ulcer patients can eat any wholesome foods they want, so long as they don't eat too much or too fast. Small, frequent meals are best.[545]

What you don't put into your stomach may be as important as what you do. Besides aspirin and other NSAIDs (which are known to eat holes in the stomach), other suspects include coffee, alcohol, and cigarettes.[546]

Uterine Fibroid Tumors

Fibroid tumors are masses of connective tissue that tend to grow on the wall of the uterus before menopause, when estrogen secretion dominates. The most common tumors of the female pelvic organs, they are rarely malignant. But they can still precipitate a hysterectomy, by causing excessive menstrual bleeding and pelvic pain. Fibroid tumors are the most common reason given, in fact, for this surgery. More than 40 percent of women over 50 have benign fibroid tumors, and from 1982 to 1984 more than half a million uteri were removed to excise them.[547]

CONVENTIONAL TREATMENT

Medical wisdom says that fibroids cannot be dissolved. Small ones may disappear by themselves after menopause, but the conventional treatment for eliminating large or painful fibroids remains surgical removal.[548] Usually, this means removal of the uterus, with or without the ovaries. One downside of this approach is that it can result in the prolapse of other organs—including the intestines, bowels, bladder, and vagina—causing pelvic pain, sexual problems, or pressure on the bowels and bladder. Hysterectomy can also have other long-term complications, including osteoporosis, bone and joint pain and immobility, chronic fatigue, urinary problems, emotional problems, depression, and increased risk of heart disease. The Nurses' Health Study found that for women who had had both ovaries removed and weren't on hormone replacement therapy, the risk of a nonfatal heart attack was twice that of other women.[549] Even when both ovaries aren't removed, in more than a third of cases the ovaries die following hysterectomy and menopause follows.[550] The abruptness of the change can also wreak havoc on hormone balance, bringing on severe hot flashes within 24 hours of the operation.

In normal women, the ovaries continue to secrete some hormones for many years after menopause.[551] One is testosterone, which encourages libido. In recent studies in the United Kingdom, 33 to 46 percent of women reported decreased sexual response after hysterectomy or oophorectomy (removal of the uterus and ovaries).[552] For some women, the cervix and uterus are also major triggers for orgasm, which are eliminated with a hysterectomy.[553]

Vicki Hufnagel, M.D., author of *No More Hysterectomies*, favors a modified surgery that can eliminate fibroids and correct uterine prolapse while preserving the uterus and ovaries. Called "female reconstructive surgery," the procedure involves a surgical resectioning of the organ. The abdomen is opened with a bikini-type incision and the uterus is lifted out for complete inspection. The tissue connected to the uterus is clamped off with a special clamp and a drug is injected to stop the flow of blood, to allow maximum surgical time without bleeding. Fibroid tumors are then removed or, in the case of prolapse, the ligaments and organs are restructured and resuspended.

Nonsurgical Alternatives: Natural Progesterone

Fortunately, even this surgery may not be necessary in the majority of cases. Hormone researcher John Lee, M.D., maintains that uterine fibroids can be both prevented and treated with *natural* progesterone cream—not the synthetic form of the hormone, but a plant derivative of a type of yam (*Pro-Gest*). Estrogen stimulates the growth of fibroids, which are common in the estrogen-dominant phase of "perimenopause" (early menopause, before menses have ceased). If estrogen levels are allowed to drop off naturally after menopause, existing uterine tumors will typically atrophy by themselves. But problems arise when estrogen is artificially supplied. Fibroid tumors will then be stimulated to grow. These fibroids usually remain nonmalignant, but they can cause excessive menstrual bleeding and pelvic pain, precipitating a hysterectomy.[554] Supplementing before menopause with natural progesterone, estrogen's antagonist, may help prevent fibroids from developing.[555]

CAUTION: Only natural progesterone works for this purpose. Synthetic progesterone is contraindicated for fibroids, since it tends to make them grow.

Surgery Avoided with Simple Cream

Dr. Lee cites the case of a former patient who telephoned to say she had developed a large fibroid tumor. Her gynecologist, concerned that its rapid growth suggested cancer, recommended immediate removal of her uterus and ovaries. Dr. Lee recommended that she try natural progesterone cream instead, and she agreed. When the woman returned to her gynecologist a month later, the tumor was about 10 percent smaller. After three months, it was 25 percent reduced; and six months later (or ten months from when she began using natural progesterone), it was gone.

The authors of this book have had similar experiences. Both were diagnosed with large fibroid tumors for which they were told surgical removal was required. In both cases, before menopause, the tumors disappeared on their own with the aid of natural remedies, including natural progesterone cream, acupuncture, homeopathy, and herbs.

OTHER NATURAL REMEDIES FOR SHRINKING FIBROIDS

Oriental herbs can also help shrink tumors. Chinese herbal products by Seven Forests useful for shrinking unwanted growths include

- *Laminaria 4* for fatty type swellings
- *Zedoria Tablets* for hard masses

- *Chih-ko* and *Curcuma* for phlegm or blood stagnation, considered in Chinese medicine to be the cause of many fibroids.

Even malignant tumors have responded to Chinese herbs. In a recent study, proteins extracted from Chinese medicinal herbs were shown to selectively injure tumor cell lines while preserving normal cell lines. Conventional cytotoxic (cell killing) chemotherapy, by contrast, kills normal along with aberrant cells.[556]

Dr. Ray Peat, developer of natural progesterone in topical cream form, observes that the heavy and irregular menstrual bleeding accompanying a uterine tumor can be a symptom of an underactive thyroid gland. He suggests that before removal of the uterus is undertaken for excessive bleeding, *thyroid therapy* should be tried.[557] (See "Hypothyroidism.")

NATURAL REMEDIES TO COUNTERACT BLEEDING AND BALANCE HORMONES

Natural remedies can also help stop the heavy bleeding that often accompanies a fibroid. One is *natural progesterone cream.*

Another is the herb *chasteberry.* German research has shown that the chasteberry plant increases luteinizing hormone, which stimulates progesterone synthesis and secretion. It not only can help regulate periods involving too frequent or too much bleeding but is a good treatment for fibroids and for inflammation of the lining of the womb. *NOTE: Chasteberry should not be used during pregnancy, since it's a strong uterine stimulant.*[558]

Other natural remedies for heavy bleeding include

- *Homeopathic Mother Tincture of Thlaspi Bursa*—take 10 drops in water every hour until bleeding slows.

- *Bleeding* (a combination homeopathic by BHI)—take 1 pill every 15 minutes as needed until bleeding slows, then 4 times daily until it stops.

- *Luvos Earth and Trillium*—take 20 drops of this herbal formula in water 3 times daily or, in cases of acute bleeding, use 50 drops in water followed by 20 drops every hour.

- *Yunnan Pai Yao*—take 2 capsules every hour until bleeding stops. This Chinese formula is highly effective both topically and orally to stop bleeding on which nothing else seems to work. It was used by Vietnamese soldiers, who put it on their wounds to avoid leaving a bloody trail when they got shot.

Once bleeding is stopped, steps should be taken to build up the blood and balance the body to avoid repeating the problem each month. (See "Anemia.") Useful remedies for toning and balancing when fibroid tumors are present include:

- *Female Tonic* by MPI—take one tablespoonful twice daily.
- *Fibrozolve* by Futurplex—take 10 drops 3 to 4 times daily.
- *Female Balancer*—take 10 drops 3 times daily.
- *Vita Gyn* by Eclectic Institute—take 4 pills twice daily for 5 days after the period.
- *Grapeseed extract*—take 1 mg per pound of body weight daily.
- *Cat's Claw*—take 2 capsules 3 times daily.

CAUTION: Although fewer than .2 percent of fibroid tumors are found to be malignant, that remains a possibility.[559] If you have symptoms suggesting fibroids—including abdominal swelling, pelvic or back pain, heavy or irregular bleeding, painful periods, constipation, pressure on the bladder, or frequent urination—see a gynecologist. While the natural remedies discussed here are safe, you should not attempt self-treatment. If you are interested in exploring natural remedies, see an Oriental medical, homeopathic, or naturopathic physician.

Uterine Prolapse

Uterine prolapse is a condition in which the uterus descends into the lower part of the vagina or, in some cases, actually outside the vaginal opening. Childbirth is considered the most common precipitating cause, since it substantially stretches the muscles of the uterus. Loss with age of the collagen that keeps the muscles elastic can also precipitate pelvic floor disorders. Heavy lifting and other exercise that causes the abdominal wall muscles to contract are a third precipitating cause.[560]

CONVENTIONAL TREATMENT

No known drug will reverse a prolapsed uterus. The conventional treatment is hysterectomy—surgical removal of the uterus—but this option has obvious drawbacks. A less drastic option that preserves the female organs is a surgical re-sectioning of the uterus called "female reconstructive surgery." Both are discussed under "Uterine Fibroid Tumors."

A mechanical stopgap measure for prolapse is the pessary, a device placed within the vagina to support the bladder, vagina, and rectum.

Kegel exercises, involving contracting and relaxing the uterine muscles, are also recommended for uterine prolapse. They may forestall the condition but won't reverse it.

NATURAL ALTERNATIVES TO SURGERY

Then can a prolapsed uterus be reversed? The authors think it can.

Uterine Prolapse Reversed without Surgery

One of the authors was scheduled for female reconstructive surgery at the age of 50 to repair a prolapsed uterus and remove a large fibroid tumor. The surgery had been recommended several years earlier, but she ignored the advice until her symptoms got so pronounced that she had to quit going for walks, which resulted in a precipitous and quite uncomfortable drop in the subject organ.

She subsequently canceled the operation, after both the prolapse and the fibroid disappeared of their own volition. She attributed this rather remarkable result primarily to the use of a three-percent natural progesterone cream (*Pro-Gest*). (See "Menopause.") Whenever she allows several days to pass without rubbing one-quarter to one-half teaspoon of this cream on her abdominal area at night, her uterus invariably drops uncomfortably. She has tried this experiment on numerous occasions over the past three years, always with the same result. She has tried switching brands but has found no over-the-counter formulation but Pro-Gest that keeps her uterus in suspension, although she can't explain why. Another product that seems to work but is available only by prescription is a six-percent natural progesterone cream made by Women's International Pharmacy in Madison, Wisconsin. She also uses a number of other natural hormone boosters, including the precursor hormones *DHEA* and *pregnenolone* and a natural estrogen cream derived from plants (*Ostaderm*). In addition, she has undergone biannual live-cell therapy, a treatment developed in Germany consisting of injections of fetal cells of animal organs. This therapy is available in Guatemala, where she lives, but has been kept off the U.S. market by the prohibitive cost of FDA approval.

Ellen also discontinued the use of all contraceptive creams, after she was advised by a practitioner that they could be contributing to the problem. She has delivered two large babies, but so have many other women who managed to avoid uterine prolapse. Contraceptive creams contain nonoxynol-9, which breaks down into nonylphenol when it comes in contact with the body. Nonylphenols are estrogen-mimicking chemicals that are toxic to the body and can disrupt its hormone balance even in very low concentrations. They are absorbed not only from contraceptive creams but from ubiquitous sources including plastic products, polystyrene food containers, detergents, personal-care products, and the polyvinyl chloride tubing through which water passes.[561]

HERBAL AND HOMEOPATHIC SUPPORT

In China, a form of the herb *black cohosh* called *Sheng Ma* is traditionally used for uterine and bladder prolapse, as well as for measles, toothache, and canker sores. Black cohosh (*Cimicifuga racemosa*) is also native to North America, where it was first used by Native Americans to ease the pain of menstruation and childbirth and to antidote rattlesnake bites. Black cohosh is an estrogenic herb that has a regulating and normalizing effect on hormone production and is contained in many formulas for balancing women's hormones. A powerful uterine tonic, it is useful for bladder and uterine prolapse and vaginal atrophy. *CAUTION: Black cohosh should not be used during abnormally heavy menstrual periods.*[562]

Other Chinese herbal formulas recommended for uterine prolapse include *Ginseng and Astragalus* and *Tang Kuei Formula*, both by Zand.

The appropriate homeopathic remedy is *Sepia*. It is used to counteract a loss of energy which leaves the body with unable to hold the organs in place or the blood in the blood vessels. The patient is not only tired but bruises easily and has hemorrhoids, varicose veins, and prolapse.

*V*aginal Dryness, Menopausal Vaginal Infections

Lack of vaginal lubrication during intercourse means hormone levels are dropping. It can be one of the first symptoms of menopause. Classic symptoms of vaginal atrophy are dryness, irritation, burning, and a feeling of pressure. There may also be a yellowish discharge. The vagina gets progressively shorter and narrower, its skin tissue thins, and its muscular layer is replaced with fibrous tissue. The vagina shrivels and shrinks and loses its flexibility, while the labia become small, colorless, and flat.[563]

The vagina also becomes susceptible to infection. This is because its thin walls lack the normal secretions that cleanse the vaginal tissues. Vaginal pH rises (meaning it becomes more alkaline instead of the normal acid), allowing undesirable bacteria to replace the friendly bacterial flora. The result can be urinary-tract infections. (See "Vaginitis," "Bladder Infection.")

CONVENTIONAL TREATMENT

For vaginal infections, *antibiotics* are usually prescribed, but since the problem in this case is the alkalinity of the vagina, the infections tend to recur, leading to long-term drug use that can be dangerous and expensive.[564] Many physicians resort to chronic suppressive therapy with *sulfonamides*, sulfa drugs that can produce complications that are life-threatening.[565]

For vaginal dryness, lubricants and moisturizers are available. A vaginal suppository called *Replens* is effective but expensive. Cheaper options are *K-Y Jelly* and *Mennen's Baby Magic*. A drawback of these products is that they contain mineral oil, which blocks pores and congests tissue, is difficult for the body to dispose of, and tends to be allergenic.

ALTERNATIVE APPROACHES

For menopausal vaginal infections, hormone treatment is an effective alternative to antibiotics. In a 1988 University of Florida Medical School study, when postmenopausal women with a history of recurrent infection and antibiotics were treated with estrogen, vaginitis was cured and urinary-tract infections went away for good. The estrogen worked by restoring the normal vaginal flora and pH.[566]

At first, the women took estrogen by mouth; but they were already past menopause and were upset by the return of their periods, painful enlargement of the breasts, and nausea. Some of the women were therefore switched to a vaginal *estrogen cream* taken twice weekly. The cream, which avoided passage through the digestive tract, proved to be just as effective as the pills without their unpleasant side effects.

European research shows that hormone therapy can help in cases not only of vaginal infection but of vaginal dryness and atrophy. In a European study reported in 1991, 20 postmenopausal women (average age 73) were treated with oral estrogen in the form of *estriol*. When their flora and epithelial ells were compared to those of 20 untreated women of similar age and 20 healthy younger women (average age 28), they more nearly resembled those of the younger women than those of the untreated postmenopausal women.[567]

A 1991 Norwegian review concluded that estriol is a safe, cheap, and effective therapy for the symptoms of estrogen deficiency after menopause, including atrophy of the vagina, urethra, and bladder, urinary tract infections, and abnormal function of the lower urinary tract. The researchers found that estriol had no metabolic effects or serious side effects at recommended doses and was safe for use long-term.[568]

Oral estriol is not available in this country, but estriol is the major estrogen component in *Ostaderm V*, an estrogen/progesterone cream derived from plants that is designed for vaginal use. David Shefrin, N.D., who uses this cream for severe atrophic vaginitis, observes, "It has always amazed me how easily the vaginal problems can be reversed. Women whose vaginas bled just with the introduction of a small speculum or from taking a Pap smear return literally after six weeks with a moist, pink, youthful vagina. Not all cases can be completely reversed in just six weeks, however. In those women with profound atrophy, the process may take a few months. Prognosis then depends on how great the loss of estrogen was and for how long. So it's very important to educate these women early on."[569]

The natural way to maintain vaginal lubrication is to remain sexually active. However, lack of vaginal lubrication can keep you from being sexually active. One option is to use natural progesterone and estrogen creams vaginally for lubrication. Another product that is petroleum-free is

Lubricating Gel by Women's Health Institute. Another natural product that studies show to be effective in relieving atrophic vaginitis is *vitamin E.* You can insert the capsules vaginally, take them by mouth, or open them up and apply the oil directly to the vaginal tissues. *Evening primrose oil* can be used in the same way.

Vaginitis, Vaginosis, Vaginal Yeast Infection

According to the National Vaginitis Association, vaginal infections (vaginitis) are the most common gynecological disorders, prompting more than ten million doctor visits annually. Types of vaginal infections include

- *Bacterial vaginosis,* the most common type of vaginitis. Bacteria are found naturally in the vagina, but this disorder results from a change in the balance of vaginal bacteria. Characterized by a milklike discharge with a fishy odor, it can precipitate pelvic infection leading to infertility or complications of pregnancy.
- *Candidiasis* (yeast infection), a relatively harmless fungal infection caused by an overgrowth of yeast cells (*candida*). Symptoms include itching, burning, and a white discharge resembling cottage cheese.
- *Trichomoniasis* (trich), a sexually transmitted disease caused by a parasite. It is characterized by a fishy odor, heavy yellow-green or gray discharge, and painful intercourse.[570]

CONVENTIONAL TREATMENT

Women commonly treat their own vaginal infections with nonprescription products. Antifungal creams such as *clotrimazole* and *miconazole,* once available only by prescription, can now be purchased over the counter. The National Vaginitis Association warns, however, that unless you've had yeast infections before and are sure of their symptoms, you should not attempt self-treatment without getting a diagnosis first, since antifungals won't cure the bacterial and parasitic infections that have similar symptoms but more hazardous outcomes. For these, it recommends prescription medications. Recurrent yeast infections can also be an indication of something more serious, such as diabetes or the HIV virus. The popular nonprescription anti-fungals can also have side effects; and even if you have a true fungal infection, the drugs don't deal with the underlying cause, so the infection is liable to recur.

ALTERNATIVE TREATMENT

To correct overgrowths of yeast and other invaders permanently, a proper acid-alkaline balance needs to be restored and maintained within the vagina. Yeast can't live in an acid environment.

One option is boric acid capsules, which increase vaginal acidity. Boric acid has been found to cure yeast infections in 98 percent of women for whom other treatments were unsuccessful. Recommended dosage is one capsule inserted vaginally every night at bedtime for a week, then two or three times a week for three more weeks. A good brand is *Y-Stat* by Bezwecken.

CAUTION: Professional advice should be sought before undertaking this treatment, since sensitive women occasionally experience some burning or watery discharge. Keep boric acid out of the reach of children, for whom it can be fatal at doses of as little as five grams.

Floral balance can also be restored with a vaginal douche containing liquid *acidophilus*.[571] Yogurt containing active lactobacillus acidophilus culture can be included in the diet as well.

Garlic is known for its antifungal properties. In laboratory experiments, its antifungal activity has proved to be greater than that of either nystatin or amphotericin B.[572] Health-food stores now sell deodorized garlic tablets that make this age-old remedy both easy to take and socially acceptable. It can be taken orally in odorless capsule form.

Other recommended supplements include *vitamins A, E, C* and *B6*, *zinc*, and *grapefruit seed extract*. An herbal combination containing a mixture of powdered *goldenseal, myrrh,* and *slippery elm* may also help.[573]

To discourage vaginal yeast, it's best to avoid foods on which yeast thrive: those containing sugar, molds, or yeasts; and aged or fermented foods, including breads made with yeast, aged cheeses, vinegar, and beer. No anticandida diet will effect a permanent cure, however, unless the underlying problem is also corrected. See "Candidiasis," "Fungal Infections."

*W*arts

Warts are the second-most common skin complaint after acne. Common warts are small, hard, round, elevated lumps, usually found on the hands. Most people get them at some time, though children and young adults are more susceptible than older adults. Caused by the human papilloma virus (HPV), they are mildly contagious and can be spread to other parts of the body. Most warts go away by themselves, but this may take awhile— months or even years.

CONVENTIONAL TREATMENT

For the impatient, there are medical remedies. Over-the-counter options usually contain *salicyclic acid* (the main ingredient in aspirin). More invasive treatments include freezing, burning or cutting off the offending growth. But these treatments can lead to scarring.[574] They also don't prevent recurrences and may encourage them. When one wart is burned or frozen off, three are liable to pop up in its place. Since the cause is a virus, the problem generally runs much deeper than the manifestation on the skin.

NATURAL ALTERNATIVES

Homeopathic treatment takes a bit longer than cutting or burning, but it's more effective over the long term. Even if you're having your warts burned off, homeopaths say homeopathic remedies should accompany them. The immediate effect will be to make the wart reappear, but then the virus will be cleared from the system.

Hannah Kroeger (Kroeger Herb Shop) makes a wart formula called *Wart* that is simple and effective. Use both orally (ten drops three times a day) and topically (one drop applied to the wart three times a day) for three to four weeks. If any change at all is seen in the wart, the remedy should be continued. If no change is seen, the remedy probably isn't going to work. In that case, constitutional remedies specific to the patient need to be selected by a practitioner. (See Chapter 3.) Likely homeopathic possibilities include *thuja* and *causticum*.

Wart Cured with Natural Treatment

A mother sought help for her 11-year-old son, who had a huge wart on his foot. The mother had tried everything, including having the wart burned off, but it had grown back. A single course of *thuja* caused the wart to vanish for good. *Silica*, an extract of the herb *horsetail* strengthens and supports healthy skin, hair, bones, and nails. Several people have reported their warts disappeared after a few weeks on silica. (*Alta Silica* tablets—1 pill 2 to 3 times daily or standardized horsetail extract.)

Endnotes

1. See disucssion under "Ulcers."

2. See A. Gaby, "Cost of Developing a New Drug Skyrockets," *Townsend Letter for Doctors* (August/September 1990), p. 523, citing "Drug R & D Costs Doubled in Decade," *American Medical News* (May 18, 1990), pp. 3, 53.

3. "Pills Don't Come with a Seal of Approval," *U.S. News & World Report* (September 29, 1997), p. 74; C. Kalb, "When Drugs Do Harm," *Newsweek* (April 27, 1998), p. 61.

4. J. Woolsey, et al., "Combatting Terrorism, Protecting Freedom," *CATO Journal* (December 1, 1996).

5. "Harper's Index," *Harper's* (December 1997), p. 17.

6. A. Melville, C. Johnson, *Cured to Death* (New York: Stein and Day, 1982), pp. 136–40.

7. E. Hess, "Drug-related Lupus," *New England Journal of Medicine* 318(22): 1460–62 (1988).

8. "Hazards of Non-practolol Beta Blockers," *British Medical Journal* 1(6060): 529 (1977); A. Melville, et al., *op cit.*, pp. 136–40.

9. See M. Castleman, *Nature's Cures* (Emmaus, PA: Rodale Press, Inc., 1996), pp. 218–10.

10. See, e.g., J. Shaw, "Aging Process and Anti-aging Effects of Chinese Herbal Medicines," *International Journal of Chinese Medicine* 1: 45–48 (1984); *Herbal Pharmacology in the People's Republic of China: A Trip Report of the American Pharmacology Delegation* (Washington, D.C.: National Academy of Sciences, 1975); J. Chen, "'Pharmacology,' Medicine and Public Health in the People's Republic of China," DHEW Publication No. (NIH) 72–67, pp. 93–108 (1972); Kiangsu New Medical College, *Pharmacopoeia of Chinese Drugs (Chung Yao Ta Zi Tien)* (Shanghai: People's Publishing House, 1977) (in Chinese).

11. *U.S. Senate Document No. 264, 74th Congress, 2nd Session, 1936.*

12. F. Batmanghelidj, M.D., *Your Body's Many Cries for Water* (Falls Church, VA: Global Health Solutions, 1995).

13. See "Suppression and Obstruction to Cure," *Townsend Letter for Doctors* (June 1995), pp. 112–13.

14. An earlier meta-analysis is discussed in D. Ullman, *The Consumer's Guide to Homeopathy* (New York: G.P. Putnam's Sons, 1995), pp. 44–46.

15. *Ibid.*, p. 344

16. *Ibid.*, p. 56.

17. R. Gerber, *Vibrational Medicine* (Santa Fe, NM: Bear & Co., 1988), pp. 206–10.

18. S. Bharija, M. Belhaj, "Acetylsalicylic Acid May Induce a Lichenoid Eruption," *Dermatologica* 177:19 (1988); S. Begley, "Don't Drink the Water?," *Newsweek* (February 5, 1990), pp. 60–61.

19. S. Roan, "Sufferers of Acne, Beware: Pimples May be Winning," *Los Angeles Times* (May 8, 1996).

20. A. Saloman, "Acne Drug Can Kill, British Doctors Warn," *Reuters* (January 18, 1996); T. Halvorson, "Warning Issued for Painkiller," *Gannet News Service* (March 7, 1995).

21. "Gray Hair and Acne," *University of California, Berkeley Wellness Letter* 4(8): 7 (1988); J. Trowbridge, M. Walker, *The Yeast Syndrome* (New York: Bantam Books, 1986).

22. A. Shalita, et al., "Isotretinoin Revisited," *Cutis* 42: 1–19 (1988).

23. E. Lammer, et al., "Retinoic Acid Embryopathy," *New England Journal of Medicine* 313: 837–41 (1985).

24. F. Tornatore, "Anti-acne Medication and Depression," *Psychopharmacology Update* (May 1, 1996); A. Shalita, et al., *op cit.*; H. Roenigk Jr., "Retinoids," *Cutis* 39: 301–05 (1987). See D. Blanc, et al., "Eruptive Pyogenic Granulomas and Acne Fulminans in Two Siblings Treated with Isotretinoin," *Dermatologica* 177: 16–18 (1988).

25. A. Shalita, et al., *op cit.*

26. "What's the Connection between Hormones and Skin?", *Pharmacy Times* (May 1989), pp. 49–51.

27. P. Boyer, et al., "Can Hormone Therapy Save Your Skin?", *Prevention* (January 1, 1997).

28. J. Trowbridge, et al., *op cit.*, pp. 301–20.

29. See D. Gates, et al., *The Body Ecology Diet* (Atlanta, GA: B.E.D. Publications, 1993).

30. For other home cosmetic ideas, see T. Jeffries, "Healthy Hints for Looking Good . . . Naturally," *Health Quest* (February 28, 1995); and T. Moore, *Kitchen Cosmetics*, reviewed in *Health Quest* (March 31, 1994).

31. *Drug Facts and Comparisons* (St. Louis: Facts and Comparisons, 1998).

32. D. Chopra, M.D., *Perfect Health: the Complete Mind/Body Guide* (New York: Harmony Books, 1990), pp. 171–75.

33. See "Growth Hormone in Elderly People," *Lancet* 337:1131-32 (1991); "Human Growth Hormone: The Fountain of Youth?" *Harvard Health Letter* 17(8): 1-3 (1992); Peter Doskoch, "Body of Evidence: Research Findings on Six Popular Anti-aging Medications and Treatments," *Psychology Today* (November 21, 1996).

34. See P. Doskoch, *op. cit.*

35. S. Moncada, et al., "Biosynthesis of Nitric Oxide from L-arginine," *Biochemical Pharmacology* 38(11): 1709–15 (1989); A. Barbul, et al., "Wound Healing and Thymotropic Effects of Arginine: A Pituitary Mechanism of Action," *American Journal of Clinical Nutrition* 37: 786–94 (1983); J. Daly, et al., "Effect of Dietary Protein and Amino-acids on Immune Function," *Critical Care Medicine* 1990 (supp. 2): 86–93.

36. J. Chen, "Pharmacologic Actions and Therapeutic Uses of Ginseng and Tang Kwei," *International Journal of Chinese Medicine* 1(3): 23–27 (1984).

37. P. Doskoch, *op. cit.*; Kathleen Doheny, "Body Watch; Beat the Clock; Supplemental testosterone. Antioxidants. [etc.]," *Los Angeles Times* (January 1, 1997).

38. P. Airola, N.D., *Are You Confused?* (Phoenix, AZ: Health Plus, Publishers, 1971), pp. 112-13, 137.

39. L. Cornaro, *Discourses on the Sober Life* (Mokelumne Hill, CA: Health Research [undated]).

40. S. Starr, "Supplements for the Brain," *Health Foods Business* (May 1997), p. 28.

41. E. Freeman, "HIV Does Not Cause AIDS," *Health Quest: The Publication of Black Wellness* (October 31, 1996).

42. S. Byrnes, "Benzene, Lubricants and AIDS," *Journal of International Health Research* (July 1996).

43. L. Horowitz, *Emerging Viruses: AIDS and Ebola—Nature, Accident or Genocide?* (Tetrahedron Publishing Group, 1996). For similar theories and supporting data, see J. Rappoport, *AIDS Inc.* (San Bruno, California: Human Energy Press, 1988), pp. 209–41; T. Bearden, *AIDS: Biological Warfare* (Greenville, TX: Tesla Publishing Co., 1988), pp. 11–17.

44. "Foulpox," *The Economist* (November 22, 1997), p. 96.

45. M. Berer, "Women and HIV/AIDS," *Contemporary Women's Issues Collection* (January 1, 1993).

46. "Zidovudine (AZT) Delays Appearance of AIDS Symptoms," *American Pharmacy* (October 1989), p. 21; J. Lublin, "Some Rodents Given High Doses of AZT Develop Cancer, AIDS Drug Maker Says," *Wall Street Journal* (December 6, 1989), p. B4; J. Wallace, "AIDS in the Workplace," *Wellcome Programs in Pharmacy* (Park Row Publishers, Inc. 1987).

47. L. Garrett, "Doubts Linger about AIDS Drug, Despite Record OK," *Newsday* (March 5, 1996).

48. "Alpha Lipoic Acid," *World News Tonight with Peter Jennings* (September 29, 1997).

49. K. Kerr, "No Magic Bullet: AIDS Researchers See Little Hope for Vaccine in a Decade," *Newsday* (May 26, 1997).

50. P. Sanders, *Health Quest* (October 31, 1996).

51. *Ibid.*

52. L. Yi, "A Report of 2 Cases of Type B AIDS Treated with Acupuncture," *Journal of Traditional Chinese Medicine* 9(2): 95–96 (1989).

53. G. Pragati, "Ayurvedic Cure for AIDS?" *India Currents* (November 30, 1994).

54. C. Osterman, "From Herbs to Ozone, AIDS Patients Seek Alternatives," *Reuters* (July 9, 1996).

55. "Plagued by Cures," *The Economist* (November 22, 1997), p. 95.

56. N. Freundlich, "Health: Fight Sneezing—Without Snoozing," *Business Week* (April 7, 1997); D. Levy, "Allergy-relief Alternatives to Seldane," *USA Today* (January 14, 1997); "Slow, and Then Too Slow; FDA Falls Short in Dealing with an Already Approved Drug," *Los Angeles Times* (Home Edition) (January 15, 1997).

57. N. Freundlich, *op. cit.*; K. Painter, "Allergy Shots Give Little Help in Asthma Battle," *USA Today* (January 30, 1997).

58. F. Batmanghelidj, M.D., *Your Body's Many Cries for Water* (Falls Church, VA: Global Health Solutions, 1995).

59. S. Squires, "Allergy Season Returns," *Washington Post Health* (April 18, 1989), pp. 6–7.

60. H. Sampson, S. Scanlon, "Natural History of Food Hypersensitivity in Children with Atopic Dermatitis," *Journal of Pediatrics* 115: 23–27 (1989).

61. R. Henig, "Who Gets Allergies?" *Washington Post Health* (May 31, 1988), p. 15.

62. See G. Maleskey, "Stuffed Up? Try These Natural Remedies," *Prevention* (September 1984), pp. 63–66.

63. T. Friend, "Alzheimer's Deaths 'Underestimated,'" *USA Today* (March 4, 1996); M. Aronson, "Alzheimer's Disease," *Colliers Encyclopedia CD-ROM* (February 28, 1996); D. Chopra, M.D., *Ageless Body, Timeless Mind* (New York: Harmony Books, 1993), p. 242.

64. J. Talan, "Alzheimer's Drug Gets Mixed Results," *Newsday* (April 6, 1994).

65. Dr. H. R. Casdorph, Dr. M. Walker, *Toxic Metal Syndrome* Garden City Park, NY: Avery Publishing Group, 1995).

66. D. Crapper, et al., "Brain Aluminum Distribution in Alzheimer's Disease and Experimental Neurofibrillary Degeneration," *Science* 180: 511–13 (1973); D. Crapper, et al., "Aluminum, Neurofibrillary Degeneration and Alzheimer's Disease," *Brain* 99: 67–80 (1976); D. Perl, A. Brody, "Alzheimer's Disease: X-ray Spectrometric Evidence of Aluminum Accumulation in Neurofibrillary Tangle-bearing Neurons," *Science* 208: 297–99 (1980); J. Candy, et al., "New Observations on the Nature of Senile Plaque Cores," in E. Vizi, et al., eds., *Regulation of Transmitter Function: Basic and Clinical Aspects* (Amsterdam: Elsevier Press, 1984), pp. 301–04; O. Bugiani, B. Ghetti, "Progressing Encephalomyelopathy with Muscular Atrophy, Induced by Aluminum Powder," *Neurobiol. Aging* 3: 209–22 (1982). See P. Altmann, et al., "Serum Aluminum Levels and Erythrocyte Dihydropteridine Reductase Activity in Patients on Hemodialysis," *New England Journal of Medicine* 317(2) :80–84 (1987).

67. C. Starr, "Aluminum and Alzheimer's," *Drug Topics* (April 17, 1989), p. 30, citing *Lancet* 1:59 (1989).

68. M. Werbach, M.D., "Does Aluminum Exposure Promote Alzheimer's?" *Nutrition Science News* (January 1998), p. 16.

69. H. Casdorph, et al., *op. cit.*, pp. 140, 162.

70. Articles summarized in "Media Events, August–October, 1990," *Dental & Health Facts* 3(4): 1 (November 1990). See S. Begley, et al., "Return of the Toxic Teeth," *Newsweek* (January 14, 1991), p. 45.

71. J. Pleva, "Mercury Poisoning from Dental Amalgam," *Journal of Orthomolecular Psychiatry* 12: 184–93 (1983); M. Vimy, et al., "Serial Measurements of Intra-oral Air Mercury: Estimation of Daily Dose from Dental Amalgams," *Journal of Dental Research* 64(8): 1072–75 (1985); R. Siblerud, "The Relationship between Mercury from Dental Amalgam and the Cardiovascular System," *Science of the Total Environment* 99: 23–35 (1990).

72. H. Casdorph, et al., *op. cit.*, p. 156, citing D. Wenstrup, et al., "Trace Element Imbalances in Isolated Subcellular Fractions of Alzheimer's Disease Brains," *Brain Research* 553: 125–31 (1990).

73. D. Eggleston, et al., "Correlation of Dental Amalgam with Mercury in Brain Tissue," *Journal of Prosthetic Dentistry* 58: 704–07 (1987); M. Nylander, et al., "Mercury Concentrations in the Human Brain and Kidneys in Relation to

Exposure from Dental Amalgam Fillings," *Swedish Dental Journal* 11: 179–87 (1987).

74. K. Sehnert, M.D., et al., "Is Mercury Toxicity an Autoimmune Disorder?" *Townsend Letter for Doctors and Patients* (October 1995), pp. 134–37.

75. T. Warren, *Beating Alzheimer's* (Garden City Park, NY: Avery Publishing Group, Inc., 1991); T. Warren, "Reversing Alzheimer's disease" [Web Page: http://www.halcyon.com/alzh9/].

76. M. Werbach, M.D., "Does Aluminum Exposure Promote Alzheimer's?" *Nutrition Science News* (January 1998), p. 16.

77. M. Zucker, "The Miracle of E," *Let's Live* (November 1997), citing the April 24, 1997, *New England Journal of Medicine*.

78. J. Birkmayer, et al., "Coenzyme Nicotinamide Adenine Dinucleotide: New Therapeutic Approach for Improving Dementia of the Alzheimer's Type," *Annals of Clinical and Laboratory Science* 26(1): 1–9 (1996).

79. *Ibid.*

80. M. Castleman, *Nature's Cures* (Emmaus, PA: Rodale Press, Inc., 1996), p. 421.

81. C. Johnston, et al., "Holotranscobalamin Levels in Plasma Are Related to Dementia in Older People," *Journal of the American Geriatric Society* 45: 779–80 (June 1997).

82. D. Williams, "More Suggestions for Alzheimer's Victims," *Alternatives* 4(22): 175 (April 1993).

83. D. Williams, "Alzheimer's Remedy Found in the Remote Mountain Villages of China," *Alternatives* 5(9): 70 (March 1994).

84. J. Sullivan, "Iron and the Sex Difference in Heart Disease Risk," *Lancet* (June 13, 1981), pp. 1293–95.

85. M. Packer, "Combined Beta-adrenergic and Calcium-entry Blockade in Angina Pectoris," *New England Journal of Medicine* 320(11): 709–18 (1989).

86. D. Waters, et al., "Limited Usefulness of Intermittent Nitroglycerin Patches in Stable Angina," *Journal of the American College of Cardiology* 13(2): 421–25 (1989).

87. *Thorne Research Abstracts* (March 10, 1995), citing *Fortschr Med* 111: 352–54 (1993) and 110: 290–92 (1992).

88. O. Fonorow, "Counterattack," *Townsend Letter for Doctors* (April 1997), p. 98; C. Morisco, et al., "Effect of Coenzyme Q10 Therapy in Patients with Congestive Heart Failure: A Long-term Multicenter Randomized Study," *Clinical Investigation* 71:S134–36 (1993).

89. M. Wolbers, "Angina: Handling the Facts and the Myths," *Your Good Health* 2(5): 21–23 (1984).

90. F. Ellis, T. Sanders, "Angina and Vegan Diet," *American Heart Journal* 93(6): 803–05 (1977).

91. P. Kuo, et al., "The Effect of Lipemia upon Coronary and Peripheral Arterial Circulation in Patients with Essential Hyperlipemia," *American Journal of Medicine* 26: 68–75 (1959).

92. C. Kilham, "Kava for Anxiety and Insomnia," *Nutrition Science News* 2(5): 232–34 (May 1997).

93. "Top 200 Drugs of 1988," *Pharmacy Times* (April 1989), p. 40.

94. W. Leary, "F.D.A. Asks Stronger Label on Sleeping Pill under Scrutiny," *New York Times* (September 23, 1989), p. 6.

95. R. Greene, "The Mellow Market," *Forbes* (October 31, 1988), p. 106.

96. D. Greenblatt, et al., "Effect of Gradual Withdrawal on the Rebound Sleep Disorder after Discontinuation of Triazolam," *New England Journal of Medicine* 317(12):722–28 (1987).

97. P. Roy-Byrne, et al., "Relapse and Rebound Following Discontinuation of Benzodiazepine Treatment of Panic Attacks: Alprazolam Versus Diazepam," *American Journal of Psychiatry* 146(7): 860–65 (1989).

98. D. Lindenberg, et al., "D,l-kavain in Comparison with Oxazepam in Anxiety Disorders. A Double-blind Study of Clinical Effectiveness," *Forschr Med.* 108:49–50, 53–54 (1990).

99. C. Kilham, *op. cit.*

100. T. Munte, et al., "Effects of Oxazepam and an Extract of Kava Roots (Piper Methysticum) on Event-related Potentials in a Word Recognition Task," *Neuropsychobiology* 27:46–53 (1993).

101. G. Lewis, "An Alternative Approach to Premedication: Comparing Diazepam with Auriculotherapy and a Relaxation Method," *American Journal of Acupuncture* 15(3):205–13 (1987); B. Brown, *Stress and the Art of Biofeedback* (New York: Harper & Row, Publishers 1977).

102. P. Fowler, "Aspirin, Paracetamol and Non-steroid Anti-inflammatory Drugs: A Comparative Review of Side Effects," *Medical Toxicology* 2:338–66 (1987).

103. "Nonsteroidal Anti-inflammatory Drugs," *Medical Letter* 25:15–16 (1983).

104. M. Langman, "Anti-inflammatory Drug Intake and the Risk of Ulcer Complications," *Medical Toxicology* 1 (Supp. 1):34–38 (1986).

105. See M. Liang, "Living with Arthritis," *Harvard Medical School Health Letter* 14(2): 5–8 (1988).

106. R. Evers, M.D., "A Successful Therapy for the Relief of Chronic Degenerative Diseases" (200 Beta St., Belle Chasse, LA 70037; undated).

107. A. Hoffer, M.D., "Arthritis," *Townsend Letter for Doctors* (December 1997), p. 104.

108. See K. Sehnert, M.D., et al., "Is mercury toxicity an autoimmune disorder?" *Townsend Letter for Doctors and Patients* (October 1995), pp. 134–37.

109. W. Price, D.D.S., *Dental Infections—Oral and Systemic* vol. 1 and *Dental Infections and the Degenerative Diseases* vol. 2 (Cleveland, OH: Penton Publishing Co., 1923). See E. Brown, R. Hansen, *The Key to Ultimate Health* (La Mirada, CA: Advanced Health Research Publishing, 1998).

110. L. Power, "Exploring the Link Between Diet, Arthritis," *Los Angeles Times* (May 6, 1986), p. 3.

111. C. Lucas, L. Power, "Dietary Fat Aggravates Active Rheumatoid Arthritis," *Clinical Research* 29(4):754A (1981).

112. M. Fabella, "Slow Down Osteoarthritis," *Health Facts* (October 1, 1996).

113. Z. Kime, M.D., *Sunlight* (Penryn, CA: World Health Publications, 1980), pp. 229–31.

114. J. Whitaker, M.D., "A Safe, Simple Treatment for Arthritis," *Human Events* (April 7, 1995).

115. J. Theodosakis, M.D., et al., *The Arthritis Cure: The Medical Miracle That Can Halt, Reverse, and May Even Cure Osteoarthritis* (New York: St. Martin's Press, 1997).

116. A. Manning, "Can Nutrient Combo Really Work Wonders on Arthritis?," *USA Today* (February 11, 1997).

117. Research summarized in J. Heimlich, *What Your Doctor Won't Tell You*, p. 156.

118. S. Stolberg, "Inhalers Linked to Cataracts," *Daily News* (Los Angeles), July 2, 1997, p. 20; W. Hines, "For Asthma Sufferers, an Encouraging View of Overcoming a Lifelong Disorder," *Washington Post Health* (April 18, 1989), p. 6; L. Thompson, "The Asthma Dilemma: With Better Treatment Available, Why Are More Patients Dying?" *id.* (August 25, 1987), pp. 12–14; "The Baffling Rise in Asthma Deaths," *Newsweek* (May 22, 1989), p. 79.

119. R. Walker, "Fungus May be Linked to Lung Disease," *Call and Post* (Cleveland) (January 19, 1995).

120. See R. Roberts, J. Sammut, *Asthma: An Alternative Approach* (New Canaan, CT: 1997); "Plagued by Cures," *The Economist* (November 22, 1997), p. 95.

121. "OTC Asthma Inhalers," *Pediatrics for Parents* (April 1, 1995); A. Buist, "Asthma Mortality: What Have We Learned?", (1989); B. Lanier, "Who Is Dying of Asthma and Why?", *Journal of Pediatrics* 115:838–40 (1989).

122. H. Silverman, et al., *The Pill Book*, 7th Ed. (New York: Bantam Books, 1996), p. 687.

123. V. MacDonald, "Asthma Steroid Can Kill, Health Officials Admit," *The Sunday Telegraph* (London) (July 20, 1997); *Nursing89 Drug Handbook* (Springhouse, PA: Springhouse Corporation, 1989), p. 470.

124. S. Stolberg, *op. cit.*; A. Rooklin, "Theophylline: Is It Obsolete for Asthma?", *Journal of Pediatrics* 115:841–45 (1989); D. DeSilver, "Powerful Drugs, Disturbing Effects," *Vegetarian Times* (August 1989), p. 24; R. Henig, "The Big Sneeze," *Washington Post Health* (May 31, 1988), pp. 12–15.

125. A. Rooklin, *op. cit.*; D. DeSilver, *op. cit.*

126. "Improper Use of Asthma Drug Suspected in Deaths," *Dallas Morning News* (November 17, 1994), p. 10A; H. Silverman, *op. cit.*, p. 100.

127. F. Foulart, "An Alternative Approach to Reversing Asthma," *Alternative and Complementary* Therapies 3(3):179–82 (June 1997), citing R. Firshein, *Reversing Asthma: Reduce Your Medications with This Revolutionary New Program* (New York: Warner Books, 1996).

128. W. Lewis, *Medical Botany* (New York: John Wiley & Sons, 1977), p. vii.

129. S. Lingling, Y. Hongying, "Effect of Needling Sensation Reaching the Site of Disease on the Results of Acupuncture Treatment of Bronchial Asthma," *Journal of Traditional Chinese Medicine* 9(2):140–43 (1989); B. Brown, *Stress and the Art of Biofeedback* (New York: Harper & Row, Publishers, 1977).

130. See G. Maleskey, "Stuffed Up? Try These Natural Remedies," *Prevention* (September 1984), pp. 63-66.

131. See R. Roberts, J. Sammut, *Asthma: An Alternative Approach* (New Canaan, CT: Keats Publishing, Inc., 1997).

132. T. Gordon, W. Kannel, "Premature Mortality from Coronary Heart Disease: The Framingham Study," *Coronary Heart Disease* 215(10):1617–25 (1971).

133. See R. Frentzel-Beyme, et al., "Mortality among German Vegetarians: First Results after Five Years of Follow-up," *Nutrition and Cancer* 11:117–26 (1988); H. Kahn, et al., "Association Between Reported Diet and All-cause Mortality," *American Journal of Epidiology* 119:775–87(1984); D. Snowdon, "Animal Product Consumption and Mortality because of All Causes Combined, Coronary Heart Disease, Stroke, Diabetes and Cancer in Seventh-day Adventists," *American Journal of Clinical Nutrition* 48:739–48 (1988); and other studies cited in E. Brown, *With the Grain* (New York: Carroll & Graf 1990).

134. S. Fallon, et al., "Diet and Heart Disease: Not What You Think," *Consumers' Research Magazine* (July 1, 1996).

135. See E. Brown, L. Walker, *The Informed Consumer's Pharmacy* (New York: Carroll & Graf, 1990).

136. *Annals of Internal Medicine* 127:501-08 (1997).

137. *Lancet* 350:1041–44, 1047–59 (October 11, 1997).

138. D. Chopra, M.D., *Perfect Health: the Complete Mind/Body Guide* (New York: Harmony Books, 1990), pp. 8–9.

139. S. Squires, "Heart Researchers Find Diet Alone Can Help," *Washington Post Health* (November 15, 1988); "It's True, You Can Reverse Heart Disease Through Vegetarianism," *Vegetarian Times* (February 1990), p. 18.

140. S. Squires, *op. cit.*

141. L. McKeown, "Vitamin E May Cut Heart Risk," *Medical Tribune* (November 26, 1992), p. 1.

142. "Crataegus—More Than the Heart?" *MediHerb Professional Newsletter* nos. 28–29, citing J. Graham, *BMJ* (November 1939), p. 951; E. Frank, et al., *Arztl Forsch* 10:3 (1956); J. Kandziora, *MMW* 111:295 (1969); M. Iwamoto, et al., *Planta Med* 42:1 (1981).

143. G. Bushkin, et al., "ALA Fights Free Radical Damage," *Nutrition Science News* (November 1997), p. 572.

144. A. Wolf, et al., "Dietary L-arginine Supplementation Normalizes Platelet Aggregation in Hypercholesterolemic Humans," *J. Am. Coll. Cardiol.* 29:479–85 (1997).

145. C. Jiang, et al., "Progesterone Induces Endothelium-independent Relaxation of Rabbit Coronary Artery in Vitro," *Eur. J. Pharmacol.* 211:163–67 (1992); K. Miyagawa, et al., "Medroxyprogesterone Interferes with Ovarian Steroid Protection Against Coronary Vasospasm," *Nature Med.* 3:324–27 (1997).

146. U. Erasmus, *Fats and Oils* (Vancouver, B.C., Canada: Alive Books, 1989), p. 252, 254.

147. T. Gower, "The New Villain in Your Veins," *Esquire* (March 1997), p. 110; L. Sroufe, M. Stewart, "Treating Problem Children with Stimulant Drugs," *New England Journal of Medicine* 289(8):407–13 (1973).

148. O. Fonorow, "Counterattåck," Townsend Letter for Doctors (April 1997), p. 98.

149. "Raynaud's Sufferers Warm to Acupuncture," *Nutritional Science News* (November 1997) p. 539.

150. R. Henig, "Courts enter the hyperactivity fray," *Washington Post Health* (March 15, 1988), p. 8.

151. *Ibid.*; L. Williams, "Parents and doctors fear growing misuse of drug used to treat hyperactive kids," *Wall Street Journal* (January 15, 1988), p. 25.

152. L. Sroufe, et al., *op. cit.*; M. McBride, "An individual double-blind crossover trial for assessing methylphenidate response in children with attention deficit disorder," *Journal of Pediatrics* 113:137–45 (1988).

153. R. Barkley, C. Cunningham, "Do stimulant drugs improve the academic performance of hyperactive children? A review of outcome research," *Clinical Pediatrics* 17:85–92 (1978); K. Gadow, "Effects of stimulant drugs on academic performance in hyperactive and learning disabled children," *Journal of Learning Disabilities* 16:290–99 (1983); J. Werry, "Drugs and learning," *Journal of Child Psychology and Psychiatry* 22:283–90 (1981).

154. A. Morgan, "Use of stimulant medications in children," *American Family Practice* 38(4):197–202 (1988); "Methylphenidate Revisited," *Medical Letter* 30(765):51–52.

155. See R. Mendelsohn, M.D., *How to Raise a Healthy Child in Spite of Your Doctor* (Chicago: Contemporary Books, Inc. 1984), pp. 205-06; L. Moll, "The link between food and mood," *Vegetarian Times* (August 1986), pp. 28-30; R. Wunderlich, M.D., D. Kalita, "Nourishing your hyperactive child to health," *Good Health* 2(5):16-19 (1984).

156. L. Moll, *ibid.*; R. Wunderlich, *ibid.*; "Hay fever's far-reaching effects," *U.S. Pharmacist* (August 1989), p. 22.

157. J. Diamond, M.D., et al., and the Burton Goldberg Group, *Alternative Medicine* (Puyallup, WA: Future Medicine Publishing, Inc., 1993), p. 546.

158. B. Van Rosen, "Paralysis," *Colliers Encyclopedia CD-ROM* (February 28, 1996); J. Brody, "Bell's Palsy Is Linked with Herpes Infection," *New York Times* (January 3, 1996), §C, p. 8.

159. D. Vergano, "The Trouble with Condoms," *Science News* 150(11):165 (1996).

160. C. Houck, "The Infection that Drives Women Absolutely Crazy," *Redbook* (May 1, 1996).

161. *Ibid.*

162. R. Morrison, *Desktop Guide*, (Albany, CA: Hahnemann Clinic Publishing, 1993), p. 338.

163. C. Danielson, et al., "Hip Fractures and Fluoridation in Utah's Elderly Population," *JAMA* 268(6):746–48 (August 12, 1992).

164. J. Reginster, et al., "Prevention of Postmenopausal Bone Loss by Tiludronate," *Lancet* (December 23/30, 1989), pp. 1469–71.

165. L. Huppert, "Hormonal Replacement Therapy," *Medical Clinics of North America* 71(1):23–39 (1987).

166. U. Barzel, "Estrogens in the Prevention and Treatment of Postmenopausal Osteoporosis: A Review," *American Journal of Medicine* 85:847–50 (1988).

167. S. Godbey, et al, "Boning Up: Old-fashioned Calcium Helps Newfangled Drugs," *Prevention* (February 1, 1997).

168. M. Abramowicz, "New Drugs for Osteoporosis," *Medical Letter* (January 1, 1996), p. 1; E. Tanouye, "Delicate Balance: Estrogen Study Shifts Ground for Women—and for Drug Firms," *Wall Street Journal* (June 15, 1995), pp. A1 ff.; R. Ochs, "Promising Drugs for Osteoporosis," *Newsday* (September 30, 1995); W. Kuznar, " New Cautions for Osteoporosis Drug," *Modern Medicine* (June 1, 1996).

169. J. Lee, "Osteoporosis Reversal: The Role of Progesterone," *International Clinical Nutrition Review* 10(3):384–91 (1990); J. Lee, "Is Natural Progesterone the Missing Link in Osteoporosis Prevention and Treatment?" *Medical Hypotheses* 35:314–16 (1991).

170. Dr. Lee feels that the beneficial effects on bone attributed to estrogen in earlier studies may have been due largely to the progesterone that accompanied it. Studies before 1976 lacked adequate measurement of bone mineral density; and in those after 1976, estrogen was routinely accompanied by a progestin. J. Lee, "Successful Menopausal Osteoporosis treatment: Restoring Osteoclast/osteoblast Equilibrium" [unpublished paper]; Tape, "Dr. John Lee Speaking on Natural Progesterone," 1992.

171. J. Lee, "Is Natural Progesterone the Missing Link . . .," *op. cit.*; J. Lee, "Osteoporosis reversal," *op. cit.* Dr. Lee notes that while these other factors were necessary to prevent bone loss, they could not alone account for the impressive results of this study. See E. Brown, L. Walker, *Menopause and Estrogen* (Berkeley, California: Frog, Ltd., 1996).

172. B. Beeley, "Profile: Alan Gaby, M.D.," *Meno Times* (March 1, 1996), citing Alan Gaby, M.D.

173. See E. Brown, L. Walker, *Menopause and Estrogen, op. cit.*.

174. B. Beeley, *op. cit.*

175. See G. Anderson, et al., "Effect of Dietary Phosphorus on Calcium Metabolism . . . ," *Journal of Nutrition* 102:1123–32 (1972); J. Froom, "Selections from current literature: Hormone Therapy in Postmenopausal Women," *Family Practice* 8(3):288–92 (1991); E. Brown, L. Walker, *The Informed Consumer's Pharmacy* (New York: Carroll & Graf, 1990), pp. 342–43.

176. N. Fuchs, "Calcium Controversy," *Townsend Letter for Doctors* (August/September 1993), pp. 906–08; "Nutritional Consequences of Antacids for Hyperacidity," *Nutrition & the M.D.* (November 1986), p. 1.

177. B. Dawson-Hughes, et al., "A Controlled Trial of the Effect of Calcium Supplementation on Bone Density in Postmenopausal Women," *New England Journal of Medicine* 323:878-83 (1990).

178. O. Epstein, et al., "Vitamin D, hydroxyapatite, and Calcium Gluconate in Treatment of Cortical Bone Thinning in Postmenopausal Women with Primary Biliary Cirrhosis," *American Journal of Clinical Nutrition* 35:426–30 (1982); "Microcrystalline Hydroxyapatite Versus Calcium Gluconate," *Meta Update* 90(3):4 (March 1990); *Townsend Letter for Doctors* (December 1990), p. 863.

179. B. Beeley, *op. cit.*

180. N. Fuchs, "Calcium Controversy," Townsend Letter for Doctors (August/September 1993), pp. 906–908.

181. J. Lieberman, O.D., Ph.D., *Light: Medicine of the Future* (Santa Fe, NM: Bear & Company Publishing, 1991), p. 70.

182. D. Lawson, et al., "Relative Contributions of Diet and Sunlight to Vitamin D State in the Elderly," *British Medical Journal* 2:303–05 (1979); M. Poskitt, et al., "Diet, Sunlight, and 25-Hydroxy Vitamin D in Healthy Children and Adults," *British Medical Journal* 1:221–23 (1979).

183. M. Holick, "Photosynthesis of Vitamin D in the Skin: Effect of Environmental and Life-style Variables," *Federation Proceedings* 46:1876–82 (1987).

184. S. Cummings, et al., "Epidemiology of Osteoporosis and Osteoporotic Fractures," *Epidemiologic Reviews* 7:178–208 (1985); J. Chalmers, et al., "Geographical Variations in Senile Osteoporosis," *Journal of Bone and Joint Surgery* 52-B:667–75 (1970); G. Lewinnek, et al., "The Significance and a Comparative Epidemiology of Hip Fractures," *Clinical Orthopaedics and Related Research* 152:35–43 (1980). See E. Brown, *With the Grain, op. cit.*

185. R. Walker, et al., "Calcium Retention in the Adult Human Male as Affected by Protein Intake," *Journal of Nutrition* 102:1297–1302 (1972); M. Hegsted, et al., "Urinary Calcium and Calcium Balance in Young Men as Affected by Level of Protein and Phosphorus Intake," *ibid.* 111:553–62 (1981).

186. R. Peat, *Nutrition for Women* (Eugene, OR: Kenogen, 1981), p. 23.

187. M. Shangold, "Exercise in the Menopausal Woman," *Obstetrics and Gynecology* 75:53S-58S (1990).

188. D. Swartzendruber, "The Possible Relationship Between Mercury from Dental Amalgam and Diseases I: Effects Within the Oral Cavity," *Medical Hypotheses* 41:31–34 (1993). See E. Brown, R. Hansen, *The Key to Ultimate Health*, (La Mirada, CA: Advanced Health Research Publishing, 1998).

189. W. Ray, et al.,"Psychotropic Drug Use and the Risk of Hip Fracture," *New England Journal of Medicine* 316:363–69 (1987).

190. J. Williams, et al., "Biliary Excretion of Aluminum in Aluminum Osteodystrophy with Liver Disease," *Annals of Internal Medicine* 104:782–85 (1986), reviewed in "Toxicologic Consequences of Oral Aluminum," *Nutrition Reviews* 45(3):72–74 (1987).

191. *Drug Facts and Comparisons* (St. Louis: Facts and Comparisons, 1998).

192. See W. Crook, M.D., *The Yeast Connection* (Jackson, TN: Professional Books 1985), pp. 291–92.

193. Quelling Candida," *Nutrition Science News* 2(5):236 (May 1997).

194. The Cardiac Arrhythmia Suppression Trial Investigators, "Preliminary Report: Encainide and Flecainide on Mortality in a Randomized Trial of Arrhythmia Suppression After Myocardial Infarction," *New England Journal of Medicine* 321(6):406–12 (1989).

195. S. Kopecky, et al., "The Natural History of Lone Atrial Fibrillation," *New England Journal of Medicine* 317(11):669–74 (1987).

196. T. Hayes, "Local Physician Cuts Carpal Tunnel Surgery Time," *Indianapolis Business Journal* 16:34 (1995).

197. J. Lieberman, *Light: Medicine of the Future* (Santa Fe, NM: Bear and Co., Publishing, 1991).

198. J. Kingham, et al., "Macular hemorrhage in the aging eye: The effects of anticoagulants," *New England Journal of Medicine* 318(17):1126–27 (1988).

199. "Long-term Vitamin C Use Decreases Cataracts," *Nutrition Science News* (January 1998), p. 10, citing *American Journal of Clinical Nutrition* (October 1997).

200. "Lutein May Halt Macular Degeneration," *Life Extension* (January 1998), p. 21.

201. See "Sexually Transmitted Diseases," *National Women's Health Report* (March 1, 1993); E. Brown, L. Walker, *The Informed Consumer's Pharmacy* (New York: Carroll & Graf, 1990).

202. S. Fallon, "Diet and Heart Disease: Not What You Think," *Consumers' Research Magazine* (July 1, 1996).

203. J. Golier, et al., "Low Serum Cholesterol Level and Attempted Suicide," *American Journal of Psychiatry* 152:419–23 (1995), discussed by Alan Gaby, M.D., in *Townsend Letter for Doctors* (December 1995), p. 21.

204. "W.H.O. Cooperative Trial on Primary Prevention of Ischaemic Heart Disease Using Clofibrate to Lower Serum Cholesterol: Mortality Follow-up: Report of the Committee of Principal Investigators," *Lancet* 2:379–85 (1980).

205. Lipid Research Clinics Program, "The Lipid Research Clinics Coronary Primary Prevention Trial results. I. Reduction in Incidence of Coronary Heart Disease," *JAMA* 251:351–64 (1984).

206. M. Frick, et al., "Helsinki Heart Study: Primary-prevention Trial with Gemfibrozil in Middle-aged Men with Dyslipidemia: Safety of Treatment, Changes in Risk Factors, and Incidence of Coronary Heart Disease," *New England Journal of Medicine* 317:1237–45 (1987). The difference in total deaths wasn't statistically significant.

207. See "Gemfibrozil and Coronary Heart Disease," *New England Journal of Medicine* 318(19):1274 (1988).

208. P. Canner, et al., "Fifteen Year Mortality in Coronary Drug Project Patients: Long-term Benefit with Niacin," *American Journal of Cardiology* 8:1245–55 (1986).

209. "Cholesterol-Drug Boost," *Newsday* (November 13, 1997).

210. "Health and Medicine," *Newsday* (November 18, 1997).

211. C. Blum, R. Levy, "Current Therapy for Hypercholesterolemia," *JAMA* 261(24):3582–87 (1989).

212. G. Cowley, "What's High Cholesterol?" *Newsweek* (November 14, 1994), p. 63.

213. See, e.g., A. Keys, et al., "The Diet and All Causes Death Rate in the Seven Countries Study," *Lancet* 2:58–61 (1981) (all-cause mortality in 12,000 men under age 60 in seven countries positively associated with saturated fat intake); and other studies cited in E. Brown, *With the Grain* (New York: Carroll & Graf 1990).

214. S. Pratt, "Body and Soy: New Study Indicates Soy-rich Diet Can Lower Cholesterol," *Chicago Tribune* (August 22, 1995).

215. L. Nicholson, "Focus on Fiber," *Center Post* 10(9):1 (1989).

216. "Psyllium and Cholesterol," *Harvard Medical School Health Letter* 13(8):1 (1988), citing *Archives of Internal Medicine* (February 1988), pp. 292–96.

217. "Mystery of High-fiber Diet Unraveled," *Washington Post* (October 26, 1987), p. A7; S. Siwolop, "Curbing Killer Choleserol," *Business Week* (October 26, 1987), pp. 122–23.

218. "Crataegus—More Than the Heart?" *MediHerb Professional Newsletter* nos. 28-29, citing J. Graham, *BMJ* (November 1939), p. 951; E. Frank, et al., *Arztl Forsch* 10:3 (1956); J. Kandziora, *MMW* 111:295 (1969); M. Iwamoto, et al., *Planta Med* 42:1 (1981).

219. "A Reliable Guide to Ten Top Natural Remedies," *Health* (October 1997), p. 69.

220. D. Buchwald, et al., "Chronic Fatigue and the Chronic Fatigue Syndrome in a Pacific Northwest Health Care System," *Annals of Internal Medicine* 123:2:81(8) (1995).

221. D. Nambudripad, *Say Goodbye to Illness* (Buena Park, CA: Delta Publishing Company, 1993), p. 287; L. Casura, "Sick of Being Patient, Part 1," *Townsend Letter for Doctors* (June 1996), pp. 36–41.

222. *American Journal of Medicine* 90:730 (1991), quoted in M. Ali, M.D., *The Canary and Chronic Fatigue* (Denville, NJ: Life Span Press, 1994), pp. 325-27.

223. L. Casura, "Sick of being patient, Part 2," *Townsend Letter for Doctors* (June 1996), pp. 54-63.

224. D. Nambudripad, *op. cit.*, pp. 312-13.

225. M. Ali, M.D., *op. cit.*

226. "Researchers Present Latest Findings on Pycnogenol," *Nutrition Science News* (July 1997), p. 308.

227. Dr. H. R. Casdorph, Dr. M. Walker, *Toxic Metal Syndrome* (Garden City Park, NY: Avery Publishing Group, 1995), pp. 151–52.

228. Sherry Rogers, M.D., *Wellness Against All Odds* (Syracuse, NY: Prestige Publishing, 1994), p. 240.

229. H. Gelb, D.M.D., *Killing Pain Without Perscription* (New York: Harper & Row, Publishers, 1980), pp. 43–44.

230. Consumer's Union, *The Medicine Show,* (New York: Pantheon Books, 1980), pp. 34–36.

231. "Late News on the Cold Front," *University of California, Berkeley Wellness Letter* 5:4-5 (1988).

232. See A. Orfuss, "Cold Sore," *Colliers Encyclopedia* CD-ROM (February 28, 1996).

233. H. Buttram, M.D., "Measles-mumps-rubella (MMR) Vaccine as a Potential Cause of Encephalitis (Brain Inflammation) in Children," *Townsend Letter for Doctors* (December 1997), p. 100.

234. J. Whitaker, *Health & Healing* (April 1995).

235. CONSENSUS Trial Study Group, "Effects of enalapril on mortality in severe congestive heart failure: Results of the Cooperative North Scandinavian Enalapril Survival Study," *New England Journal of Medicine* 316(23):1429–35 (1987); J. Cohn, et al., "Effect of vasodilator therapy on mortality in chronic congestive heart failure:

Results of a Veterans Administration Cooperative Study," *New England Journal of Medicine* 314:1547–52 (1986).

236. M. Packer, "Do Vasodilators Prolong Life in Heart Failure?" *New England Journal of Medicine* 316:1429–35 (1987); "Vasodilators for Chronic Congestive Heart Failure," *Medical Letter* 30(758):13–14 (1988).

237. See T. Smith, "Digitalis: Mechanisms of action and clinical use," *New England Journal of Medicine* 318(6):358–65 (1988); K. Butler, et al., *The Best Medicine* (San Francisco: Harper & Row, 1985), pp. 464–71.

238. *Thorne Research Abstracts* (March 10, 1995), citing *Fortschr Med* 111:352–54 (1993) and 110:290–92 (1992).

239. C. Morisco, et al., "Effect of Coenzyme Q10 Therapy in Patients with Congestive Heart Failure: A Long-term Multicenter Randomized Study," *Clinical Investigation* 71:S134–36 (1993).

240. D. Chopra, M.D., *Perfect Health: the Complete Mind/Body Guide* (New York: Harmony Books, 1990), pp. 8–9.

241. "Constipation," *Colliers Encyclopedia CD-ROM* (February 28, 1996).

242. J. Whitaker, "The natural cure for constipation.," *Human Events* (August 12, 1994).

243. C. Inlander, "Is It Time to Get Off the Bran Wagon?," *People's Medical Society Newsletter* (February 1, 1995).

244. *Ibid.*

245. B. Hunter, "Beneficial Bacteria (Bifidobacteria)," *Consumers' Research Magazine* (January 1, 1996).

246. S. Gilbert, "Eight Drugstore Remedies that Can Make You Sick," *Redbook* (February 1, 1996).

247. K. Doheny, "Ahem! Now That We Have Your Attention, Read About Coughing," *Los Angeles Times*, "Life & Style," p. 2 (March 5, 1997).

248. See D. Zimmerman, *Essential Guide to Nonprescription Drugs* (New York: Harper & Row, 1983), pp. 113–15

249. S. Satel, J. Nelson, "Stimulants in the Treatment of Depression: A Critical Overview," *Journal of Clinical Psychiatry* 50(7):241–49 (1989).

250. *Ibid.*; "Advances in the Diagnosis and Management of Depression (II)," *American Pharmacy* (February 1988), pp. 33–37.

251. S. Roan, "Dangerous Combinations," *Newsday* (January 14, 1997).

252. C. Starr, "Introducing Wellbutrin, a One-of-a-kind Antidepressant," *Drug Topics* (August 7, 1989); "Advances in the Diagnosis and Management of Depression," *op. cit.*; G. Cowley, et al., "The Promise of Prozac," *Newsweek* (March 26, 1990), pp. 38–41.

253. G. Null, "Prozac, Eli Lilly and the FDA," *Townsend Letter for Doctors* (March 1993), pp. 1 ff.; "A Prozac Backlash," *Newsweek* (April 1, 1991), pp. 64–67.

254. D. Manders, "The Curious Continuing Ban of L-tryptophan: The Serotonin Connection," *Townsend Letter for Doctors* (October 1992), pp. 880–81; Citizens for Health, "Prepare for the Worst: FDA Propaganda Ready to Barrage Media," *ibid.* (August/September 1993), pp. 860–61.

255. R. Podell, "Inositol Found Effective for Depression and Panic-Anxiety," *Nutrition Science News* (October 1996), p. 18.

256. W. Poldinger, et al., "A Functional-dimensional Approach to Depression," *Psychopathology* 24:53–81 (1991).

257. S. Miller, "A Natural Mood Booster," *Newsweek* (May 5, 1997), p. 74; C. Jones, "St.-John's-Wort Gets New Attention," *Nutrition Science News* (September 1997), p. 436.

258. M. Shangold, "Exercise in the menopausal woman," *Obstetrics and Gynecology* 75:53S-58S (1990); R. Peat, *Nutrition for Women* (Eugene, OR: Kenogen, 1981), p. 92.

259. "PMS? Let 'Em Eat Carbs," *Vegetarian Times* (March 1990), p. 17.

260. A. Stoll, "Choline in the Treatment of Rapid-cycling Bipolar Disorder," *Biol. Psychiatry* 40:382–88 (1996).

261. R. Henig, "Beyond insulin," *New York Times Magazine* (March 20, 1988), pp. 50–51.

262. "Plagued by Cures," *The Economist* (November 22, 1997), p. 95.

263. A. Thorburn, et al., "Slowly digested and absorbed carbohydrate in traditional bush-foods: A protective factor against diabetes?" *American Journal of Clinical Nutrition* 45:98–106 (1987); B. Karlstrom, et al., "Effect of leguminous seeds in a mixed diet in non-insulin-dependent diabetic patients," *Diabetes Research* 5:199–205 (1987).

264. See J. Lauerman, "Diabetes: How Scary Is It?", *Cosmopolitan* (May 1, 1994).

265. G. Johnson, et al., *Harvard Medical School Health Letter Book* (Cambridge, Massachusetts: Harvard University Press, 1981); T. Pollare, H. Lithell, et al., "A Comparison of the Effects of Hydrochlorothiazide and Captopril on Glucose and Lipid Metabolism in Patients with Hypertension," *New England Journal of Medicine* 321:868–73 (1989).

266. See "The Second Generation Oral Sulfonylureas: Glyburide and Glipizide," *American Pharmacy* NS28(10):55–59 (1988); R. Campbell, "Clinical Use of Insulin: Side Effects & Dosing Factors," *Pharmacy Times* (November 1988), pp. 154-63.

267. M. Billingham, et al., "Lipoprotein Subfraction Composition in Non-insulin-dependent Diabetes Treated by Diet, Sylphonylurea, and Insulin," *Metabolism* 38(9):850–57 (1989).

268. T. Byfield, "Developing Diabetes," *Body Bulletin* (August 1, 1996).

269. J. Anderson, K. Ward, "High-Carbohydrate, High-fiber Diets for Insulin-treated Men with Diabetes Mellitus," *American Journal of Clinical Nutrition* 32:2312–21 (1979).

270. L. Nicholson, "Focus on fiber," *Center Post* 10(9):1, 7 (1989). See E. Brown, *With the Grain* (New York: Carroll & Graf 1990).

271. R. Rizek, E. Jackson, "Current Food Consumption Practices and Nutrient Sources in the American Diet," in *Animal Products in Human Nutrition* (New York: Academic Press 1982), pp. 150–51; C. Adams, *Nutritive Value of American Foods in Common Units* (Washington D.C.: Agricultural Research Service, USDA 1975); J. Gear, et al., "Biochemical and Haematological Variables in Vegetarians," *British Medical Journal* 1:1415 (1980); K. West, *Epidemiology of Diabetes and Its Vascular Lesions* (New York: Elsevier North-Holland 1978); D. Snowdon, "Animal Product Consumption and Mortality Because of All Causes Combined, Coronary Heart

Disease, Stroke, Diabetes, and Cancer in Seventh-day Adventists," *American Journal of Clinical Nutrition* 48:739–48 (1988).

272. T. Friend, "Chromium Test on Diabetics 'Spectacular'," *USA Today* (June 10, 1996); J. Carper, "Chromium, the Forgotten Fuel," *USA Weekend* (January 12, 1997) .

273. "Alpha Lipoic Acid Lowers Diabetes Risk," *Let's Live* (November 1997), p. 4, citing *Metabolism* 46:763-68 (1997).

274. "Silymarin May Help in Diabetes," *Let's Live Nutrition Insights* (November 1997), p. 9.

275. See D. Richard, *Stevia: Nature's Sweet Secret* (Bloomingdale, IL: Blue Heron Press, 1996).

276. Zane Kime, M.D., *Sunlight* (Penryn, CA: World Health Publications, 1980), pp. 39-41, 58-62.

277. A. Levin, "Diarrhea in Infants and Young Kids: Oral Rehydration and Homeopathy," *Health Facts* (June 1, 1994).

278. See D. Hussar, "New Drugs of 1988," *American Pharmacy* (March 1989), pp. 25-52.

279. See D. Zimmerman, *The Essential Guide to Nonprescription Drugs* (New York: Harper & Row, Publishers 1983), pp. 237-49.

280. D. Zimmerman, *op. cit.*

281. I. Salam, et al., "Randomised Trial of Single-dose Cirpfloxacin for Travellers' Diarrhoea," *Lancet* 344: 1537-9 (December 1994).

282. A. Levin, "Diarrhea in Infants . . .," *op. cit.*

283. B. Wood, "Apples for Diarrhea," *Pediatrics for Parents* (November 1, 1993).

284. The study involved 81 Nicaraguan children, aged six months to five years, who were randomly assigned to receive either a homeopathic remedy or a placebo. Those in the treatment group received one of 18 different homeopathic remedies normally prescribed for acute diarrhea, depending on the child's specific symptoms and traits (a departure from the standard study, which requires uniform doses of a single treatment). The children were also given oral rehydration. A. Levin, *op. cit.*

285. B. Hunter, "Beneficial Bacteria (Bifidobacteria)," *Consumers' Research Magazine* (January 1, 1996).

286. M. Kline, et al., "Acidophilus for Sertraline-induced Diarrhea," *American Journal of Psychiatry*, 151:1521-22 (1994).

287. G. Gates, et al., "Effectiveness of Adenoidectomy and Tympanostomy Tubes in the Treatment of Chronic Otitis Media with Effusion," *New England Journal of Medicine* 317(23):1444-51 (1987); W. Crook, "Pediatricians, Antibiotics, and Office Practice," *Pediatrics* 76(1):139-40 (1985).

288. G. Gates, et al., *op. cit.*; J. Paradise, "Otitis Media in Infants and Children," *Pediatrics* 65(5):917 (1980); J. Paradise, C. Bluestone, "Adenoidectomy and Chronic Otitis Media," *New England Journal of Medicine* 318(22):1470 (1988); P. Lorentzen, P. Haugsten, "Treatment of Acute Suppurative Otitis Media," *Journal of Laryngology and Otology* 91:331-40 (1977).

289. G. Gates, et al., *op. cit.*; T. McGill, et al., "A Seven-year-old Japanese-American Boy with Persistent Right-ear Drainage Despite Antibiotic Therapy," *New England*

Journal of Medicine 316:1589-97 (1987). The widespread use of antibiotics for treating ear infections is based on only a handful of studies, and their results have been questioned. See, e.g., W. Crook, *op. cit.*; M. Diamant, B. Diamant, "Abuse and Timing of Use of Antibiotics in Acute Otitis Media," *Archives of Otolaryngology* 100:226-32 (1974).

290. *The Medical Advisor* (Alexandria, Virginia: Time-Life Books, 1996), pp. 641-42.

291. M. Diamant, et al., *op. cit.*

292. W. Crook, *op. cit.*

293. E. Mandel, et al., "Efficacy of Amoxicillin with and Without Decongestant-antihistamine for Otitis Media with Effusion in Children," *New England Journal of Medicine* 316(8):432–37 (1987).

294. E. Cantekin, et al., "Lack of Efficacy of a Decongestant-antihistamine Combination for Otitis Media with Effusion ('Secretory' Otitis Media) in Children: Results of a Double-blind, Randomized Trial," *New England Journal of Medicine* 308:297–301 (1983).

295. M. Casselbrandt, et al., "Otitis Media with Effusion in Preschool Children," *Laryngoscope* 95:428–36 (1985); J. Lous, M. Fiellau-Nikolajsen, "Epidemiology of Middle Ear Effusion and Tubal Dysfunction," *Int. J. Pediatr. Otorhinolaryngoly* 3:303–17 (1981).

296. The Endometriosis Association, Milwaukee, "Facts and Figures on Endometriosis," *U.S. Pharmacist*, p. 42 (February 1993).

297. *Drug Facts and Comparisons*, 1993 edition (St. Louis: Facts and Comparisons), pp. 2549–52.

298. "Natural Tampons: An Alternative to Dioxin-Bleached Products," *Health Foods Business* (June 1997), p. 22.

299. *Planta Medica* (August 1993).

300. L. McTaggart, ed., *What Doctors Don't Tell You* 5(10):1–3 (January 1995).

301. "Ten Best Air-Cleaning Plants," *Catalist* (July/August, 1994), p. 26.

302. M. Rumelt, "Blindness from Misuse of Over-the-counter Eye Medications," *Annals of Ophthalmology* 20:26–30 (1988).

303. F. Fraunfelder, S. Meyer, "Systemic Side Effects from Ophthalmic Timolol and Their Prevention," *Journal of Ocular Pharmacology* 3(2):177–84 (1987); J. Siwek, "Excess Eyedrops," *Washington Post Health* (October 6, 1987), p. 21.

304. J. Siwek, *ibid.*

305. J. Lieberman, O.D., Ph.D., *Light: Medicine of the Future* (Santa Fe, NM: Bear & Company Publishing, 1991), pp. 152–54, citing W. Allen, "Suspected Carcinogen Found in 14 of 17 Sunscreens," *St. Louis Post Dispatch* (March 9, 1989).

306. J. Kruse, "Should Fever Be Treated?" *Washington Post Health* (March 7, 1989), p. 11; T. Rosenthal, D. Silverstein, "Fever: What to Do and What Not to Do," *Postgraduate Medicine* 83(8):75–84 (1988).

307. See J. Dobowy, et al., "Inhibition of Postpyrogenic Increase of Phagocytic and Killing Activity of Neutrophils by Nonsteroid Antiinflammatory Drugs," *Archivum Immunologiae et Therapiae Experimentalis* 36(3):295–301 (1988); E. Kiester Jr., "A

Little Fever is Good for You," *Science* (November 1984), pp. 168-73; T. Rosenthal, et al., *op. cit.*

308. T. Rosenthal, et al., *op. cit.*; J. Kruse, *op. cit.*

309. "Acetaminophen Doesn't Help Chicken Pox Sufferers," *American Pharmacy* NS29(11):13 (November 1989).

310. D. Jaffe, et al., "Antibiotic Administration to Treat Possible Occult Bacteremia in Febrile Children," *New England Journal of Medicine* 317 (19):1175–80 (1987).

311. T. Rosenthal, et al., *op. cit.*; H. Kai, et al., "Heat, Drugs, and Radiation Given in Combination is Palliative for Unresectable Esophageal Cancer," *International Journal of Radiation Oncology, Biology, and Physics* 14(6):1147–52 (1988); H. Bicher, et al., "Microwave Hyperthermia as an Adjunct to Radiation Therapy: Summary Experience of 256 Multifraction Treatment Cases," *ibid.* 12:1667–71 (1986); F. Storm, "Clinical Hyperthermia and Chemotherapy," *Radiologic Clinics of North America* 27(3):621–27 (1989); Prof. Werner Zabel, cited in K. Ally, "Cancer Defeated by Body's Own Defenses," *Tidskrift for Halsa* (Sept. 9, 1975).

312. "Researchers Present Latest Findings on Pycnogenol," *Nutrition Science News* (July 1997), p. 308.

313. P. Fisher, et al., "Homeopathic Treatment of Primary Fibromyalgia [in French]," *Homeopathic Francaise* 79:15–22 (1991).

314. J. Whitaker, M.D., "Getting the Jump on Colds and Flu," *Human Events* (December 16, 1996).

315. De Flora, et al., "Attenuation of Influenza-like Symptomatology and Improvement of Cell-mediated Immunity with Long-term N-acetylcysteine Treatment," *Eur. Respir. J.* 1:1535–41 (1997), reported in *Life Extension* (January 1998), p. 25.

316. J. Ferley, et al., "A Controlled Evaluation of a Homeopathic Preparation in the Treatment of Influenza-like Syndromes," *British Journal of Clinical Pharmacology* 27:329–35 (1989).

317. S. Fishkoff, "A Berry Good Idea to Cure the Flu," *Jerusalem Post* (January 19, 1996).

318. P. Phillips, "New Drugs for the Nail Fungus Prevalent in Elderly," *JAMA* 276(1):12–13 (July 3, 1996).

319. R. Wild, "A Skeptic's Guide to Sports Medicine," *Men's Health* (April 1, 1996).

320. A. Levin, "The New Gallbladder Surgery: Too Much, Too Soon," *Health Facts* (March 1, 1993).

321. *Ibid.*; F. Fessenden, "A Closer Look: The Rewards and Hidden Risks of Laparoscopy," *Newsday* (November 3, 1996).

322. M. Murray, et al., *Encyclopedia of Natural Healing* (Rocklin, CA: Prima Publishing, 1991), p. 325.

323. C. SerVaas, "Dr. Denis Burkitt: A Passion for Preventing Disease," *Saturday Evening Post* (March 1, 1995).

324. J. Carper, *The Food Pharmacy* (New York: Bantam Trade Paperback Books, 1989), p. 275.

325. P. Pitchford, *Healing with Whole Foods* (Berkeley: North Atlantic Books, 1993), p. 283.

326. "Heliobacter Pylori," *Nutrition Science News* (September 1997), p. 452.

327. See E. Brown, L. Walker, *The Informed Consumer's Pharmacy* (New York: Carroll & Graf, 1990).

328. "Worried Sick: Hassles and Herpes," *Science News* (December 5, 1987), p. 360; H. Nelson, "Sensitive Armor," *Los Angeles Times* (September 19, 1988), p. II:3.

329. "Sexually Transmitted Diseases," *National Women's Health Report* (March 1, 1993); "Cosmo's Guide to Sexual Wellness," *Cosmopolitan* (September 1, 1994); "Interferon for Treatment of Genital Warts," *Medical Letter* 30(770):70–92 (1988).

330. B. Sardi, "Glaucoma" [a three-part series], *Townsend Letter for Doctors & Patients* (November 1995), p. 64; *ibid.* (December 1995), p. 46; *ibid.* (January 1996), p. 52.

331. G. Johnson, S. Goldfinger, *Harvard Medical School Health Letter Book* (Cambridge, MA: Harvard University Press, 1981), pp. 364–68; J. Francois, "Corticosteroid Glaucoma," *Metabolic Ophthalmology* 2:3–11 (1978); R. Mohan, et al., "Steroid Induced Glaucoma and Cataract," *Indian Journal of Ophthalmology* 37:13–16 (1989); J. Henahan, "Study Shows Link Between Facial Steroids, Secondary Glaucoma," *Ophthalmology Times* (October 1, 1993), p. 32.

332. B. Sardi, *op. cit.*

333. F. Fraunfelder, S. Meyer, "Systemic Side Effects from Ophthalmic Timolol and Their Prevention," *Journal of Ocular Pharmacology* 3(2):177–84 (1987).

334. P. O'Dea, "Glaucoma therapy: The Pharmacist's Role in Compliance," *American Pharmacy* (September 1988), pp. 38–42.

335. B. Sardi, *op. cit.*, citing "Weighing the Evidence for Glaucoma Treatment," *Ocular Surgery News* (July 15, 1988), pp. 33-37; F. Jay, et al., "Early Trabeculectomy Versus Conventional Management in Primary Open-angle Glaucoma," *British Journal of Ophthalmology* 72:881–89 (1988).

336. F. Fraunfelder, et al., *op. cit.*; F. Fraunfelder, et al., "Systemic reactions to ophthalmic drug preparations," *Medical Toxicology* 2:287–93 (1987).

337. F. Stocker, "New Ways of Influencing the Intraocular Pressure," *New York State Medical Journal* 49:58–63 (1949).

338. B. Sardi, *op. cit.*

339. "Sexually Transmitted Diseases," *National Women's Health Report* (March 1, 1993); E. Brown, L. Walker, *The Informed Consumer's Pharmacy* (New York: Carroll & Graf, 1990).

340. F. Mathews, et al., "Gout," *Colliers Encyclopedia CD-ROM* (February 28, 1996).

341. See W. Robertson, et al., "The Effect of High Animal Protein Intake on the Risk of Calcium Stone-formation in the Urinary Tract," *Clinical Science* 57:285–88 (1979); W. Robertson, et al., "Prevalence of Urinary Stone Disease in Vegetarians," *Eur. Urol.* 8:334–39 (1982); I. Pave, "So You Thought Gout Was a Thing of the Past?" *Business Week* (October 5, 1987), p. 129.

342. M. Howe, "Hair Loss," *Country Living* (July 1, 1995); J. Balch, M.D., et al., *Prescription for Nutritional Healing* (Garden City Park, NY: Avery Publishing Group, 1990).

343. "Myth: There's a Cure for Male Pattern Baldness," *University of California Berkeley Wellness Letter* 5(2):8 (1988); "Minoxidil: A Few of the Questions You're Likely to Hear," *American Pharmacy* NS28(11):47–50 (1988); D. Fischer, "The Bald Truth," *U.S. News & World Report* (August 4, 1997).

344. R. Ochs, "Headaches: The Causes of and Cures for a Painful Malady That Afflicts Millions," *Newsday* (September 29, 1996).

345. N. Regush, et al., "Migraine Killer," *Mother Jones* (September 19, 1995).

346. T. Maugh II, "Nose Drops of Anesthetic Ease Migraines, Study Finds," *Los Angeles Times* (July 24, 1996).

347. "Feverfew," *Vegetarian Times* (November 1988), p. 15; J. Carper, "Can Herbs Heal You?," *USA Weekend* (July 13, 1997).

348. "Doctor Discovers Aspirin-free Headache Cure," *Vegetarian Times* (April 1987), p. 10; J. Carper, *The Food Pharmacy* (New York: Bantam Trade Paperback Books, 1989), p. 275.

349. "The Natural Way to Get Relief," *Redbook* (February 1, 1996).

350. "Herbal Aspirin Relieves Pain," *Catalist* (July/August 1994); "Magnesium Boosts Energy, Helps Migraines," *Let's Live Nutrition Insights* (November 1977), p. 6.

351. B. Brown, *Stress and the Art of Biofeedback* (New York: Harper & Row, Publishers, 1977); R. Ochs, *op. cit.*

352. See E. Brown, R. Hansen, *The Key to Ultimate Health* (La Mirada, CA: Advanced Health Research Publishing, 1998).

353. E. Infante, "A New Fight Over Common Lice Drug," *USA Today* (September 13, 1994).

354. W. Martin, "Reducing Deaths from Heart Attacks and Cancer," *Townsend Letter for Doctors* (January 1998), p. 72.

355. J. Scott, "Heart Drugs Do Equally Well in Study," *Los Angeles Times* (April 4, 1989), V:1,6.

356. J. Carey, "Genentech: A David that comes on like Goliath," *Business Week* (October 30, 1989), p. 165; "Heart Attacks: The First Few Hours," *Harvard Medical School Health Letter* 13(11):5–8 (1988).

357. J. Scott, *op. cit.*; "Study Questions Value of Biotech Drug," *Los Angeles Times* (March 9, 1990), p. D2.

358. J. Justice, S. Kline, "Analgesics and Warfarin: A Case that Brings Up Questions and Cautions," *Postgraduate Medicine* 83(5):217–20 (1988); See K. Butler, L. Rayner, *The Best Medicine* (San Francisco: Harper & Row, Publishers, 1985), pp. 464–71.

359. "Aspirin After Myocardial Infarction," *Lancet* i:1172–73 (1980); W. Fields, et al., "Controlled Trial of Aspirin in Cerebral Ischaemia," *Stroke* 8:310–16 (1977); Canadian Cooperative Study Group, "A Randomised Trial of Aspirin and Sulfinpyrazone in Threatened Stroke," *New England Journal of Medicine* 299:53–59 (1978); A. Leaf, P. Weber, "Cardiovascular Effects of N-3 Fatty Acids," *New England Journal of Medicine* 318(9):549–57 (1988); "Fish Oil Pills: Jumping the Gun," *University of California, Berkeley Wellness Letter* 3(5):1 (1987).

360. *British Medical Journal* 314:634-38 (March 1, 1997).

361. O. Fonorow, "Counterattack," *Townsend Letter for Doctors* (April 1997), p. 98.

362. W. Martin, "Reducing Deaths from Heart Attacks and Cancer," *Townsend Letter for Doctors* (January 1998), p. 72.

363. See E. Brown, R. Hansen, *The Key to Ultimate Health* (La Mirada, CA: Advanced Health Research Publishing, 1998); E. Brown, L. Walker, *The Informed Consumer's Pharmacy* (New York: Carroll & Graf, 1990).

364. J. Klotter, "Chemical contributors to Gulf War Syndrome," *Townsend Letter for Doctors & Patients* (June 1997), p. 27; A. Gaby, "Toxic Chemicals: The Effect of Cumulative Exposure," *ibid.*, p. 31.

365. Dr. H. Casdorph, Dr. M. Walker, *Toxic Metal Syndrome* (Garden City Park, NY: Avery Publishing Group, 1995), p. 126, citing G. Wenk, et al., *Neurotoxicology* 3:93–99 (1982); and J. Bjorksten, "Dietary Aluminum and Alzheimer's Disease," *Science of the Total Environment* 25:81–84 (1982).

366. *Medical Hypotheses* 82(9):265-82.

367. D. Williams, "Cleaning House," *Alternatives* 4(12):97-100 (1992).

368. See N. Clarke, et al., "Treatment of Occlusive Vascular Disease with Disodium Ethylene Diamine Tetra-acetic Acid (EDTA)," *American Journal of Medical Science* 239:732 (1960); N. Clarke, et al., "Treatment of Angina Pectoris with Disodium Ethylene Diamine Tetra-acetic Acid," *ibid.* 232:645 (1956); C. Lamar, "Chelation Therapy of Occlusive Arteriosclerosis in Diabetic Patients," *Angiology* 15:379 (1964).

369. R. Evers, M.D., "A Successful Therapy for the Relief of Chronic Degenerative Diseases" (200 Beta St., Belle Chasse, LA 70037; undated).

370. R. Keith, et al., "Utilization of Renal Slices to Evaluate the Efficacy of Chelating Agents for Removing Mercury from the Kidney," *Toxicology* 116:67–75 (January 1997).

371. S. Ziff, et al., *Dental Mercury Detox* (Orlando, Florida: Bio Probe, Inc., Publisher), pp. 37–40.

372. Y. Omura, et al., *Acupuncture Electrotherapy Research* 21(2):133–60 (1996).

373. G. Bushkin, et al., "ALA Fights Free Radical Damage," *Nutrition Science News* 2(11):572 (November 1997).

374. D. Ullman, *The Consumer's Guide to Homeopathy* (New York: Dorling Kindersley, 1995), p. 56.

375. A. Levin, "A Primer on Hemorrhoids," *Health Facts* (June 1, 1993).

376. See J. Kaufman, et al., *Over the Counter Pills That Don't Work* (New York: Pantheon Books, 1983), p. 144; Consumers Union, *The Medicine Show* (New York: Pantheon Books, 1980), pp. 136–39.

377. A. Fisher, *Contact Dermatitis* (Philadelphia: Lea and Febiger 1973), pp. 42, 312, 313; North American Contact Dermatitis Group, "Epidemiology of Contact Dermatitis in North America," *Archives of Dermatology* 108:537–40 (1973).

378. Consumers Union, *op. cit.*; J. Kaufman, et al., *op. cit.*

379. A. Levin, *op. cit.*

380. S. Guttmacher, et al., *op. cit.*; N. Kaplan, "Non-drug treatment of hypertension," *Annals of Internal Medicine* 102:359-73 (1985).

381. M. Weinberger, "Diuretics and Their Side Effects," *Hypertension* 11 (Supp II):II-16—II-20 (1988), citing W. Kannel, et al., "Hypertension, Antihypertensive Treatment and Sudden Death," *CVD Epidemiol. Newsletter* 37:34 (1985), and T, Morgan, et al., "Failure of Therapy to Improve Prognosis in Elderly Males with Hypertension," *Med. J. Aust.* 2:27–32 (1980).

382. T. Pollare, H. Lithell, et al., "A Comparison of the Effects of Hydrochlorothiazide and Captopril on Glucose and Lipid Metabolism in Patients with Hypertension," *New England Journal of Medicine* 321:868-73 (1989).

383. M. Weinberger, *op. cit.*

384. See Hypertension Detection and Follow-up Program Cooperative Group, "Five-year Findings of the Hypertension Detection and Follow-up Program," *JAMA* 242(23):2562-71 (1979); E. Brown, L. Walker, *The Informed Consumer's Pharmacy* (New York: Carroll & Graf, 1990), chapter 12.

385. Multiple Risk Factor Intervention Trial Research Group, "Multiple Risk Factor Intervention Trial," *JAMA* 248(12):1465-77 (1982).

386. A. Helgeland, "Treatment of Mild Hypertension: A Five Year Controlled Drug Trial. The Oslo Study," *American Journal of Medicine* 69:725-32 (1980). See I. Holmes, et al., "Treatment of Mild Hypertension with Diuretics: The Importance of ECG Abnormalities in the Oslo Study and in MRFIT," *JAMA* 251(10):1298-99 (1984).

387. J. Wikstrand, "Initial Therapy for Mild Hypertension," *Pharmacotherapy* 6(2):64–72 (1986), citing G. Olsson, N. Rehnqvist, "Reduction of Non-fatal Reinfarctions in Patients with a History of Hypertension by Chronic Postinfarction Treatment with Metoprolol," *Acta Medica Scandinavica* (1986), and J. Wikstrand, et al.," Antihypertensive Treatment with Metoprolol or Hydrochlorothiazide in Patients Aged 60–75 years: Report from a Double-blind International Multicenter Study," *JAMA* (1986).

388. "Magnesium in human nutrition," *Nutrition & the M.D.* 14(11):1-3 (1988).

389. M. Weinberger, *op. cit.*

390. *Ibid.*

391. Medical Research Council Working Party on Mild to Moderate Hypertension, "Adverse Reactions of Bendrofluazide and Propranolol for the Treatment of Mild Hypertension," *Lancet* 8246:539–43 (1981).

392. R. Ochs, "A High-Tension Drug Study," *Newsday* (October 22, 1996); R. Ochs, "Hypertension Drug Fuels Debate," *Newsday* (September 11, 1996).

393. R. Mikkelsen, "Study Links Drugs with Cardiac Risk," *Reuters* (September 30, 1995).

394. B. Hunter, "Should Everyone Cut Back on Sodium?" *Consumers' Research Magazine* (February 1, 1995).

395. F. Batmanghelidj, M.D., *Your Body's Many Cries for Water* (Falls Church, VA: Global Health Solutions, Inc., 1995), chapter 6.

396. T. Maugh II, "Diet Alone Found to Lower Blood Pressure," *Los Angeles Times* (April 177, 1997). For full details, see the Internet at http://dash.bwh.harvard.edu.

397. *Ibid.*

398. O. Lindahl, et al., "A Vegan Regimen with Reduced Medication in the Treatment of Hypertension," *British Journal of Nutrition* 52:11–20 (1984).

399. S. Briggs, "Magnesium—A Forgotten Mineral," *Nutrition Science News* (September 1997), p. 430.

400. B. Hunter, *op. cit.*

401. R. Siblerud, "The Relationship Between Mercury from Dental Amalgam and the Cardiovascular System," *Science of the Total Environment* 99:22-35 (1990); See E. Brown, R. Hansen, *The Key to Ultimate Health* (La Mirada, CA: Advanced Health Research Publishing, 1998).

402. N. Kaplan, "Non-drug Treatment of Hypertension," *Annals of Internal Medicine* 102:359–73 (1985).

403. See C. Patel, K. Datey, "Relaxation and Biofeedback Techniques in the Management of Hypertension," *Angiology* 27(2):106–13 (1976).

404. *Ibid.*; K. Datey, et al., "'Shavasan'—a Yogic Exercise in the Management of Hypertension," *Angiology* 20:325-33 (1969); N. Kaplan, *op. cit.* Simple relaxation also works, but not as well. See, e.g., R. Jacob, et al., "Relaxation Therapy for Hypertension: Comparison of Effects with Concomitant Placebo, Diuretic, and Beta-blocker," *Archives of Internal Medicine* 146:2335–40 (1986).

405. H. Benson, M.D., *The Relaxation Response* (New York: William Morrow and Co., 1975), pp. 99-102.

406. S. Fahrion, et al., "Biobehavioral Treatment of Essential Hypertension: A Group Outcome Study," *Biofeedback Self Regul.* 11(4):257–77 (1986).

407. C. Patel, et al., *op. cit.*; compare R. Jacob, et al., *op. cit.* See also C. Patel, M. Carruthers, "Coronary Risk Factor Reduction Through Biofeedback-aided Relaxation and Meditation," *Journal of the Royal College of General Practitioners* 27:401–05 (1977), a British study investigating the effects of meditation and relaxation reinforced by biofeedback.

408. See N. Kaplan, *op. cit.*

409. G. Mancia, et al., "Effects of Blood Pressure Measurement by the Doctor on Patient's Blood Pressure and Heart Rate," *Lancet* 2:695–98 (1983).

410. B. Eskin, et al., "The Disease in Disguise," *Good Housekeeping* (April 1, 1995); J. Lippert, "The Disease Doctors Ignore," *Redbook* (August 1, 1994).

411. J. Lippert, "The Disease Doctors Ignore," *Redbook* (August 1, 1994).

412. J. Lee, "Osteoporosis Reversal: The Role of Progesterone," *International Clinical Nutrition Review* 10(3): 384–91 (1990). Compare J. Franklyn, et al., "Long-term Thyroxine Treatment and Bone Mineral Density," *Lancet* 340:9–13 (1992), finding no significant difference in bone mineral density between patients on thyroid treatment and controls. Evidently, thyroid supplementation itself is not detrimental; it is excess thyroid that does harm.

413. R. Peat, *Nutrition for Women* (Eugene, OR: Kenogen, 1981) pp. 16–21.

414. "What Causes Heartburn? What Can I Do about It?" *University of California, Berkeley Wellness Letter* 3(9):8 (1987); L. Altman, M.D., "Scientists Track Clues Linking Bacterium to Stomach Disorders," *New York Times* (January 3, 1989), p. C3.

415. See "Nutritional consequences of Antacids for Hyperacidity," *Nutrition & the M.D.* (November 1986), p. 1.

416. H. Silverman, *The Pill Book* (New York: Bantam Books, 1996).

417. A. Wade, ed., *Martindale: The Extra Pharmacopoeia*, 29th ed. (London: The Pharmaceutical Press, 1989), pp. 891, 1547.

418. D. Zimmerman, *The Essential Guide to Nonprescription Drugs* (New York: Harper & Row, Publishers 1983), pp. 237–49.

419. See J. Williams, et al., "Biliary Excretion of Aluminum in Aluminum Osteodystrophy with Liver Disease," *Annals of Internal Medicine* 104:782-85 (1986), reviewed in "Toxicologic Consequences of Oral Aluminum," *Nutrition Reviews* 45(3):72–74 (1987); H. Casdorph, M. Walker, *Toxic Metal Syndrome* (Garden City Park, NY: Avery Publishing, 1995).

420. "Aluminum and Orange Juice," *U.S. Pharmacist* (April 1989), p. 30, citing *Lancet* 2:849 (1988); A. Bakir, et al., "Hyperaluminemia in Renal Failure: The Influence of Age and Citrate Intake," *Clinical Nephrology* 31(1):40–44 (1989).

421. R. Lasser, et al., "The Role of Intestinal Gas in Functional Abdominal Pain," *New England Journal of Medicine* 293:524-26 (1975); *Federal Register* 47:486 (January 5, 1982).

422. T. Gossel, "Antiflatulence Agents," *U.S. Pharmacist* (August 1989), pp. 18 ff.

423. A. Lange, "Homeopathy for Childhood Ear Infections," *Nutrition Science News* (October 1996), p. 40; A. Chambers, "Drugs Increasing Health-care Costs," *Getting the Most for Your Medical Dollar* (August 1, 1995).

424. R. Weiss, "Common Staph Bacteria Found Resisting Powerful Antibiotic," *Washington Post* (August 22, 1997), p. A02.

425. W. Crook, "Pediatricians, Antibiotics, and Office Practice," *Pediatrics* 76(1):139–40 (1985).

426. M. Walker, "Olive Leaf Extract," *Nutrition Science News* (January 1998), p. 18.

427. "H_2O_2 in Farming," *ECHO Newsletter* III(II):8–16 (Summer 1989); W. Forest, "AIDS, cancer cured by hyper-oxygenation," *Health Freedom News* (June 1989), pp. 27–37; "Ozone kills all viruses," *Coastal Post* (July 27, 1987), p. 19.

428. J. Lieberman, *Light: Medicine of the Future* (Santa Fe, NM: Bear & Co., 1990) pp. 141–43.

429. *Vegetarian Times* (June 1997), pp. 78–79.

430. "What's Worse . . . The Insect Bite or the Insect Repellant?" *Townsend Letter for Doctors & Patients* (July 1997), p. 154; "Insect Repellants," *Medical Letter* (May 19, 1989), pp. 45–46; "Are Insect Repellants Safe?" *University of California, Berkeley Wellness Letter* (June 1988), p. 7; "Prevention and Treatment of Insect Stings," *Pharmacy Times* (April 1989), pp. 33–38; C. O'Neill, "The big sting," *Washington Post Health* (June 28, 1988), p. 22.

431. G. Cowley, "Melatonin mania," *Newsweek* (November 6, 1995), pp. 60-63.

432. C. Kilham, "Kava for Anxiety and Insomnia," *Nutrition Science News* 2(5):232-34 (May 1997).

433. D. McCree, "The Appropriate Use of Sedatives and Hypnotics in Geriatric Insomnia," *American Pharmacy* NS29(5):49–53 (1989).

434. See S. Gilbert, "Eight Drugstore Remedies that Can Make You Sick," *Redbook*, (February 1, 1996).

435. T. Gossel, "OTC Relief of Itching," *U.S. Pharmacist* (July 1989), pp. 33–40; P. Parish, *Medicines* (London: Penguin Books, 1989), pp. 270–72.

436. T. Gossel, *op. cit.*; D. Zimmerman, *Essential Guide to Nonprescription Drugs* (New York: Harper & Row, Publishers, 1983), pp. 449–71.

437. See A. Convery, "Home Health Remedies that Doctors Recommend," *Cosmopolitan* (November 1, 1996), citing Jonathan Wright, M.D., and herbalist Jude Williams.

438. "Frequent Fliers Saying Fresh Air Is Awfully Thin at 30,000 Feet," *New York Times* (June 6, 1993), section 1, p. 1.

439. W. Leary, "F.D.A. Asks Stronger Label on Sleeping Pill Under Scrutiny," *New York Times* (September 23, 1989), p. 6.

440. R. Becker, M.D., *Cross Currents* (Los Angeles: Jeremy P. Tarcher, Inc., 1990), p. 70.

441. See B. Arnot, "The Lowdown on Lyme Disease," *Good Housekeeping* (June 1, 1995).

442. H. Aldercreutz, et al., "Dietary Estrogens and the Menopause in Japan," *Lancet* 339:1233 (1992); Y. Beyenne, "Cultural Significance and Physiological Manifestations of Menopause: A Biocultural Analysis," *Culture, Med. Psychiatry* 10:58 (1986).

443. R. Rubin, "Estrogen Anxiety," *U.S. News & World Report* (April 4, 1994), p. 60.

444. The increased risk was 41% for women on HRT vs. 32% for women on estrogen alone. G. Colditz, et al., "The Use of Estrogens and Progestins and the Risk of Breast Cancer in Postmenopausal Women," *New England Journal of Medicine* 332:1589-93 (June 15, 1995).

445. S. Whitcroft, et al., "Hormone Replacement Therapy: Risks and Benefits," *Clinical Endocrinology* 36:15–20 (1992); N. Lauersen, M.D., *PMS: Premenstrual Syndrome and You* (New York: Simon & Schuster, 1983).

446. S. Roan, "Study Urges Use of 2nd Hormone in Estrogen Therapy," *Los Angeles Times*, Home Edition Part A, p. 1 (February 7, 1996).

447. See E. Brown, L. Walker, *Menopause and Estrogen* (Berkeley: Carroll &Graf, 1996).

448. M. Key, "Data on Estrogens in Soybeans May Make ERT More Acceptable," *Cancer Biotechnology Weekly* (October 23, 1995), p. 10; E. Braverman, et al., "Natural Estrogen and Progesterone: Research Indicates Health Benefits of Natural vs. Synthetic Hormones," *Total Health* (October 1991), p. 55.

449. J. Chen, "Pharmacologic Actions and Therapeutic Uses of Ginseng and Tang Kwei," *International Journal of Chinese Medicine* 1(3):23–27 (1984).

450. D. Bensky, et al., *Chinese Herbal Medicine: Materia Medica* (Seattle: Eastland Press, 1986), p. 476.

451. E. Duker, et al., "Effects of Extracts from *Cimicifuga racemosa* on Gonadotropin Release in Menopausal Women and Ovariectomized Rats," *Planta Medica* 57:420–24 (1991).

452. P. Holmes, *The Energetics of Western Herbs* (Boulder, Colorado: Artemis, 1989), pp. 471–73.

453. K. Keville, "A Total Approach to Fighting PMS," *Vegetarian Times* (August 1986), pp. 40 ff.

454. B. Borho, "Therapy of the Menopausal Syndrome with Mulimen—Results of a Multicentre Post-marketing Survey," *Biological Therapy* 10(2):226–29 (1992).

455. Lita Lee, "Estrogen, Progesterone and Female Problems," *Earthletter* 1(2):1–4 (June 1991).

456. H. Aldercreutz, et al., *op. cit.*

457. G. Wilcox, et al., "Oestrogenic Effects of Plant Foods in Postmenopausal Women," *British Medical Journal* 301(6757):905–06 (1990).

458. L. Barbach, Ph.D., *The Pause* (New York: Penguin Books, 1993), p. 174, citing S. Weed, *Menopausal Years.*

459. N. Shaw, et al., "A Vegetarian Diet Rich in Soybean Products Compromises Iron Status in Young Students," *Journal of Nutrition* 125:212–19 (1995).

460. See, e.g., A. Hain, et al., "The Control of Menopausal Flushes by Vitamin E," *British Medical Journal* 7:9 (1943).

461. G. Burton, et al, "Comparison of Free Alpha-tocopherol & Alpha-tocopheryl Acetate as Sources of Vitamin E in Rats and Humans," *Lipids* 23:834–40 (1988).

462. See L. Barbach, *op. cit.*; J. Balch, M.D., et al., *Prescription for Nutritional Healing* (Garden City Park, NY: Avery Publishing Group, 1990), p. 241.

463. L. Nachtigall, M.D., et al., *Estrogen* (New York: Harper Collins Publishers, 1991), p. 75; J. Balch, M.D., et al., *op. cit.*

464. L. Vorhaus, "Infectious Mononucleosis," *Colliers Encyclopedia CD-ROM* (February 28, 1996); A. Rochell, "Chronic Fatigue Syndrome is Still a Mystery," *The Atlanta Journal and Constitution* (March 27, 1996).

465. D. Zimmerman, *Essential Guide to Nonprescription Drugs* (New York: Harper & Row, Publishers, 1983), p. 558.

466. "Myth: Carbonated Beverages Relieve Nausea," *University of California, Berkeley Wellness Letter* 3(4):8 (1987).

467. "Ovarian Cysts—Surgery Not Always Necessary," *Health Facts* (December 1, 1996), citing *British Medical Journal* (November 2, 1996).

468. N. Hellmich, "Obesity Getting Worse, Especially in Kids," *USA Today* (March 7, 1997), p. 1; L. Brody, "The Diet Years," *Los Angeles Times* (February 1, 1996).

469. R. Abcarian, "A Growing Body of Evidence," *Los Angeles Times* (July 16, 1997).

470. J. Talan, et al., "Popular Diet Pills Recalled," *Newsday* (September 16, 1997).

471. E. Bravo, "Phenylpropanolamine and Other Over-the-counter Vasoactive Compounds," *Hypertension* 11 (Supp. II):II-7—II-10 (1988); R. Glick, et al., "Phenylpropanolamine: An Over-the-counter Drug Causing Central Nervous System Vasculitis and Intracerebral Hemorrhage," *Neurosurgery* 20(6):969–74 (1987)

472. CNN (June 3, 1997).

473. J. Whitaker, "How to Win the Weight Loss Battle," *Human Events* (June 3, 1994).

474. "Sweetener, Brain Tumors Linked?" *The Atlanta Journal* (November 5, 1996); "Olestra: Just Say No," *University of California at Berkeley Wellness Letter* 12(5):1–2 (February 1996).

475. "Deciphering the Grapefruit Juice Effect," *Science News* 151:327 (May 24, 1997).

476. M. Rhodes, "America's Top 6 Fad Diets," *Good Housekeeping* (July 1, 1996).

477. B. Jensen, D.C., *Tissue Cleansing Through Bowel Management* (Escondido, CA: Bernard Jensen, D.C., 1981).

478. J. Barilla, "Natural Remedies Show Effectiveness," *Health News & Review* (June 1, 1995).

479. S. Squires, "Happy 100th, Aspirin," *Los Angeles Times* (August 13, 1997).

480. "Toxicity of Nonsteroidal Anti-inflammatory Drugs," *Medical Letter* 25:15–16 (1983).

481. E. Neus, "Got a Cold? Is There a Pill Safe to Take?" *Gannett News Service* (January 18, 1995).

482. "Elderly Users," *Vegetarian Times* (May 1989), p. 13.

483. J. Barilla, *op. cit.*

484. See Consumers Union, *The Medicine Show* (New York: Pantheon Books, 1980), pp. 25–26.

485. M. Kapp, "Placebo Therapy and the Law: Prescribe With Care," *American Journal of Law and Medicine* 8(4):371 (1982).

486. See P. Sanberg, Richard Krenna, *Over-the-Counter Drugs: Harmless or Hazardous?* (New York: Chelsea House Publishers 1986), pp. 96–98.

487. B. Brown, *Stress and the Art of Biofeedback* (New York: Harper & Row, Publishers 1977); H. Benson, M.D., *Beyond the Relaxation Response* (Times Books 1984); A. Kusuma, et al., "Acupuncture Analgesia in Tonsillectomy," *Alternative Medicine* 1(1):69–74 (1985); "Pain Control, Part II: Cancer," *Harvard Medical School Health Letter*, 14(9):1–3 (1989); J. Barilla, *op. cit.*

488. See D. Kotz, "How Safe is Your Water?" *Good Housekeeping* (November 1, 1995); "Study Says 2 Million a Year Suffer Water-borne Illness," *All Things Considered* (NPR) (July 17, 1994).

489. K. Krzystyniak, et al., "Approaches to the Evaluation of Chemical-Induced Immunotoxicity," *Environmental Health Perspectives* (December 1, 1995).

490. "Pneumonia," *Tennessee Tribune* (October 23, 1996).

491. D. Williams, "The Forgotten Hormone," *Alternatives for the Health Conscious Individual* 4(6):41–46 (December 1991).

492. G. Robinson, et al., "Problems in the Treatment of Premenstrual Syndrome," *Canadian Journal of Psychiatry* 35:199–206 (1990), citing studies.

493. M. Whitehead, et al., "The Role and Use of Progestogens," *Obstetrics and Gynecology* 75(4):59S–76S (1990).

494. J. Lee, M.D., "Slowing the Aging Process with Natural Progesterone," (Sebastipol, California; unpublished research paper).

495. L. Dennerstein, et al., "Progesterone and the Premenstrual Syndrome: A Double Blind Crossover Trial," *British Medical Journal* 290:1617–21 (1985).

496. See R. Peat, "Progesterone: Essential to Your Well-being," *Let's Live* (April 1982); "Dr. John Lee speaking on Natural Progesterone, 1992," audiotape (Sebastopol, California); L. Dusky, "Progesterone: Safe Antidote for PMS," *McCall's* (October 1990), pp. 152–56.

497. B. Goldin, et al., "Estrogen Excretion Patterns and Plasma Levels in Vegetarian and Omnivorous Women," *New England Journal of Medicine* 307:1542–47 (1982); "Less Fat, More Grain Can Ease Breast Pain," *Vegetarian Times* (May 1989), p. 11; "PMS? Let 'Em Eat Carbs," *ibid.* (March 1990), p. 17.

498. D. Duston (AP), "Calcium Seems to Help Women Deal with PMS," *Brownsville Herald* (Texas), September 3, 1991, p. 14; S. Thys-Jacobs, et al., "Calcium Supplementation in Premenstrual Syndrome, a Randomized Trial," *Journal of General Internal Medicine* 4:183–89 (1989).

499. A. Gaby, "Calcium and Premenstrual Syndrome," *Townsend Letter for Doctors* (October 1992), p. 810.

500. L. Stains, "Escape Middle-age Prostate Woes (Benign Prostatic Hyperplasia)," *Prevention* (February 1, 1997).

501. "Prostate Enlargement," *Encyclopedia of Natural Medicine*, pp. 480–86.

502. T. Geier, "The Prostate Showdown," *U.S. News & World Report* (September 2, 1996).

503. S. Foster, "Saw Palmetto Comes of Age," *Health Foods Business* (December 1996), p. 35.

504. "A Man's Guide to Healthy Living," *Wellness Advocate* (December 1994).

505. D. Steinman, "Enlarged Prostate? Try Tree Bark," *Natural Health* (July/August 1994), p. 44.

506. "A Man's Guide to Healthy Living," *op. cit.*

507. *Ibid.*

508. J. Raloff, "Radical Prostates," *Science News* 151(8):126–27 (February 22, 1997); Aged Garlic Could Slow Prostate Cancer," *ibid.* (April 19, 1997).

509. L. Stains, *op cit.*

510. *The Medical Advisor* (Alexandria, VA: Time-Life Books, 1996), pp. 872–73.

511. "Herpes Could Cause Alzheimer's," *Reuters* (January 23, 1997).

512. J. Hatem, et al., "Sinusitis: More Antibiotic Resistance and More Surgery," *Health Facts* (December 1, 1993), citing *Annals of Internal Medicine* (November 1, 1992).

513. J. Hatem, et al., *ibid.*

514. S. Berne, *Creating Your Own Personal Vision* (Santa Fe, NM: Color Stone Press, 1994).

515. See V. Beral, et al., "Malignant Melanoma and Exposure to Fluorescent Light at Work," *Lancet* 2:290–92 (1982); B. Pasternak, et al., *ibid.* 1:704 (1983); D. Rigel, et al, *ibid.* 1:704 (1983).

516. "Is the Sunscreen Craze Actually Causing More Skin Cancer?" *Alternatives* (April 1993), p. 2.

517. Z. Kime, M.D., *Sunlight* (Penryn, California: World Health Publications, 1980).

518. D. Sullivan, "Better Diet, Healthier Skin," *Health* (November 1996), pp. 44–46.

519. "Milk Thistle May Thwart Skin Cancer," *Nutrition Science News* (July 1997), p. 317; "Ginger May Curb Skin Cancer," *Let's Live Nutrition Insights* (November 1997), p. 9.

520. See D. Zimmerman, *Essential Guide to Nonprescription Drugs* (New York: Harper & Row, Publishers 1983), pp. 449–71.

521. J. McEnaney, "Herbal Concentrates, Extracts Wave of the Future," *Filipino Reporter* (December 7, 1995).

522. R. Podell, M.D., "Creatine Improves Athletes' Short-Term Performance," *Let's Live* (September 1997), p. 428.

523. G. Gates, et al., "Effectiveness of Adenoidectomy and Tympanostomy Tubes in the Treatment of Chronic Otitis Media with Effusion," *New England Journal of Medicine* 317:1444–51 (1987).

524. A. Bisno, "Acute Rheumatic Fever: Forgotten but Not Gone," *New England Journal of Medicine* 316(8):476–78 (1987).

525. S. Holmberg, G. Faich, "Stroptococcal Pharyngitis and Acute Rheumatic Fever in Rhode Island," *JAMA* 250(17):2307–12 (1983).

526. "Recognizing a Stroke May Limit Damage," *New Pittsburgh Courier* (May 7, 1997).

527. "The Latest on the Heart Beat: New Treatment and Prevention Options," *The Jewish Week* (Jan 24, 1997).

528. K. Khaw, E. Barrett-Connor, "Dietary Potassium and Stroke-associated Mortality," *New England Journal of Medicine* 316(5):235–40 (1987). Advocates of drug therapy point to a significant drop in stroke deaths in the years since drug treatment has been aggressively pursued. The trouble with this theory is that the drop actually began *before* the drugs became popular. See N. Kaplan, "Non-drug Treatment of Hypertension," *Annals of Internal Medicine* 102:359–73 (1985). Khaw, et al., propose another explanation: the drop may be linked to the increased consumption of potassium-rich fruits and vegetables occurring at the same time.

529. H. Trowell, "Hypertension and Salt," *Lancet* (July 22, 1978), p. 204.

530. F. Furlow, "Vital Vitamins?" *Psychology Today* 30(2):22 (March 1997).

531. A. Chen, "Effective Acupuncture Therapy for Stroke and Cerebrovascular Diseases," *American Journal of Acupuncture* 21(2):105–14 (1993).

532. W. Hoffmann-Axthelm, *History of Dentistry* (Chicago: Quintessence Publishing Co., Inc., 1981), pp. 334–35.

533. "Morphine's Actions Outside the Brain," *Science News* (May 24, 1997), p. 322.

534. D. Ullman, *The Consumer's Guide to Homeopathy* (New York: Dorling Kindersley, 1995), p. 344, note 1.

535. "Sexually Transmitted Diseases," *National Women's Health Report* (March 1, 1993); "Cosmo's Guide to Sexual Wellness," *Cosmopolitan* (September 1, 1994); E. Brown, L. Walker, *The Informed Consumer's Pharmacy* (New York: Carroll & Graf, 1990).

536. W. Price, D.D.S., *Dental Infections—Oral and Systemic* [vol. 1] and *Dental Infections and the Degenerative Diseases* [vol. 2] (Cleveland, OH: Penton Publishing Co., 1923).

537. H. Gelb, D.M.D., *Killing Pain Without Prescription* (New York: Harper & Row, 1980), pp. 43–44.

538. "Toxic Shock Syndrome," *Iris: A Journal About Women* (December 1, 1994); C. Drinkall, "Toxic Shock Syndrome," *Colliers Encyclopedia CD-ROM*, 28 Feb 1996.

539. H. Spiro, "Peptic Ulcer," *Colliers Encyclopedia CD-ROM* (February 28, 1996).

540. M. Lane, et al., "Recurrance of Duodenal Ulcer After Medical Treatment," *Lancet* (May 21, 1988), pp. 1147–49.

541. M. Sax, "Clinically Important Adverse Effects and Drug Interactions with H_2-receptor Antagonists: An Update," *Pharmacotherapy* 7 (6 Pt 2):110–15S (1987); J. Weber, et al., "How Glaxo's Eager Beavers Chewed up Tagamet's Lead," *Business Week* (October 10, 1988), pp. 40–41; J. Aymard, et al., "Haematological Adverse Effects of Histamine H_2-receptor Antagonists," *Medical Toxicology* 3:430–48 (1988); S. Smith, M. Kendall, "Ranitidine *Versus* Cimetidine: A Comparison of Their Potential to Cause Clinically Important Drug Interactions," *Clinical Pharmacokinetics* 15:44–56 (1988).

542. *Ibid.*; J. Aymard, et al., *op. cit.*

543. M. Driks, et al., "Nosocomial Pneumonia in Intubated Patients Given Sucralfate as Compared with Antacids or Histamine type 2 Blockers: The Role of Gastric Colonization," *New England Journal of Medicine* 317(22):1376–1382 (1987).

544. B. O'Reilly, "Why Doctors Aren't Curing Ulcers," *Fortune* (June 9, 1997); A. Levin, "Bacteria as the Cause of Peptic Ulcer Disease," *Health Facts* (August 1, 1994).

545. See "Diet Therapy of Peptic Ulcer Disease," *Nutrition & the M.D.* 14(2):1–2 (1988), citing *Gut* 27:2329 (1986), *J. Lab. Clin. Med.* 100:296 (1982), *J. Clin. Gastroenterol.* 3 (Supp 2):45 (1981), *Gastroenterology* 89:366 (1985) and 90:1617 (1986); J. Gaska, et al., *op. cit.*; A. Rydning, et al., "Prophylactic Effect of Dietary Fibre in Duodenal Ulcer Disease," *Lancet* (October 2, 1982), pp. 736–39 (1982); "Myth: A Bland, Milky Diet Can Help Prevent or Cure Ulcers," *University of California, Berkeley Wellness Letter* 3(10):8 (1987).

546. "Diet therapy of peptic ulcer disease," *Nutrition & the M.D.* 14(2):1-2 (1988).

547. V. Hufnagel, M.D., *No More Hysterectomies* (New York: Penguin Books, 1989), pp. 108, 117; L. Nachtigall, M.D., et al., *Estrogen* (New York: Harper Collins Publishers, 1991), p. 192.

548. V. Hufnagel, *op. cit.*, p. 124.

549. G. Colditz, et al., "Menopause and the Risk of Coronary Heart Disease in Women," *New England Journal of Medicine* 316(18):1105–10 (1987).

550. V. Hufnagel, *op. cit.*, citing *Arch. Gynaekol* 35:1 (1989).

551. See, e.g., M. Kobayashi, et al., "Immunohistochemical Localization of Pituitary Gonadotrophins and Estrogen in Human Postmenopausal Ovaries," *Acta Obstetrica et Gynecologica Scandinavica* 72:76–80 (1993).

552. L. Zussman, et al, "Sexual Response after Hysterectomy-oophorectomy: Recent Studies and Reconsideration of Psychogenesis," *American Journal of Obstetrics and Gynecology* 140(7):725–29 (1981).

553. A. Kinsey, *Sexual Behavior in the Human Female* (Philadelphia: W.B. Saunders Co., 1953).

554. S. Lark, M.D., *Menopause Self Help Book* (Berkeley, California: Celestial Arts, 1990, 1992), pp. 220–21; V. Hufnagel, M.D., *op. cit.*; J. Lee, M.D., "Slowing the Aging

Process with Natural Progesterone" (Sebastopol, California; unpublished research paper).

555. J. Lee, *ibid.*

556. S. Tsao, et al., "Toxicities of Trichosanthin and Alpha-momorcharin, Abortifacient Proteins from Chinese Medicinal Plants, on Cultured Tumor Cell Lines," *Toxicon* 28(10):1183–92 (1990).

557. R. Peat, *Nutrition for Women* (Eugene, Ore.: Kenogen, 1981), p. 17.

558. P. Holmes, *The Energetics of Western Herbs* (Boulder, Colorado: Artemis, 1989), pp. 471–73.

559. V. Hufnagel, *op. cit.*, p. 108.

560. C. Harris, "Doctors Still Prescribe Drugs that Don't Mix," *Gannett News Service* (April 30, 1996).

561. T. Colburn, et al., *Our Stolen Future* (New York: Penguin Books, 1996).

562. "Herbal Wisdom," *Meno Times* (September 1, 1996).

563. M. Beard, "Atrophic vaginitis: Can It Be Prevented as Well as Treated?" *Postgraduate Medicine* 91(6):257–60 (1992).

564. *Ibid.*; D. Shefrin, et al., *op. cit.*

565. M. Privette, et al., "Prevention of Recurrent Urinary Tract Infections in Postmenopausal Women," *Nephron* 50:24–27 (1988). See also J. Baldassarre, et al., "Special Problems of Urinary Tract Infection in the Elderly," *Medical Clinics of North America* 75(2):375–90 (1991).

566. M. Privette, *ibid.*

567. I. Milsom, et al., "Vaginal Immunoglobulin A (IgA) Levels in Post-menopausal Women: Influence of Oestriol Therapy," *Maturitas* 13(2):129–35 (1991).

568. B. Eriksen, et al., "Urogenital Estrogen Deficiency Syndrome: Investigation and Treatment with Special Reference to Hormone Substitution," *Tidsskrift for den Norske Laegeforening* 111(24):2949–51 (1991). See also U. Molander, et al., "Effect of Oral Oestriol on Vaginal Flora and Cytology and Urogenital Symptoms in the Post-menopause," *Maturitas* 12(2):113–20 (1990); D. Gerbaldo, et al., "Endometrial Morphology After 12 Months of Vaginal Oestriol Therapy in Post-menopausal Women," *Maturitas* 13(4):269–74 (1991).

569. D. Shefrin, et al., *op. cit.*

570. A. Hardie, "Women Seek Irritation Relief—Now," *The Atlanta Journal and Constitution* (April 24, 1997). For a free booklet, "Women's Guide to Vaginal Infections," write the National Vaginitis Association, 117 S. Cook St., Suite 315, Barrington, IL. 60010.

571. "Yeast Infections," *MidLife Woman* (January 1, 1994).

572. See W. Crook, M.D., *The Yeast Connection* (Jackson, TN.: Professional Books, 1985), pp. 291–92.

573. "Vaginal Yeast Infections," *National Women's Health Report* (May 1, 1995).

574. *The Medical Advisor* (Alexandria, VA: Time-Life Books, 1996), pp. 872–73.

_A_ppendix:
Natural Remedy Health Advisor

CONDITION	REMEDY	TYPE OF REMEDY	COMPANY	DIRECTIONS FOR USE
Abscess	Gun Powder 6x	single homeopathic	Boiron	3 to 5 pellets 3 times daily
	Pyrogenium 6x	single homeopathic	Dolisos	3 to 5 pellets 3 times daily
topical for	Black Ointment	herbal drawing salve	Nature's Way	apply topically twice daily
to promote healing	Calendula 6X	single homeopathic	Boiron	2 pills 3 times daily
Acne	Acne Gel	homeopathic gel	Nelson	apply to clean face twice daily
oral for	Margarite Acne Pills	Chinese patent	People's Republic	take 5 pills 2 times daily
Acne Rosacea	Bioptron Light	special light	Swiss Tech	to face 4 min, twice daily
Aging	Green Tea	single herb	Jarrow	2 capsules twice daily
	Ginkgo Biloba + OPC	herb combination	Jarrow	1–2 pills twice daily
Alcohol Abuse	Nux Vomica 30c	single homeopathic	Boiron	2 pills 2 to 3 times daily
	Kuduz	single herb	Nature's Plus	1 capsule 2 to 3 times daily
Allergies	Aller Total	combination remedy	Apex	10 drops 4 times daily
Anger	Relaxed Wanderer	Chinese herbal	K'an	3 pills 2 to 3 times daily
	Anger Release	homeopathic combination	Apex	2 pills 4 times daily

387

CONDITION	REMEDY	TYPE OF REMEDY	COMPANY	DIRECTIONS FOR USE
Anemia	Precious Pills	Chinese patent	Planetary Formulas	8 pills 3 times daily
Angina	Cactus	homeopathic combination	Marco Pharma	10 drops 3 times daily
Anxiety	5 Flower Essence	flower essence	FES	4 drops 4 times daily
	Skullcap and Oats	single herb	Eclectic	2 droppersfuls 3 times daily
	Nutrizac	herbal combination	Nature's Plus	1 pill 3 times daily
Arrhythmia	Cactus	herbal combination	Marco Pharma	20 drops in water up to 3 times daily
Arthritis	Cosamin DS	herbal combination	Nutramax	2 pills in A.M., 1 in P.M.
	CM Plus	cetyl myristoleate	Longevity Science	2 capsules 3 times daily
topical for	Arthritis Cream	homeopathic cream	CompliMed	daily
	Zeel Cream	homeopathic cream	Heel	apply twice daily
	Arthritis Cream	homeopathic cream	CompliMed	apply 2 to 3 times daily
Asthma	Black Currant Seed Oil	single herb	Natrol	2 pills up to 4 times daily
Atherosclerosis	Viscum	single herb	Marco Pharma	3 pills 3 times daily
Attention Deficit	GABA	homeopathic combination	Deseret	10 drops 3 times daily
Back Pain	Specific Lumbaglin	Chinese patent	Peace Medicine	2 capsules 3 times daily
Bladder infection	Uri Control	homeopathic combination	BHI	1 pill every hour × 4, then 4 times a day
	Cranberry 1000	herbal combination	Nature Plus	2 pills 3 times daily
	Tao Chih Pien	Chinese patent	Tianjin	4 pills twice daily

Condition	Remedy	Type of Remedy	Company	Directions for Use
Bone Spurs	Calcium Absorption	homeopathic combination	BioForce	2 tablets before each meal
Broken Bones	Symphytum 6x or 30x	single homeopathic	Boiron	3 to 5 pellets 3 times daily
	Comfrey Poultice	single herb	Now	topically, twice daily
Bronchitis	Trauma	homeopathic combination	CompliMed	10 drops 4 times daily
	Ping chuan	Chinese patent	Sing-Kyn	10 pills 3 times daily
	Dulpumon	homeopathic combination	CompliMed	10 drops 4 times daily
Bruises	Trauma	homeopathic combination	CompliMed	10 drops 4 times daily
topical for	Wan Hua Oil	Chinese patent	Guangzhou	apply twice daily
	Trauma One	homeopathic cream	Nutrition Now	apply 2–3 times daily
Burns	Cantharis 6x	single homeopathic	Boiron	2 pills 4 times daily
topical for	Ching Wan Hung	Chinese patent	Great Wall	apply twice daily
Candida Albicans	Mycocan Combo	homeopathic combination	PHP	10 drops 4 times daily × 1 week
Canker sores	Borax 6x	single homeopathic	Boiron	3 to 5 pellets 3 times daily
Carpal tunnel syndrome	Tin Tzat	Chinese patent	Hang Lam	5 pills 4 times daily
	Pro-Gest Cream	herbal cream	Transitions	apply ¼ tsp daily
Cataracts	Raynaudin	combination product	Ecological Formulas	2 capsules daily
Chemical Detox	Exchem	homeopathic combination	Apex	10 drops 3 times daily
Chicken pox	Varicella	single homeopathic	Dolisos	one dose at onset
Cholesterol, high	Ultra guggulow	herbal combination	Doctors Best	2 to 3 tablets daily

389

Condition	Remedy	Type of Remedy	Company	Directions for Use
Cholestrol, high	Grapefruit fiber	herbal combination	Now	one tablespoon twice daily
Chronic Fatigue	Brucella	German homeopathic	Staufen	1 ampule every 3 days
	Adrenal/Spleen	homeopathic combination	CompliMed	10 drops 4 times daily
Cold Sores, topical for	Calendula/Hypericum	combination ointment	Boiron	apply twice daily
Cold, onset of	Cold & Flu Solution	homeopathic combination	Dolisos	1 tablet every hour × 4
	Yin Chiao	Chinese patent	Tian Jin	3 tablets 3 times daily
	Elderberry C 1000	herb/vitamin combination	Zand	2 tablets 3 times a day
Colic	Gripe Water	herb combination	Abbigle	1–2 tablespoonful as needed
	Cocyntal	homeopathic combination	Boiron	1 liquid dose pack as needed
Constipation	Sankaijo	Chinese patent	Sato Pharmaceutical	take each night at bedtime
Cough	Chestal	cough syrup	Boiron	1 teaspoonful 4 times daily
	Cough	homeopathic combination	Bioforce	10 drops 4 times daily
Cuts/Sores, topical for	Calendula Gel	homeopathic gel	Boiron	apply twice daily
Depression	Nutrizac	herbal combination	Nature's Plus	1 capsule 3 times daily
	Magnesium	mineral supplement	Twin Labs	500mg 2 to 3 times daily
Detox	Lymphonest	homeopathic combination	Nestmann	25 drops in water 3 times daily
Diabetes	Syzygium Jamb 30x	single homeopathic	Dolisos	10 drops 3 times a day
	Diabetrol	combination remedy	CardioVas Research	1 capsule before meals
	Chromium Picolinate	trace mineral	Various	1 capsule with breakfast and lunch

Condition	Remedy	Type of Remedy	Company	Directions for Use
Diarrhea	Diarrmed	homeopathic combination	CompliMed	10 drops 3 times daily
Dry Skin	Evening Primrose	herbal oil	Efamol	2600mg at bedtime
Ear Aches	Elderberry C 500	herb/vitamin combination	Zand	1–2 pills 3 times daily
	ABC	homeopathic combination	Marco Pharma	5 drops every 15 min, then 4 times daily
	Elderberry C 1000	herb/vitamin combination	Zand	1–2 pills 3 times daily
	Chamilla	homeopathic combination	Boiron	1 pill every hour × 4, then 4 times daily
Edema	parsley	single herb	Nature's Herbs	2 capsules 3 times daily
Endometriosis	Pro-Gest Cream	herbal cream	Transitions	¼ teaspoonful daily
Excess Bleeding	Trillium	herbal combination	Marco Pharma	mix with Luvos
	Luvos Earth	mineral earth	Marco Pharma	Take every hour as needed
Eye care	Eye	homeopathic combination	BHI	1 pill 3 times daily
	OPC-3	single herb	Jarrow	100mg/day
Fear	Phosphorus	single homeopathic	Boiron	3 pills twice a day
Fever	Fever Reducer	homeopathic combination	B&T	1 every hour, as needed
	Belladonna 6x	single homeopathic	Standard	2 every hour, up to 5 doses
	Zhong Gan Ling	Chinese patent	Zand	as directed on package
Fibroids	Fibrosolve	homeopathic combination	Apex	10 drops 3 times
	Female Balance	homeopathic combination	Apex	10 drops 3 times

Condition	Remedy	Type of Remedy	Company	Directions for Use
Fibromyalgia	Malic Acid Plus	combination formula	Pain & Stress Center	2 pills 3 times daily
	Proanthenols	antioxidant combination	Life Plus	100mg daily
	Lyprinex	oil combination	Life Plus	2–4 pills 4 times daily
Flu, first stage of	Cold & Flu Solution Plus	homeopathic combination	Dolisos	1 every hour × 4, then 4 times daily
Food Poisoning	Salmonella	German homeopathic	Staufen	1 ampule every 2–3 days
Fungal Infection	Fungisode	homeopathic combination	Molecular Biologicals	10 drops 3 times daily
Gallbladder	Li Dan Formula	herbal combination	Kan	4 to 6 pills 3 times daily
	Liver/gallbladder	homeopathic combination	Complimed	10 drops 3 times daily
Gas/Bloating	Gasalia	homeopathic combination	Boiron	1 every 15 min if needed, up to 4 times
	Vermicin	homeopathic combination	Complimed	10 drops 3 times daily
Gout	cherry juice	herbal concentrate	Knudsen	drink 1 glass daily
Grief	Ignatia 30X	single homeopathic	Boiron	3 pills twice a day
	5 Flower Essence	flower essence	FES	4 drops 4 times daily
	Skullcap and Oats	herbal combination	Eclectic	2 droppersful to calm, or for sleep
Hangover	Nux Vomica	single homeopathic	Boiron	3 to 5 pellets every hour × 5
Headache	Headache	homeopathic combination	Bioforce	2 pills 3 times daily
Head lice	Tea Tree Oil	herbal oil	Thursday Plantation	apply to scalp, then shampoo

Condition	Remedy	Type of Remedy	Company	Directions for Use
Heart, strengthen	Cactus	herbal combination	MarcoPharma	20 drops in water up to 3 times daily
Heavy Metal Poisoning	Co Enzyme Q-10	nutritional supplement	Jarrow	100–200mg daily
	Mercury Antitiox	homeopathic combination	Apex	5–10 drops 3 times daily
Hemorrhoids	Fargelin	Chinese patent	United Pharmacy	3 pills 3 times daily
topical for	Hemorrhoid Cream	homeopathic cream	Nelsons	apply twice daily
Hepatitis	Hepatitis A	homeopathic nosode	Staufen	1 ampule every 3 days, right to left
	Heptatica	herbal combination	Marco Pharma	30 drops in water 3 times daily
	Ultimate Green	herbal combination	Nature's Secret	one packet daily
High Altitude	Cellular Oxygenator	homeopathic combination	PHP	10 drops 4 times daily
High Blood Pressure	Hawthorne Berry	single herb	Jarrow	2 capsules twice daily
Hypothyroidism	Thyroid	homeopathic combination	CompliMed	10 drops 3 times daily
Immune System	Jarrow Pak Plus	vitamin/herb combination	Jarrow	one packet daily
	Thymactive	homeopathic combination	NF Formulas	10 drops 3 times daily
Incontinence	Ginseng and Astragalus	herbal combination	Zand	1 droppersful in water, 3 times daily
	Sepia	single homeopathic	Boiron	2 pills 3 times daily
Indigestion	Gastrica	homeopathic combination	Complimed	10 drops 3 times daily
	Curing Formula	Chinese patent	Zand	1 vial after meals

Condition	Remedy	Type of Remedy	Company	Directions for Use
Infections, bacterial	Bacticin	homeopathic combination	CompliMed	10 drops 4 times daily
	Gun Powder 6x	single homeopathic	Dolisos	3 pills 2 to 5 times daily
Inflammation	Inflammation	homeopathic combination	BHI	1 tablet 4 times daily
Insect bites	Biting Insects	homeopathic combination	Molecular Biological	5 drops 3 times daily
Insomnia	Skullcap & Oats	herbal combination	Eclectic	1 dropperful at 7 P.M. and repeat at bedtime
	Passiflora 6x	single homeopathic	Boiron	2 pills at 7 P.M. and repeat at bedtime
Jet Travel	Melatonin 12x	single homeopathic	Dolisos	2 pills 3 times daily
	Geopathic Stress	homeopathic combination	Deseret	10 drops, in water sip during flight
Kidney	Kidney Liquessence	homeopathic combination	PHP	one teaspoonful twice daily
Kidney Stone	Passwan	Chinese herb formula	Zand	2 droppersfuls in water 3 times daily
Knee pain	Arth-X-Plus	herbal combination	Trace Min Research	2 pills 3 times daily
Laryngitis	Laryngitis Pills	Chinese patent	Szechuan	10 pills 3 times daily
Leg Cramps	Calcium Absorption	homeopathic combination	Bioforce	2 pills 3 times daily
	AB Calm	mineral supplement	A to B Calm	1 packet before bed
Liver Detox	Hepatica	herbal extracts	MPI	30 drops in water 3 times daily
	Ultimate Greens	herbal combination tablets	Nature's Secret	1 or 2 packets daily

Condition	Remedy	Type of Remedy	Company	Directions for Use
Low Energy for Men	Four Ginsengs	herbal combination	Natrol	2 with lunch
Low Energy for Women	Adrenal/spleen	homeopathic combination	CompliMed	10 drops 4 times daily
Lyme Disease	Borrelia	German homeopathic	Staufen	1 ampule every 3 days
Lymphatic Drainage	Mucus Dissolver	homeopathic combination	PHP	10 drops 3 times daily
Menstrual problems	Pro-Gest Cream	herbal cream	Transitions	¼ teaspoonful daily
Migraine	Migramed	homeopathic combination	CompliMed	10 drops 3 times daily
	Mygrafew	single herb	Nature's Way	1–2 pills 2–3 times daily
Motion Sickness	Travel Sickness	Homeopathic combination	Dolisos	2 pills every hour as needed
	Sea Band	wrist band	Sea Band Int'l.	wear on wrists
Nails	VegeSil	single herb	Flora	1 to 3 capsules daily
	Calcium Absorption	homeopathic combination	Bioforce	2 pills 3 times daily
Neck Pain	Spinaflex	homeopathic combination	CompliMed	10 drops 3–4 times daily
Nervousness	Calms	homeopathic combination	Hyland	1–2 tablets 3 times daily as needed
Nose Bleeds	Skullcap and Oats	herbal combination	Eclectic	2 droppersful up to 4 times daily
	Bleeding	homeopathic combination	BHI	2 pills every 15 min
Osteoporosis	Pro-Gest Cream	herbal cream	Pro Tech	¼ teaspoonful daily
	Calcium Absorption	homeopathic combination	Bioforce	2 pills 3 times daily
Ovarian cysts	Ovaruallkystom	German homeopathic	Staufen	1 ampule every 3 days
Pain	Trauma	homeopathic combination	CompliMed	10 drops every hours, as needed

Condition	Remedy	Type of Remedy	Company	Directions for Use
Pancreas	Pancrease Total M-17	homeopathic combination	Apex	10 drops 3 times daily
Parasite Protocol	Para A	herbal combination	Marco Pharma	2 to 3 droppersful 3 times daily
Parasites	Vermicin	homeopathic combination	CompliMed	10 drops 3 times daily
PMS	Hsiao Yao Wan	Chinese patent	Lanzhou Fo Chi	8 pills 3 times daily
	Natural Phases	homeopathic combination	Boiron	1 pill 3–4 times daily
Pneumonia	Pneumonia M	German homeopathic	Staufen	1 ampule every 2–3 days
	Ping Chuan	Chinese patent	Sing-Kyn	10 pills 3 times daily
	Elecampane	single herb	various	25 drops in water 4 times daily
Poison oak, poison ivy	Contact Allergies	homeopathic combination	Molecular Bio	10 drops 4 times daily
Prostate Enlargement	Saw palmetto + pygeum	herbal combination	Jarrow	1 capsule 3 times daily
	Pumpkin seed oil	herbal extract	Hains	2 capsules 2 to 3 times daily
Psoriasis, oral for	Squalene	shark liver oil	Japan Health	2 pills 2 to 3 times daily
topical for	Shark Liver Oil	topical oil	Squalene	apply small amount to affected area
Rashes	Armadillo Pills	Chinese patent	United	4 pills 3 times daily
Scars	Scargo	herbal combination	Home Health	apply twice daily
Sciatica	Sciatica Pills	Chinese patent	People's Republic	5 to 10 pills 3 times daily
Sex Drive	Jasmine	gem elixir	Botanical Alchemy	4 drops 4 times daily
Sinusitis	Peptostrep	homeopathic nosode	Staufen	1 ampule every 3 days
	Be Yin Lin	Chinese patent	Sansum	3 pills 3 times daily

CONDITION	REMEDY	TYPE OF REMEDY	COMPANY	DIRECTIONS FOR USE
Sports Endurance	Redimax	homeopathic combination	BHI	1 tablet 4 times daily
	Endurox	herbal combination	Pacific Health	2 before exercise
Stage Fright	Gelsenium 30X	single homeopathic	Boiron	2 pills every 2 hours
	5 Flower Essence	flower essence	FES	4 drops 4 times daily
Stomach Ulcers	Fare You	Chinese patent	Qiaoguang	2 tablets 3 times daily
	Campylobacter Pylori	German homeopathic	Staufen	1 ampule every 3 days
Strep Throat	Lymphatic	homeopathic combination	BHI	1 pill 5 times daily
	Inflammation	homeopathic combination	BHI	1 pill 5 times daily
Stress	Rescue Remedy	flower essence	Bach Flowers	4 drops 4 times daily
	Skullcap and Oats	herbal combination	Eclectic	1–2 droppersful 4 times daily
	Lavender Oil	essential oil	John Steele	1–2 drops as needed
	Stress-X	herb/vitamin combination	Trace Min Research	2 pills 3 times daily
Stretch Marks	Scargo	herbal oil	Home Health	apply twice daily
Stroke	Alpha Lipoic Acid	nutritional supplement	Jarrow	250 to 500mg daily
Tooth Infection	Bacticin	homeopathic combination	CompliMed	10 drops 3–4 times daily
	Corynebacterium	German homeopathic	Staufen	1 ampule as directed
	Gun Powder 6x	single homeopathic	Dolisos	3 pills 4 times daily
	Pyrogenium 6x	single homeopathic	Dolisos	3 pills 4 times daily
Trauma, topical for	Arnica Gel	homeopathic gel	Boiron	apply twice daily

Condition	Remedy	Type of Remedy	Company	Directions for Use
Uterine Prolapse	OstraDerm V	vaginal herbal cream	Bezwecken	1/4 tsp vaginally 3 times per week
	Sepia	single homeopathic	Boiron	2 pills 3 times daily
Vertigo	Vertigo Drops	homeopathic combination	Molecular Bio	10 drops 3 to 4 times daily
Virus	Virus	homeopathic combination	Dolisos	1 every hour × 4 hours
Warts	Wart	homeopathic combination	Kroeger	10 drops 3 times daily
Wounds	Calendula	topical herb extract	Boiron	apply topically twice daily

Index